# Perinatal Development

A Psychobiological Perspective

# BEHAVIORAL BIOLOGY

## AN INTERNATIONAL SERIES

*Series Editors*

**James L. McGaugh**

*Department of Psychobiology*
*University of California*
*Irvine, California*

**John C. Fentress**

*Department of Psychology*
*Dalhousie University*
*Halifax, Canada*

**Joseph P. Hegmann**

*Department of Zoology*
*The University of Iowa*
*Iowa City, Iowa*

*A list of books in this series is available from the publisher on request.*

# Perinatal Development
## A Psychobiological Perspective

Edited by

**Norman A. Krasnegor**
Human Learning and Behavior Branch
Center for Research for Mothers and Children
National Institute of Child Health and Human Development
National Institutes of Health
Bethesda, Maryland

**Elliott M. Blass**
Department of Psychology
Johns Hopkins University
Baltimore, Maryland

**Myron A. Hofer**
Department of Psychiatry
Columbia University College of Physicians and Surgeons
and Department of Developmental Psychobiology
New York State Psychiatric Institute
New York, New York

**William P. Smotherman**
Laboratory for Psychobiological Research
Departments of Psychology and Zoology
Oregon State University
Corvallis, Oregon

1987

ACADEMIC PRESS, INC.
**Harcourt Brace Jovanovich, Publishers**
Orlando   San Diego   New York   Austin
Boston   London   Sydney   Tokyo   Toronto

iv

Figure 3, page 232, reprinted by permission from McCormick & Thompson, "Cerebellum: Essential involvement in the classically conditioned eyelid response," *Science, 223,* 296–299, January 20, 1984, © AAAS.

Figure 8, page 240, modified by permission of the publisher from *Principles of Neural Science,* edited by E. R. Kandel and J. H. Schwartz, page 338. Copyright 1981 by Elsevier Science Publishing Co., Inc.

ACADEMIC PRESS, INC.
Orlando, Florida 32887

*United Kingdom Edition published by*
ACADEMIC PRESS INC. (LONDON) LTD.
24–28 Oval Road, London NW1 7DX

Library of Congress Cataloging in Publication Data

Perinatal development.

    (Behavioral biology)
    Includes index.
    1. Infants—Development—Congresses.  2. Psychobiology,
Experimental—Congresses.  I. Krasnegor, Norman A.
II. Series: Behavioral biology (New York, N. Y. : 1978)
[DNLM: 1. Child Behavior.  2. Child Development.
3. Infant, Newborn—psychology.  4. Perinatology.
WS 420 P4404]
RJ134.P47  1987    599'.0334    86-26543
ISBN 0—12—445910—2 (hardcover) (alk. paper)
ISBN 0—12—445911—0 (paperback) (alk. paper)

PRINTED IN THE UNITED STATES OF AMERICA

87 88 89 90    9 8 7 6 5 4 3 2 1

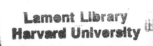

# Contents

**3**  Behavioral Characteristics of Emerging Opioid Systems
       in Newborn Rats
*Elliott M. Blass and Priscilla Kehoe*

**4**  The Role of Sensory Modality in the Ontogeny of
       Stimulus Selection
*Norman E. Spear and Juan C. Molina*

**5**  Neonatal Preference for Mother's Voice
*William P. Fifer*

**III**  **Neural Substrates of Behavioral Plasticity**

**6**  Development of Olfactory Specificity in the Albino Rat:
       A Model System
*Gordon M. Shepherd, Patricia E. Pedersen, and Charles A. Greer*

Contents

**14** Biologic and Behavioral Factors Underlying the Onset
and Maintenance of Maternal Behavior in the Rat

*Jay S. Rosenblatt*

**15** Maternal Influences on the Developing Circadian
System

*Steven M. Reppert, Marilyn J. Duncan, and David R. Weaver*

**V   Social and Emotional Development**

**16** Psychobiologic Consequences of Disruption in
Mother–Infant Relationships

*Seymour Levine*

# Preface

This volume consists of 19 chapters devoted to selected topics on the psychobiological bases of behavioral development. What sets this work apart from others is its emphasis on the perinatal period. The chapters presented discuss exciting new approaches to the interdisciplinary study of behavior during gestation and in the early postnatal period of development. A second feature of interest is that the contents include comparative aspects of development. Results are presented on perinatal development in rat, monkey, and human offspring. In addition, the book exposes the reader to the ideas, perspectives, and findings of a leading group of psychobiologists and neurobiologists who specialize in research on biological and behavioral mechanisms evident in the perinatal period that are necessary for normative behavioral development to proceed.

This book should be of interest to developmental psychologists, developmental neurobiologists, and those investigators interested in sensory, cognitive, and social/emotional development. The researchers and clinicians working in the field of neonatology should also find the volume of interest, since it presents data on the linkages between biological and behavioral mechanisms that may be involved in the diagnosis and treatment of babies born at risk. Finally, the work provides basic scientific underpinnings for the emerging field of research and practice known as behavioral pediatrics. As such, the book may be of immediate use as a contribution to the syllabus for medical and doctoral-level courses that focus on pediatric psychology, behavioral medicine, or child development.

The book was inspired by a conference sponsored by the Human Learning and Behavior Branch of the National Institute of Child Health and Human Development, held at the Xerox Center, Leesburg, Virginia, in September 1985. However, the contents were written and submitted independently of the meeting. The contributions are original manuscripts presented in the form of peer-reviewed scholarly chapters. As such, the book may be viewed as a useful new addition to the growing literature of developmental psychobiology.

# Acknowledgments

In addition to being subjected to the editors' scrutiny, each chapter was reviewed anonymously by other readers, whose names we make known here by way of grateful acknowledgment: Stephen Brake, Marie-Claire Busnel, Patricia Pedersen, and Edwin Rubel.

# I

# INTRODUCTION

NORMAN A. KRASNEGOR
*Human Learning and Behavior Branch*
*Center for Research for Mothers and Children*
*National Institute of Child Health and Human Development*
*National Institutes of Health*
*Bethesda, Maryland 20205*

Just a little over 25 years ago the modern era began for the subdiscipline of medicine known as neonatology. This field of research and practice has as its objective the investigation and care of babies born at risk (including risk for developmental disabilities) due in large part to premature birth and/or intrauterine growth retardation (IUGR). To deal with the unique difficulties related to the care of such tiny, immature beings, neonatologists established the neonatal intensive care unit (NICU). This specialized environment is staffed by highly trained physicians, nurses, and other health care providers whose job it is to diagnose and treat their patients with a wide array of high technology tailored for and scaled to the neonate.

Over the course of this quarter century, clinicians and researchers, who respectively treat and study these babies, have made remarkable advances that have substantially reduced morbidity and mortality in this population. With these changes has come the gradual recognition that further improvement in outcome demands a multidisciplinary approach. Such a strategy includes gaining knowledge of both biologic and behavioral development. This is so because during the immediate postnatal period there is a dynamic interplay between an organism's biologic heritage and its behavior that is necessary for achieving successful adaptation to the new environment outside the womb.

Based upon this awareness, scientists have begun to focus their attention on that aspect of ontogeny known as the perinatal period. This phase of development includes the time span that, in the human offspring, extends from the 28th week of gestation to the end of the first postnatal month. Researchers are interested in this phase because it is then that studies of biologic and behavioral interactions have a good chance of uncovering basic processes thought to be necessary for normative development to proceed on course. Recent work has investigated prenatal learning and behavioral development during the first hours and days after birth.

What is unique about this inquiry is its scientific strategy for asking sophisticated behavioral questions. This includes an appreciation for the measurement of biologic and behavioral variables and their interaction with methodological rigor in the context of the same experimental protocol. Emerging from this approach is an exciting literature on integrative psychobiology that is shedding new light on mechanisms that underpin learning, cognition, and social and affective development. Of particular importance are the contributions made by the field to the basic understanding of mechanisms that govern mother–child interactions. These findings have great relevance for clinical issues relating to this relationship as it emerges during development.

The ideas and data contained in this book are at the cutting edge of research or perinatal behavioral development. The work presented provides excellent examples both of the range and breadth of studies conducted and of innovative methodological approaches needed to address the complex questions inherent in an interdisciplinary strategy. The volume is divided into five parts: (I) Introduction, (II) Comparative Perinatal Learning, (III) Neural Substrates of Behavioral Plasticity, (IV) Parent–Infant Interaction, and (V) Social and Emotional Development.

**Comparative Perinatal Learning**

This part contains five chapters organized around the central theme of interdisciplinary approaches for studying learning prior to and just after birth. The first offering, by Jeffery Alberts, who at the time of this writing is editor of the premier journal, *Developmental Psychobiology,* addresses a central issue for perinatal development, namely, early learning. He approaches his subject from the perspective of *ontogenetic adaptation* and shows how this concept relates to the ethologist's idea of an organism's *niche.* He illustrates these relationships by describing empirical studies from his laboratory on the development of independent ingestion in rat pups. The chapter, which is both an essay at the metalevel of discourse on development and a data-rich empirical work, succeeds in both informing and stimulating the reader. His proposals for future directions of research offer clear paths for exploring the ideas that he has so clearly articulated.

The Alberts chapter is followed by that of William Smotherman and Scott Robinson. The work described provides an overview of the authors' systematic body of research designed to investigate prenatal behavioral development in the fetal rat. Smotherman and his colleagues have pioneered investigations into the learning capacity of the rat fetus using classical conditioning and operant paradigms. The studies detail the innovative methodologies that have been developed to gain this unique "window" on the heretofore unknown aspect of the rat's behavioral development. The studies are important because they provide new information about the ontogeny of the timetable for certain categories of learning. The data complement the work of others (e.g., Hall, Chap. 8 in this volume) who are studying similar learning mechanisms in rat pups during the first few days after birth. Smotherman's research is also significant because it may provide neurobiologists with a way to gestationally date the functional integrity of the rat fetus's developing brain.

The chapter by Elliott Blass and Priscilla Kehoe describes their research on the relationship of the endogenous opiate system to behavioral development of the rat pup. They demonstrate through a series of well-executed experiments how behavioral responses to isolation are mediated in part by the opioid system. The evidence for this control is impressive due to the methodological approach, which employs sophisticated pharmacological, biologic, and behavioral measurement to ascertain the functional dependency. The work is important because it provides strong evidence for central mechanisms that can exert control over behaviors emerging during the perinatal period.

Blass and Kehoe's chapter is followed by that of Norman Spear and Juan Molina, which explores the ontogeny of learning and memory in infant rats. What is unique about the work is the harmonious combination of theoretical analysis and meticulous experimentation they used to pose and answer questions about sensory coding and learning. The tour de force inherent in the many parametric studies successfully elucidates the concept of *intermodal transfer,* which they demonstrate is evident as early as the fourth postnatal day in rat pups. This work is important because parallel studies on the same phenomenon are now being conducted on human infants. The animal model herein described thus has the potential for complementing these investigations and illuminating mechanisms that may underpin both sets of observations. The authors also describe studies which illustrate how infant rats may encode experience in ways that are different from adults. These studies have major implications for gaining an understanding of the differences in what is learned by infants and adults.

In the next chapter William Fifer describes his pioneering work on maternal voice preference by human babies during the first two postnatal days. The capacity for the neonate to discriminate the mother's voice from that of another woman so early in life suggests that experience and learning about it occur prenatally. Work by DeCasper, Fifer's colleague, is suggestive of the fetus's ability both to hear complex rhythms presented to it during gestation and to distinguish such stimuli from novel ones on the first postnatal day. Fifer hopes to use his measures of nonnutritive sucking to study premature babies and discover what if any differences there are between them and full-term babies. His studies also have the potential for revealing processes involved in early attachment, learning, and perception in the neonate.

## Neural Substrates of Behavioral Plasticity

This part of the book contains five chapters grouped as a unit because they all address the development of neural substrates involved in the ontogeny and organization of behavior during the perinatal period. The first chapter in this section is authored by Gordon Shepherd, Patricia Pedersen, and Charles Greer. Its focus is upon the neuroanatomic development of the olfactory system in the albino rat. While this work does not present substantive data on the relationship between sensory learning and the ontogenesis of the neural substrate for olfaction, it does have major implications for those scientists who study early learning. This is so because many psychobiologists have recognized the importance of olfaction in the development of feeding, attachment, and social behavior. It is clear, for example, that the olfactory system is sufficiently well developed functionally during gestation to support learning based on odor cues (see Smotherman and Robinson, Chap. 2 in this volume). The superb neuroanatomic studies reported in this chapter will undoubtedly form the basis for future research that combines behavioral and anatomic approaches to elucidate functional brain/behavior mechanisms that subsume olfactory-based learning as well as social and emotional development.

The next chapter, by Michael Leon, Robert Coopersmith, Suzanne Lee, Regina Sullivan, Donald Wilson, and Cynthia Woo, describes an exciting approach to investigating neural and behavioral mechanisms that may underlie early learning. Specifically, he and his co-workers report on their studies of the neural bases for the acquisition of olfactory preference in neonatal rat pups. They combined methodological approaches that involve the behavioral induction of a preference for a particular odor with 2-DG autoradiographic neural mapping to assess the effects of such experience upon brain activity. The chapter exemplifies the cutting edge research, now possible due to technological innovation in conjunction with an interdisciplinary strategy, that is the hallmark of the best of contemporary developmental psychobiology.

An interdisciplinary approach is also taken by Warren Hall, who reports on the brain/behavior relationships involved in motivation, reward, and learning during perinatal development of rat pups. Hall's studies complement the work of Blass, Smotherman, and Alberts (described above) on early learning and that of Leon regarding the use of 2-DG autoradiography. This brain probe allows an investigator to sample activity of discrete central nervous system (CNS) structures during relevant behavioral situations. When the 2-DG autoradiographic analysis is completed, Hall can map those brain loci which are substantively involved during a particular behavioral task (e.g., a rewarded response such as paddle pushing). Further, his studies are providing an assessment of where neural activation occurs and its amount. His pioneering work should provide a much deeper understanding of basic mechanisms that subsume learning.

The role of experience in brain development is the focus of the next contribution, by William Greenough. He details studies designed to assess the question of whether mechanisms that govern CNS synaptogenesis early in life differ from those that control similar processes in the mature brain. Greenough is an acknowledged pioneer in the study of neural plasticity and is currently a leader of this field, which is crucial for gaining a basic understanding of mechanisms that link brain/behavior development. His research suggests that a critical difference between early and late brain development may be the type of information that is stored at different times during ontogenesis.

The part's final chapter, contributed by Richard Thompson, focuses upon his elegant studies designed to identify and localize CNS memory circuits that subsume associative learning in the mammalian brain. The search for the "engram," as Lashley described it, has occupied many talented researchers during this century. Thompson and his co-workers have employed a wide array of neuroscience approaches that include unit recordings, anatomic tracing, microstimulation, and various lesion techniques to track down this elusive goal. The chapter complements Greenough's in that both address the issue of storage of information in the brain. Basic results in this domain are essential for characterizing mechanisms that provide the substrate for learning.

**Parent–Infant Interaction**

Included in this part are five chapters which have as their central theme the biologic and behavioral factors involved in establishing and maintaining parent–offspring relationships. The first presentation is that of Myron Hofer, a well-known and respected intellectual leader in the field of developmental psychobiology. He reviews his many important contributions to the literature that demonstrate the rodent mother as a regulator of pups' physiological and behavioral functioning early in development. Hofer's work emphasizes the importance of olfaction in early development especially as it influences attachment between the mother and pup. He also provides data on the interaction between the olfactory and somatic senses that may elucidate olfactory-based social behavior.

The next three presentations focus upon the neural and hormonal control of what researchers term *maternal behavior*. In the first of these, Michael Numan reviews his and other workers' recent data that focus upon the identification and analysis of circuits and pathways thought to be involved in maternal behavior. His chapter provides a summary of relevant evidence that implicates the medial preoptic area (MPOA) of the basal telencephalon as a crucial substrate in the rat brain for regulating aspects of maternal behavior. His overview also describes studies that implicate the necessary role of estrogen's action upon the MPOA to facilitate maternal behavior. Finally, he presents data that suggest how MPOA input to the ventral tegmental area (VTA) is crucial for activating motor patterns involved in maternal behavior. The work is significant because it provides basic outlines for the necessary brain structures that mediate behaviors expressed by the female rat which increase the probability that her offspring will survive to maturity.

Cort Pedersen and Arthur Prange also describe central mechanisms for the control of maternal behavior in female rats. Their thesis suggests that the hormone oxytocin plays a crucial role in the onset of maternal behavior. Intracerebroventricular infusion of oxytocin in nulliparous rats was found to increase the frequency of maternal behavior. This effect was found to be estrogen dependent, dose related, and highly specific to oxytocin. The chapter summarizes the authors' and others' data on the function of this centrally acting posterior pituitary hormone for initiating care of the young.

Jay Rosenblatt, one of the doyens of developmental psychobiology, also reviews the literature on maternal behavior. His focus is upon a number of hormones that have been experimentally linked to parental behaviors in the rodent. His cogent overview provides a summary of the evidence that implicates roles for estrogen, progesterone, oxytocin, and prolactin in guiding female behaviors that sustain pups. He also distinguishes between three phases in the organization of maternal behavior: the prepartum phase, the transitional phase, and the postpartum phase. He argues that hormonal control is much more improtant during the prepartum phase than the postpartum one. During this latter aspect of the process, stimulation from the pups is thought to increasingly exert control over the behaviors of the female that insure the pups' survival.

The last chapter in this part describes the exciting work of Steven Reppert, Marilyn Duncan, and David Weaver on the maternal rat's influence in establishing the circadian rhythm of her offspring during gestation. Reppert (who is both a psychobiologist and a pediatrician by training) and his co-workers have systematically studied the role of the maternal superchiasmatic nuclei in setting the biologic clock of her fetus. The work to date suggests that the light–dark cycle of the maternal environment entrains the fetal clock via a process mediated by hormonal messengers that encode the appropriate rhythms. He also describes studies that elucidate postnatal development of these biologic rhythms in the neonatal rat pup.

## Social and Emotional Development

In this, the final part of the volume, four chapters are grouped around the themes of development of social dyadic relationships between the primate mother and her offspring and affective development related to shyness in infant monkeys and young children. Seymour Levine, a progenitor of this discipline, describes his research on the role played by social variables in the modulation of the infant monkey's psychological and biologic response to stress. His work investigates the impact of familiar social partners upon the neuroendocrinologic and behavioral reactions of infant monkeys to separation from the mother. A central hypothesis inherent in Levine's line of investigation is that uncertainty activates the pituitary-adrenal system, while reduction of uncertainty has the effect of dampening or eliminating system reactivity. He and his co-workers believe that stable and familiar social relationships engender predictability in the environment. This influences the certainty–uncertainty continuum and, thereby, an organism's capacity to adapt to stress.

Leonard Rosenblum's contribution focuses upon the relationship of the physical and social environments as the framework within which to study the emergence of maternal behavior and its relation to the developing infant. He reviews studies on the emergence of mother–infant and peer social relationships in several species of monkey. A large part of his

chapter is devoted to a description of his research on the impact of foraging demand upon mother–infant interactions and in turn the influence of
altered mothering on the affective development of the infant. The chapter
nicely complements Levine's in that both demonstrate the power of social
factors in shaping the behavior of infant primates during their formative
development.

The final two chapters address the emergence of stable individual differences in temperament associated with response to novel and/or challenging situations. The first presentation by Stephen Suomi reviews relevant findings on this topic from the existing literature. He then describes
his research designed to tease out genetic and maternal influences on
individual differences. His work demonstrates that there is a genetic basis
for the temperament-related behaviors of interest. This finding is particularly strong when the infant is studied in situations where it is challenged
in the absence of a caretaker (biologic mother or foster mother). In the
presence of the caretaker, however, he finds that the infant monkey's
behavior is much more influenced by the reactivity status of the caretaker.

Jerome Kagan, well known as a developmental psychologist, and his
colleagues Steven Reznick and Nancy Snidman provide an overview of
their findings to date on children who, as in Soumi's primate model,
demonstrate stereotypical temperamental responses to unfamiliar situations. They describe longitudinal studies of two cohorts of children labeled, respectively, as *inhibited* or *uninhibited*. They summarize with
clarity the differences between these two groups in psychophysiological
profile (heart rate, pupillary dilation, and muscle tension), neuroendocrine responsivity (as measured by salivary cortisol and urinary norepinephrine), and behavioral response to challenge in unfamiliar situations.
Kagan's and Soumi's data together provide unique and interesting comparative evidence for the relative influences exerted by inheritance and
experience in developmentally relevant behavior.

In summary, this volume provides a selection of studies that illustrate
the salience of developmental psychobiology as a perspective within
which to discover basic processes that govern normal development. The
work presented also demonstrates the unique contribution that this hybrid
field can make to furthering understanding of how to better care for babies
born at risk for developmental disabilities.

# II

## COMPARATIVE PERINATAL LEARNING

# 1

# Early Learning and Ontogenetic Adaptation

JEFFREY R. ALBERTS
*Department of Psychology*
*Indiana University*
*Bloomington, Indiana 47405*

The perinatal period in mammalian life is dramatic and fascinating; from the womb of the female emerges a strange and unfamiliar creature, quite unlike the adults that spawned it. The newborn animal is naive to the ways of its new and potentially hostile world. The infant has a lot to learn. Whether, when, how, how much, and at what rate the immature mammal *can* learn are fundamental and seemingly simple questions. In the present chapter, I will show that these have *not* been simple questions to answer. Much has been accomplished, however, and it is appropriate to assess some of the trends in this area and consider some possibilities for the future.

Early learning is believed to be of potentially special importance because it is seen as laying down the foundation upon which future behavior, experience, and learning will depend. It is customary to view learning as a means of adding plasticity to an organism's behavioral repertoire. Without the capacity to acquire and express novel behavior, all actions and reactions would have to be "hard-wired" into an organism.

Empirical studies of learning (and memory) in the developing animal have been a regular, albeit episodic, feature of the empirical literature during the past 30–40 years. The recent resurgence of interest in the topic has been dramatic, and progress has been impressive. Many have felt the need for additional or alternate conceptual frameworks, and the present essay will turn to special consideration of one of these: the perspective of ontogenetic adaptation, which has been gaining popularity in recent years (Adolph, 1968; Alberts, 1986; Anokhin, 1964; Galef, 1981b; Oppenheim, 1981; West & King, 1987), largely as it applied to basic conceptualizations

Perinatal Development:
A Psychobiological Perspective

11

of development. In the present essay I will address issues of adaptationist interpretations in general and their relevance to studies of learning in particular.

The organization of this chapter is as follows. First I will discuss a number of general trends that have emerged in the study of early learning. One purpose of this brief review is to highlight areas where more attention should be directed; the framework of ontogenetic adaptation will emerge as one such area.[1] To set the stage for an adaptive analysis of early learning, I will discuss meanings of various uses of the term *adaptation*. This discussion will then focus on ontogenetic adaptation and the related idea of niches during development. The development of ingestion will be used for illustrative examples. The chapter will then turn specifically to a report of investigations from my laboratory in which learning phenomenon was studied as a putative ontogenetic adaptation. The success of this analysis will be assessed, along with some suggestions for future research of this kind.

## I.  Trends in the Study of Early Learning

### A.  Capacity and Rate of Early Learning

As recently as the 1960s, one prevailing view was that the capacity to learn emerges as a landmark event in the postnatal development of many organisms. Evidence for postnatal onset of learning ability was derived from reports of unsuccessful attempts to find evidence of habituation (Scott & Marston, 1950) and to condition even simple reflexes such as leg flexion in newborn dogs (Cornwall & Fuller, 1961; James & Cannon, 1952). In contrast to studies in which young animals failed to learn, there was a spate of more recent ones in which learned responses were acquired by newborn and immature infants (see Campbell & Coulter, 1976). It is now acknowledged that newborns, even those with undeveloped nervous systems and immature sensory-motor apparatus, can learn.

Yet, even with demonstrations of basic learning competence, there remained the assumption that very young organisms may not learn as quickly as their older counterparts (Zimmerman & Torrey, 1965). This is

---

[1] The present chapter is not intended as a review or exhaustive examination of the pertinent literature. Indeed, to meet the editorial guidelines for the book, I have limited the historical, conceptual, and empirical topics and the citations within each topic. The chapter is intended to give an overview of a relatively new, vital, synthetic approach to learning in a developmental context.

the issue of rate. In order to compare accurately the rate of learning in young, very immature animals with rates in older ones, it is necessary to use tasks that can be performed with equal ease at all ages. One of the earliest well-controlled studies tested the ability of rats 30–700 days of age to escape shock by jumping to safety or to approach food in a maze. Both tasks were learned as fast or faster by the younger rats (Stone, 1929). Campbell (1967) and others (Campbell & Coulter, 1976; Lipsitt, 1971; Rovee-Collier, 1984) have reviewed critically a rather large number of studies in which simple tasks have been compared across ages. Generally speaking, when differences in motivation, or in task-relevant perceptual or motor abilities, are not obvious contributors to age-related deficits, rate or capacity of learning has not been found to be a major part of developmental milestones.

## B. Early Learning and Earlier Learning

During the past decade or so, there have been numerous convincing demonstrations of learning in immature infants. Lipsitt (1971) provided dramatic and influential findings that very young human infants can be habituated to novel stimuli and that they can be conditioned readily with both Pavlovian and operant paradigms. Compared to the human infant, most rodents are born at a much earlier point in their neural, sensory, and behavioral maturation, so it was even more startling when reports of very early learning in infant rodents began to appear.

Rudy and Cheatle (1977) found that 3-day-old rat pups learned an odor aversion after a single pairing of LiCl toxicosis with an olfactory conditioned stimulus (CS). Johanson and Hall (1979) devised an ingenious appetitive task in which a pup could obtain pulses of milk into its mouth by probing upward into the paddle. They showed that 1-day-old rat pups could discriminate between two paddles on the basis of odor and learn to respond selectively to the paddle bearing the proper discriminative stimulus.

The march into earlier developmental time has continued, bringing learning contingencies into the womb. For instance, Pedersen and Blass (1982) injected into the amnionitic fluid small quantities of citral, an olfactory stimulus. Newborns showed distinct behavioral reactions specifically controlled by citral. Meanwhile, Smotherman and his associates (see chap. 2) have introduced novel taste/odor cues into the amniotic fluid of rats and then made direct, systemic injections into the fetuses in utero. Several days later, during early postnatal life, LiCl-injected pups show specific aversions to the amniotic stimulus not seen in pups that received odor-paired saline injections in utero.

Although it was not the primary goal of these studies to identify the onset of learning, there nevertheless has been a trend to investigate earlier and earlier stages of development and to demonstrate the learning abilities in each previously untested stage of immaturity. As stimuli and responses have been increasingly refined for early ontogenetic studies, the successful demonstrations of early learning have become more abundant.

## C. Ethological Contributions

Ethological traditions of research have facilitated analyses of early learning. I use the term *ethological* broadly, to include perspectives on animal behavior that attune us to the animal's *Umwelt* (perceptual world), the stimulus control of behavior, and functional or adaptive aspects of behavior as it appears in the natural habitat. Research strategies derived from the ethological tradition have, I think, instilled in experimental psychologists an enhanced awareness of the stimuli which can be applied and manipulated most successfully in studies of learning. This awareness has infiltrated developmental investigations where researchers have made analyses based on naturally occurring stimuli, combined with detailed considerations of the development of perception (Alberts, 1984; Aslin, 1984). Similarly, the ethological tradition has fostered a greater regard for the animal's natural behavioral repertoire.

The net result of these influences has been a shift in the kinds of stimuli and responses used by experimenters in studies of early learning. For instance, with infant rats, it has become increasingly common to use as CSs odors and as reinforcers heat, milk infusions, or merely the opportunity to grasp a nipple. Naturally occurring responses such as approach, sniffing, rooting, probing, and huddling are increasingly common behavioral measures. Coincident with these methodological variations has been a rash of new findings, many revealing previously unsuspected learning and memory abilities in the immature infant (Campbell, 1984).

## D. Learning as an Object of Analysis

The empirical investigation of learning has its historical roots in old philosophical inquiries concerning the nature of mind and related ontological questions. Nonhuman animals were introduced into studies of learning by Darwin (1871) and Romanes (1884) to establish commonalities and continuities across species. This tradition has been maintained over the intervening decades, as seen in the prevailing emphases on generality of laws of learning. Indeed, some learning abilities and mechanisms are demonstrably similar in organisms that are dissimilar in most other ways.

Johnston (1985) calls this the "psychological tradition in learning," and I suggest that this tradition has fostered some pervasive and profoundly influential assumptions.

The search for general laws of learning is historically coupled with the criterion of cross-species similarities in learning. Within this tradition, learning is regarded as an "ability" that can be "possessed" by organisms. The organism thus becomes a vessel, vehicle, or holder of this ability or thing called learning. There are two, related implications. First, learning assumes the conceptual status of an *object*. Second, as a separable entity or object, learning can, for purposes of experimentation, be separated for analysis from the animal that possesses it. To the extent that we think of the organism as a possessor of learning, it seems advantageous to abstract this object called learning to see most clearly its pure, basic attributes.

The psychological tradition, as I have characterized it, encourages us to separate learning from the organism, as though it were a discrete, removable object. This disembodied learning is then dissected, evaluated, and modeled as a discrete process or hierarchical assemblage of learning processes. It is necessary to emphasize that learning is *not* an object; it has no properties independent of the organism that displays it. When we "see" learning, we actually observe a regular change in a profile of behavior that we label as *learning*. I believe that the biological concept of adaptation is a construct relevant to the study of learning in general and the role of early life in particular.


## II.  Ontogenetic Adaptation: The Perspective

### A.   Meanings of Adaptation

Adaptation is a biological concept that provides a functional framework for recognizing and interpreting the organization of living systems. To say that an organism is adapted means that it is organized in relation to some aspect or aspects of its environment. The concept of adaptation is mostly precisely and powerfully applied in the context of evolutionary theory and, as such, has been a unifying force in the fields of ecology, physiology, anatomy, and behavior.

Nevertheless, there are various uses of the term *adaptation,* and much confusion persists. The brief survey below is based on a particularly lucid discussion by Pittendrigh (1958), which has been expanded, critically examined, and further developed by other theorists, such as Williams (1966) and Gould and Lewontin (1978). Adaptation refers to the following:

1. A fitting, functional relationship between organism and environment. There is a basic and important asymmetry in this organism–environment relationship: The organism is adapted to the environment, not vice versa. There is implicit reference to an historical process of change that leads to this form of adaptation.

2. Specific features of the organism which serve a proximate end or function such as feeding, temperature regulation, territorial defense, water balance, etc. These are phenotypic features that serve some functional role in the life of an animal. This use of the term *adaptation* refers to an organismic feature—and its presumed function of purpose—not the way it got there.

3. Adjustments, usually physiological, that occur during an organism's lifetime. Seasonal changes in fur thickness or fat deposition and the enhancement of oxygen-carrying capacity in the blood of organisms that dwell at high attitudes exemplify this usage. Because these adjustments are considered to be shaped by the immediate environment and are expressed solely by the exposed individual, there is no implication of genetic change or heritability of the resultant phenotype.

4. Most precisely and powerfully and most important for the present essay, the usage as in contemporary evolutionary parlance: change in genotype. This type of adaptation explicitly indicates that historical process has been at work. Williams (1966) has carefully distinguished between an *evolutionary adaptation*—which denotes a feature shaped by natural selection for the function it now performs—and an *adaptive response*—which denotes a feature that enhances current fitness, regardless of its historical precursors. This is the distinction between historical genesis and current utility, which was, in fact, recognized and discussed by Charles Darwin (1871). I will return to discuss further the term *adaptation* and its interpretation. At this point, however, we shall consider a special combination of terminology, the idea of ontogenetic adaptation.

## B.  Adaptation during Development

The terminological marriage of *ontogenetic* and *adaptation* yields a valuable and stimulating perspective. It places adaptation in a developmental context (and vice versa). In recent years, the perspective of *ontogenetic adaptation* has been discussed and applied with increasing frequency (e.g., Alberts, 1985; Alberts & Gubernick, 1984; Galef, 1981b; Gould, 1977; Oppenheim, 1981), for it can enhance our understanding of embryology, postnatal development, and evolution.

What are the distinguishing features of this perspective? First, ontogenetic adaptation is an ecological concept, meaning that it places the developing animal into a *functional context*. In the parlance of ecology, this context is the animal's *niche*. The developing mammal occupies a distinct sequence of niches: a prenatal niche in the mother's uterus; an early postnatal niche that includes a milk-providing teat borne on an attendent parent; and subsequent niches in which further stages of differentiation involve a spectrum of distinct physical and social settings (Alberts & Cramer, 1986; Alberts & Gubernick, 1984; Galef, 1981b). There is a profile of anatomical, physiological, and behavioral transformations that corresponds in time and in form to the sequence of ingestive niches encountered by the developing rat.

West and King (1987) have written an eloquent piece on the *ontogenetic niche* as a determinative force in shaping phenotype. Niches, they argue, are inherited as surely as are genes, parents, and other features of the environment. The ontogenetic niche includes diverse factors such as parental behavior, species-typical olfactory cues, local traditions, nests, or feeding sites that are passed to subsequent generations. These sources of stimulation may be repeated in sequential generations yet are not specified by a heritable trait (see Alberts, 1984; Arnold, 1980). These nongenetic forms of inheritance are termed *exogenetic legacies* and are cast as a potent evolutionary force (West & King, 1987).

In its strictest evolutionary form, the perspective of ontogenetic adaptation is based on the assumption that natural selection can operate on *each point in development* (Williams, 1966). This is an important idea because it directs our attention to specialized responses of the organism to specific environmental challenges. Furthermore, we can ask about the historical process by which this adaptive response came about. Again, Williams's analysis can be applied. In this view, it is illuminating to discriminate between ontogenetic responses and susceptibilities. Both are based on cause-and-effect relations between organism and environment, but a *response* shows the property of unique biological, organization, whereas *susceptibility* results from the absence of this property.

The idea of ontogenetic adaptation suggests that each stage of development is a form of completeness, rather than an approximation of the final adult goal. Although this idea is not new, it does represent a departure from mainstream thought. Oppenheim (1981) argues that early in this century there emerged a "primary concern with developmental traits as precursors or antecedents of adult characteristics" (p. 354). And this concern, until quite recently, overshadowed prior perceptions that, in addition to being the pathway to adulthood, each antecedent stage is an organized entity.

C.  Ontogenetic Adaptations Reflected in
    the Development of Ingestion

To illustrate the perspective of ontogenetic adaptation, I will apply it to the vital activity ingestion. This analysis is also germane to the forthcoming treatment of learning, later in this essay.

### 1. Four Ingestive Niches

Like most mammals, the Norway rat encounters during its postnatal development four separable, sequential feeding niches. Each niche can be defined by the form of available nutrient and the pups' mode of ingestion. The four ingestive niches involve, sequentially: (a) prenatal, (b) obligate suckling, (c) weaning (suckling and feeding), and (d) solid food ingestion.

Prenatal ingestion is by infusion of nutrients through the shared maternal–fetal blood supply and placenta. Behaviorally, the pup is a passive recipient. The transition to the extrauterine environment requires immediate adoption of active, oral ingestion. The gastrointestinal system is abruptly challenged by a novel substance, mother's milk. Sampling of solid food begins during the third postnatal week ingestion. The weanling briefly inhabits dual ingestive niches, ingesting milk by suckling and food by independent feeding. The solid food niche requires new preingestive behavior, novel oral movements, and gut absorption of different and varied substances.

### 2. Sequential Adaptations

The perspective of ontogenetic adaptation reveals that in each of these ingestive niches the developing animal displays a corresponding profile of proximate adaptation. That is, development can be characterized by a sequence of stages of adaptive organization, functionally articulated in relation to the ontogenetic niche. During the perinatal period, these niches tend to be dramatically different, and the adaptive adjustments displayed by the infant are correspondingly stunning. The development of ingestion is not merely the final attainment of the adult mode of feeding. Independent feeding is but one in a sequence of distinct, elaborately organized stages.

Stages of ontogenetic adaptation are composed of constellations of adaptive adjustments on multiple levels of organization (sensory, behavioral, anatomical, physiological). Successful stagewise transitions depend on coordinated and integrated readjustments, often drastic in extent. Together, not additively, these integrated, multileveled synergies of ele-

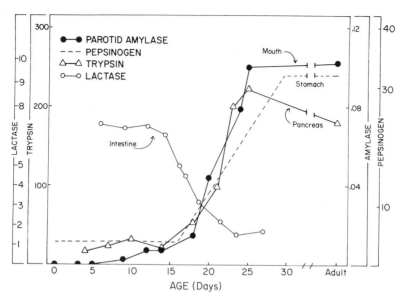

**Fig. 1.** Summary of enzyme changes in the rat's mouth, stomach, intestine, and pancreas that correlate with dietary constituents of the suckling and feeding niches and with the timing of the pup's ontogenetic transition from nursing to feeding. The data shown in this composite figure were collected in numerous separate studies reviewed by Henning (1981).

ments comprise an *adapted organism*. Pittendrigh (1958) emphasized that animals are not bundles of discrete, separable adaptations. The organism is the adaptation. Natural selection operates on individuals, not on individual adaptations.

Much as the pup's early behavior is specialized for finding, grasping and sucking on a teat, the infant gastrointestinal system is structurally and histochemically specialized for the digestion and absorption of milk. During weaning, the epithelium loses its adaptations for the liquid diet of infancy and simultaneously acquires the epithelial adaptations for adult ingestion. Figure 1 is a composite based on separate studies of age-related digestive enzyme changes in the rat. I selected these data because they show biochemical changes in the rats' mouth, stomach, pancreas, and intestine. A startlingly coherent pattern is readily apparent: The age-related changes in enzyme levels are tightly correlated. Specifically, the intestinal enzyme lactase, which is important for the breakdown and absorption of lactose, the major carbohydrate in mother's milk, shows a sudden and dramatic decline, beginning around Day 15, just prior to the onset of weaning (Galef, 1971; Thiels & Alberts, 1985). It has been suggested that this decrease in intestinal lactase renders mother's milk less utilizable and thus contributes to the accretion of a net energy deficit in the pup (Lieberman & Lieberman, 1978; Rozin, 1976) and accelerates incorporation of additional nutrient sources into the diet (Thiels & Alberts, 1985). Coincident with the decline in milk-related digestion is a coordinate surge in the digestive mechanisms that assist in the utilization of a solid-foods diet. These changes appear simultaneously in the pup's mouth, stomach, pancreas, and intestine. This physiological profile is a stunning example of an adaptive shift that corresponds to a change in ingestive niche.

## III.  The Role of Learning in Ontogenetic Adaptation

I believe that there is a viable tradition in the physiological literature in which to integrate the sequences of physiological transformation, such as those described above, into a dynamic picture of ontogenetic adaptation. In contrast, there has been relatively little effort to integrate *behavioral development* into this picture of adaptation, and the perceived role of learning has been even more meager. In the coming sections I will attempt to alter this tradition. There are numerous data indicating that a variety of *experience-sensitive mechanisms* are essential components of the pup's adaptation to each ontogenetic niche. The role of learning can be found both within each niche and in the successful transition from one niche to the next.

My goal in this discussion is twofold. First, I will describe a variety of ways in which learning is part of the pup's adaptation to its sequence of ontogenetic niches, particularly with regard to the development of ingestion. Second, I will describe one portion of a program of investigation from my laboratory which is guided by the assumptions and emphases of the perspective of ontogenetic adaptation.

### A.   Learning as Adaptation for Ingestion

#### 1.   Learned Aspects of Nipple Recognition and Suckling

Nipple seeking in rat pups is controlled by olfactory cues. Anosmic pups cannot find a nipple and suffer inanition (see Alberts, 1981, for review). If the mother's nipples are thoroughly washed, suckling is prevented (Teicher & Blass, 1976). The behavior can be reinstated by painting the cleansed nipples with pup saliva but not with other biological substances such as urine or milk (Teicher & Blass, 1977).

Studies of the sensory control of suckling have provided major insights into learned aspects of early behavior. The olfactory cue for the first nipple attachment is amniotic fluid (Teicher & Blass, 1977), which is deposited on the mother's nipples through self-licking that occurs during the interbirth intervals (Roth & Rosenblatt, 1967). This was a most profound discovery, for it pointed to a thread of chemical continuity connecting the prenatal and postnatal environments. In its new postnatal world, the pup has available at least one cue that it can recognize, and there is evidence that this recognition is *acquired* during prenatal life.

Pederson and Blass (1982) manipulated the pups' prenatal environment so that amniotic fluid did not elicit nipple attachment but another, arbitrary odor would. Nipple attachment by neonatal rats was "reassigned" to the odor of citral (lemon scent). The ability to substitute or reassign an arbitrary stimulus to the control of this essential, adaptive behavior indicates that the potency of the "normal" amniotic stimulus is not rigidly predetermined. It is learned. The precise nature of this learning process remains unclear and may involve a combination of associative and nonassociative processes. It is clear, however, that it is an experience-based mechanism.

### a. Nipple Recognition as Adaptation.

All newborn mammals need a nipple and mother's milk. The sensory-motor events underlying nipple seeking, recognition of the teat, and nursing have obvious vital, adaptive significance. The nursing sequence is adaptive in several ways. With reference to the above meanings, nipple recognition is adaptive because it reflects an overall, fitting functional relationship between pup and lactating dam (Meaning 1) and because it serves a vital, proximate purpose (Meaning 2).

The *means* of nipple recognition provides some additional insights into the nature of these mechanisms of adaptation. In a previous essay (Alberts, 1985), I analyzed nipple recognition by rat pups as an example *congenital recognition* because it is present at birth. Nevertheless, there is no evidence for the existence of a heritable mechanism that specifies a "tuned" perceptual system (see Alberts, 1985, for a discussion of congenital versus predetermined recognition).

Congenital recognition of nipple odors may be an example of a more general type of *susceptibility* rather than a specific adaptive mechanism. Recall that a "response" shows the property of unique biological organization and susceptibility results from the absence of this property (Williams, 1966). If the identification cue for nipples can be reassigned, then the relation between the identification cue and receptor is not unique and would appear to be based on an experience-sensitive susceptibility rather than a highly selected receptor. The results of Pedersen and Blass's (1982) perinatal odor-stimulation manipulation point strongly to an interpretation of ontogenetic susceptibility. Leon (chap. 7) provides a neurobiological view of possible synaptic events in the olfactory bulbs that might transduce such kinds of olfactory induction.

Additional advances have been made in the study of other forms of neonatal learning relevant to ingestive behavior of rats. Brake, Sullivan, Sager, and Hofer (1982) used jaw muscle electromyogram (EMG) recordings to characterize and quantify sucking under different schedules of milk delivery. A particularly dramatic demonstration of early ingestive learning is a study of appetitive conditioning in 1-day-old rat pups (Johanson & Hall, 1979). Neonates were equipped with an intraoral cannula through which milk could be infused. To receive milk, these newborns learned to press either of two overhead paddles, made discriminable with different spice scents.

Similar kinds of results have been obtained with classical conditioning paradigms in which olfactory cues are paired with intraoral infusions of milk. The results of such tests show that conditional olfactory and auditory stimuli can evoke stereotyped food-related responses from pups (Johanson & Teicher, 1980; Rudy & Hyson, 1982).

## 2. Learned Aspects of Weaning

Weaning, the transition from dependence on mother's milk to independent ingestion of solid food, is one of the great commonalities across mammalian development. Through the process of weaning, the infant leaves the niche of infancy and enters a new realm of independence. To accomplish the transition or transitions, the developing mammal undergoes a melange of histological, enzymatic, hormonal, and behavioral changes, some of which were mentioned earlier. The behavioral changes involved in weaning are no less profound than the renowned physiological ones, yet little attention has been afforded to behavior. Preliminary analyses of behavioral aspects of weaning are quite exciting, and learning has been implicated at several points in the process.

Rat pups that have never eaten or sampled solid food nevertheless can learn about the properties of food. Studies of initial food selection—the pup's first bite—show that rats initially select the same diet eaten by their mother during lactation. Milk carries cues that the pup can recognize in food, and these cues guide their initial food selections (Galef, 1981a). Galef and his associates have scrutinized the problem of how the weanling pup chooses safe (nonpoisonous) foods and avoids ingesting dangerous ones. The results of these studies show that pups have a strong tendency to follow adults to the colony's feeding sites, where they begin to eat the same foods that the adults are eating. Thus, the pups can benefit directly from the adults' prior experiences. It was shown, however, that the pups do not learn to avoid a food that the adults avoid; instead they learn to feed on the same, safe foods that adults consume.

In another recent set of experiments, rat pups were reared in cages that permitted access to food by the mother but not the pups. These pups lived solely on mother's milk. At 22 days of age or more, these food-naive pups were offered brief (2-hr) periods of access to two dietary concoctions which were similar in texture, consistency, and palatability but either were calorically void or contained carbohydrate (1 kcal/gm). Each diet was sweetened with saccharin and contained a distinctive, artificial, food odor. After sampling each substance, pups rapidly formed a preference for the "food" (calorie diet). Moreover, in another test, pups continued to eat the calorie-paired flavor even as part of an acaloric mixture, thus showing evidence of associative learning in early food recognition (Melcer & Alberts, 1985).

## B.  A Novel Approach to Early Learning and Ontogenetic Adaptation

I shall next discuss two aspects of a program of experimentation that has been conducted in my laboratory in which we combined an empirical analysis with a framework of ontogenetic adaptation. This led to a set of *predictive hypotheses* derived from an adaptationist interpretation which were *tested* in the laboratory. I will then discuss a case for a fresh view of the role of learning during early development, namely, some implications of ontogenetic adaptation as a conceptual influence on the study of early learning.

### 1.  Blockade of Toxiphobia: The Phenomenon

Prior to the initiation of our experiments, there had been numerous reports that rat pups can learn food-related responses to novel odors and tastes paired with illness (see Alberts & Gubernick, 1984, for summary). In contrast to numerous previous studies, we discovered that preweanling rats showed *no evidence* of learning a taste toxiphobia when a novel milk-borne CS was delivered *during a nursing episode* and paired with a lithium chloride injection (Martin & Alberts, 1979). We refer to this absence of aversion as *blockade of toxiphobia*. The critical difference underlying our results and those from other studies was that pups displaying this blockade were engaged in nutritive suckling (i.e., they were at work in their ingestive niche) during training.

In one typical procedure, pups were equipped with a tongue cannula used to deliver the flavored-milk CS. The cannula permitted control of the quantity, timing, and placement of CS delivery on the tongue of a freely moving rat. Pups from 10 to 22 days old were given oral infusions, via the tongue cannula, of geraniol-flavored milk (the CS) either while *suckling* the nipples of an anesthetized dam or while in the presence of the dam but *not suckling* (i.e., off nipple). The use of an anesthetic prevented milk letdown (Lincoln, Hill, & Wakerly, 1973). Animals were injected with lithium chloride or saline following milk delivery. On either Day 22 or 24, pups were given a choice between three otherwise acceptable diets, one of which (Diet G) contained the flavor CS. Toxiphobia is shown by suppressed intake of Diet G relative to the two other test diets (familiar, safe Purina Rat Chow and a novel diet, Purina Chow flavored with acetophenone).

Figure 2 summarizes the results of the food preference test. Older, weanling-aged pups (21–22 days old), injected with LiCl, avoided Diet G whether the milk CS was delivered while nursing or off nipple (Fig. 2, right panel). In contrast, the younger, preweanling pups that received the CS while suckling *did not show* taste toxiphobia to Diet G (Fig. 2, left and middle panels). Preweanlings trained identically, but not while suckling (i.e., off nipple), exhibited robust, single-trial conditioned aversions to Diet G (Fig. 2, left and middle panels).

Conditioned taste aversions in the preweanling pups are apparently blocked by suckling. Pups that received the flavor CS during a nursing episode lacked a toxiphobic response to the CS, whereas pups given the CS outside the suckling context showed robust aversions. The blockade or nursing-related toxiphobia disappears by 20 days of age. Weanling pups displayed clear aversions to food containing the CS experienced while nursing. Although rat pups do not acquire nursing-related taste aversions in a nursing context, it is clear that neonatal rats learn other kinds of contingencies while nursing (Brake, 1981) and that the suckling act itself, even without nutritive consequences, is rewarding (Amsel, Burdette, & Letz, 1976; Kenny & Blass, 1977).

*a. Empirical Analysis of the Blockade.* We considered several mechanistic explanations for the young pup's blockade of toxiphobia. We rejected the hypothesis that infant rats cannot discriminate the flavored-milk CS, because littermate control animals in all age groups trained off nipple acquired taste aversions (Martin & Alberts, 1979). In addition, preweanlings trained while suckling evidenced a heightened preference

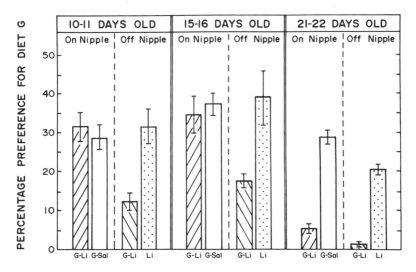

**Fig. 2** Preferences for a flavored test diet (G) in pups given a three-choice food test at weaning. During training, pups received oral infusions of flavored milk either while attached or not attached to a nipple of an anesthetized dam. From Martin & Alberts (1979).

for the food containing the flavor CS, indicating clearly that the pups were obtaining information about the CS (see Martin & Alberts, 1979, for discussion of this observation). Kehoe and Blass (1986) have evidence of topographical sensitivity for tastes on the tongue of the pup, but the pattern of our results do not seem to be determined by such regional sensitivity.

We were also concerned that age-related differences in the manner and position in which nipples are held in the pups' mouths could result in differences in taste receptor stimulation. Nipples of an anesthetized dam were implanted with small, metallic pegs, and rays were made during suckling episodes, so that the nipple location could be visualized in the mouths of suckling pups of different ages. Nipples were held in similar position, providing no support for such age-related differences.

We were concerned with the *generality* of the blockade. The results of the ensuing investigations indicated that the blockade of toxiphobia pertains to olfactory cues as well as to taste stimuli. But all cues may not equally be susceptible. Conditioning of a tactile CS (air puff) and an exteroceptive unconditioned stimulus (US) (subcutaneous shock) was not blocked when training was conducted during suckling (Alberts & Gubernick, 1984). We suggested that the blockade appears to be specific to aversive associations involving chemical cues and ingestive consequences. The blockade of learning by nursing did not extend to a radically different aversive learning situation involving a nonchemical CS (air puff) and a nonvisceral US (electric shock). In addition, it appears that suckling does not prevent the formation of *positive associations,* such as preferences for tastes (Bronstein & Crockett, 1976; Galef & Henderson, 1972) and odors (Brake, 1981) experienced while nursing.

In addition to our interest in the generality of the blockade phenomenon, we have explored the mechanisms underlying the blockade and its developmental dissolution. We examined various components of the nursing episode necessary and sufficient to account for the presence of the blockade in pups less than 20 days of age. Contextual cues, such as siblings and familiar nest cues, can affect learning and performance by preweanling rat pups (e.g., Smith & Spear, 1978). We have found, however, that the presence of siblings and familiar or unfamiliar nest cues did not interfere with the acquisition of odor aversions in pups that either received milk or no milk during training off nipple (Alberts & Gubernick, 1984).

**b. Blockade of Toxiphobia as Ontogenetic Adaptation: Preliminary Analyses and Predictions.** From the perspective of ontogenetic adaptation, we have come to appreciate a variety of morphological and physiological changes that co-occur with entry into different ingestive niches during development. Is it possible to view behavior and, more specifically, *learned aspects of behavior* in the same adaptive context? I think that it is possible and that there are both heuristic and empirical benefits to be gained from the enterprise.

The blockade phenomenon is divisible into two aspects. First is the blockade itself, namely, the lack of toxiphobia exhibited by young pups (less than 20 days of age) that receive the taste-illness pairing during a nursing episode. The second significant aspect is the *absence* of the blockade in pups older than 20-days that receive the identical CS-US pairings while they nurse.

*i. The Age-related Dissolution of Learning Strategy.* The perspective of ontogenetic adaptation does not contain emphasis on age-related changes per se. Instead, it directs our attention toward contextual changes that typically occur during development. In the case of the blockade phenomenon, we were struck by the correlation between weaning and the transitional changes in the blockade. Specifically, we noted that the blockade was intact in preweanling pups (<20 days) and disappeared as pups grew older. In the context of the pups' ontogenetic niches, the blockade operates while the infant lives as an obligate suckler, subsisting in the ingestive niche where mother's milk is the sole nutritive source. By the third postnatal week, the rat pup has entered the next niche, the weaning niche, in which there are available sources of nutrients other than mother's milk.

From an evolutionary perspective, we might expect some learning strategies to change during development as different niches are encountered. While the infant rat inhabits a feeding niche in which it is an obligate suckler, there are no possible benefits to be gained from learning or expressing an aversion to a maternally associated ingestive cue. The costs of avoiding nursing-related stimuli are great. At this stage, the preweanling might even be "protected" from acquiring or expressing aversions to maternal food cues. The weanling, in contrast, inhabits a niche in which it can acquire and utilize nutritive resources in addition to mother's milk. The weanling possesses the behavioral and physiological adaptations for consumption of such foods. In this sense, the weanling can "afford" to avoid mother's milk.

We have identified more precisely the stimulus conditions that are necessary and sufficient to obtain the blockade of toxiphobia. It is still not apparent, however, why young rat pups (<20 days of age) should fail to learn taste aversions while suckling, whereas pups just a few days older (>20 days of age) show suckling-related taste aversions under identical circumstances. There is no evidence that the sub-20-day-old has limited sensory, learning, or memory abilities. Indeed, pups in the various littermate control groups learned and demonstrated clear aversions, so long as they were not suckling during training. We also find a pattern of results interpreted as suggesting that *aversion learning* which involves *ingestion* will not be *expressed* by rat pups. That is, contrary to our initial conceptualizations, learning per se is *not* blocked. Indeed, pups can learn numerous kinds of associations during nursing (see Brake, 1981; Gubernick & Alberts, 1984; Kenny & Blass, 1977). Similarly, we have found several lines of evidence that pups *are learning* about the tastes in their mouths during suckling, but they cannot express taste-related aversions when the taste stimulus is associated with a nursing episode *prior* to 20 days of age (Gubernick & Alberts, 1984).

We conclude, therefore, that the nursing-related blockade of toxiphobia and the dissolution of this blockade are two learning strategies. These strategies alter the manner in which information is integrated and the way in which the learning is expressed. The concept of learning at the heart of this interpretation is different from that of the psychological tradition discussed at the beginning. We view these changes in learning strategy as part of an overall pattern of adaptation to two different ingestive niches. Specifically, we first worked with the view that the blockade of toxiphobia while nursing is an ontogenetic adaptation related to the feeding niche occupied by the infant rat. It is significant that the developmental dissolution of the blockade of learning by nursing coincides with reduction in the maternal milk supply and the weanling pup's exploitation of alternate food resources.

We asked whether manipulations which delayed weaning (i.e., no access to food other than mother's milk) might postpone the acquisition of nursing-related taste aversions beyond an age when such aversions would normally emerge. Conditions which subsequently permit weaning (i.e., access to alternate food sources) might allow acquisition of suckling-related flavor aversions (Gubernick & Alberts, 1984).

*ii. Delayed Weaning.* We imposed a delay of weaning by denying pups access to food and water sources other than mother's milk. Delayed weaning was accomplished in specially constructed cages that allowed mothers, but not pups, access to food and water. Pups were trained on Day 26 in our standard taste aversion procedures, and aversion learning was assessed in a three-choice food test on Day 29 (Gubernick & Alberts, 1984).

We found that 26-day-old pups without prior experience with food (delayed weaning) *did not demonstrate* a taste aversion to a suckling-related cue that had been paired with toxicosis. The delayed weaning procedure did not interfere with the pup's ability to learn and remember the taste aversion, because delayed-weaning pups trained identically, but not while suckling, displayed aversions to Diet G (Fig. 3, left panel). Normally weaned animals displayed taste aversion learning in both the on-nipple and off-nipple condition (Fig. 3, right panel). The apparent blockade of learning by delayed-weaning pups was eliminated by giving pups just 4 hr experience with solid food 2–3 days prior to training (Gubernick & Alberts, 1984).

Weanling-aged pups reared exclusively on mother's milk provided no evidence of learning a conditioned taste aversion in a nursing context. Brief experience with food prior to conditioning seemingly induces a transformation in the pups' taste aversion learning: Pups that have ingested food express aversions to CSs experienced while suckling.

*iii. Blockade of Acquisition or Expression?* On the basis of these data, we could not determine whether delayed weaning produced pups that failed to *acquire* conditioned taste aversions while nursing or failed to *express* the learned aversion. This raised the issue of a learning-performance distinction. If delayed-weaning pups failed to learn an aversion while suckling, then pups exposed to food *after* training should not show aversions to Diet G. If, however, experience with nonmaternal food resources permits the expression of a previously learned conditioned aversion, acquired while nursing, then delayed-weaning pups exposed to food

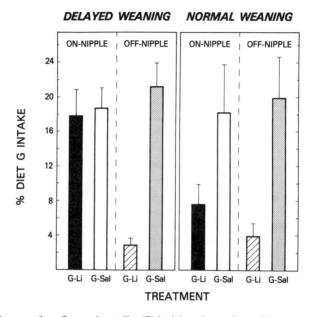

**Fig. 3** Preferences for a flavored test diet (G) in delayed-weaning and in normal-weaning rat pups given a three-choice food test on Day 29 postpartum. Pups were trained on Day 26 with oral infusions of geraniol-flavored milk either attached or not attached to a nipple of an anesthetized dam. From Gubernick & Alberts (1984).

*after* training on nipple should subsequently avoid food containing the flavor CS (Diet G). We found that a brief, 4-hr exposure to food 2 days *after* training on nipple resulted in *aversions* to Diet G (Gubernick & Alberts, 1984). Thus, a short period of ingestion, even after taste aversion conditioning, appears to eliminate the blockade.

Delayed-weaning pups trained while nursing learn aversions to the flavored milk CS but fail to express the aversion unless they experience food. Because experience with food either several days prior to training *or* after training can turn off the blockade, we must conclude that the blockade by nursing is related to a failure to *express* rather than to *acquire* a learned association, at least in the older, weanling-aged animal.

*iv. Early Weaning.* Acquisition of taste aversion learning while nursing does not occur until later in development. Exposure to alternate food is a crucial experiential mechanism underlying the ontogenetic transition in the weanling's learning strategy. Experience with nonmaternal food resources permits the *expression* of a learned aversion. Experience with food might function differently in the young preweaning than in older weanling-aged rats. Pups trained at younger ages and tested after weaning had extensive experience with food but failed to show an aversion (Martin & Alberts, 1979), suggesting the possible involvement of maturational changes in acquisition of nursing-related taste aversions. We examined whether experience with food affected acquisition or expression of taste aversion learning while suckling in younger rats (Melcer, Alberts, & Gubernick, 1985).

Pups were prematurely weaned onto solid food, without access to mother's milk. On Day 13 pups were separated from their mother and were reared together with their littermates in an incubator. Powdered food and water were provided ad libitum, and body weights were taken daily to assess growth. Pups were trained on Day 16 in our standard taste aversion paradigm (with an almond-flavored milk CS) and were given a two-choice food test on Day 21. Pups prematurely weaned onto solid food failed to display an aversion to the CS experienced while suckling and paired with illness. Pups trained off nipple avoided the food containing the flavor CS.

Prematurely weaned pups had access to only one food source, namely, solid food. Since experience with alternate food sources (milk and solid food) resulted in expression of nursing-related taste aversions in older pups (as already described), we provided alternate foods to prematurely weaned pups by giving them brief, daily access to mother's milk. These prematurely weaned animals also failed to show an aversion. The premature weaning procedures did not produce learning deficits related to nursing since prematurely weaned pups trained on nipple at 20 days of age (when suckling-related aversions normally emerge) displayed aversions.

Ingestive experience with solid food appears to function differently at two stages in development. During the stage of normal obligatory dependence on maternal resources, the preweanling's experience with food seemingly has no effect on the acquisition of taste aversion learning while suckling. The same experience with food in the older weanling rat pup does not affect learning per se but permits the *expression* of suckling-related taste aversions. The acquisition of aversions during nursing is apparently dependent in part upon some as of yet unidentified process.

## IV. Overview and Prospectus

Learning is an important but neglected element in the sequence of ontogenetic adaptations that sustains continuity throughout the stages of differentiation comprising the development of early behavior. Viewed as part of the fabric of adaptation, learning is woven into numerous facets of early adjustments, and it provides the foundation and guides the trajectory for subsequent development.

In the present chapter, I focused on various roles of learning in the ontogenetic adaptations for ingestion. The developmental physiology of ingestion has long been characterized as a sequence of stage-appropriate specializations of digestion, but we have been slow to include behavioral development in this view and even more negligent about the role of learning. I argue that too often learning is "disembodied" and thus removed from the behaviors and behavioral contexts that it serves. The perspective of ontogenetic adaptation places learning in a functional context and reveals a sequence of stage-appropriate changes that correspond to other remarkable developmental transformations of the animal.

I discussed the ontogenetic transformation of learning while nursing as part of the weanling's adaptation to the developmental change in feeding niche (Alberts & Gubernick, 1984; Gubernick & Alberts, 1984). The acquisition and expression of nursing-related conditioned taste aversions does not occur until Day 20 postpartum (Martin & Alberts, 1979). The developmental dissolution of the blockade of learning by nursing coincides with reduction in the maternal milk supply and the weanling pup's exploitation of alternate food resources. Learned aspects of toxiphobia apparently can be switched on and off as a function of the niche the pup inhabits. Some aspect or aspects of feeding experience constitute the "switch" that changes the pup's strategy.

From an adaptive framework, perhaps the blockade is not seen in older pups because of their experience with solid food and the availability of nutritive alternatives other than mother's milk. A prediction that arose from this perspective was the delaying or preventing learning about alternate foods would preserve the blockade in pups more than 20 days of age. This prediction was confirmed (Gubernick & Alberts, 1984). A related prediction that early weaning would also hasten the disappearance of the blockade did not receive empirical support (Melcer *et al.,* 1985).

Thus far, the use of adaptive perspectives has increased the range and variety of empirical questions that we can ask and has enhanced the overall interpretive framework for development and behavior. Certainly, the search for adaptive and mechanistic explanations are not mutually exclusive. They are complementary enterprises. Learning should be included in our adaptive and our mechanistic analyses of ingestive behavior (Alberts & Gubernick, 1984).

## A.   Future Directions

Recent achievements, catalyzed by the perspective of ontogenetic adaptation, have brought us to a point at which further conceptual sophistication is needed. Earlier in this chapter considerable attention was de-

voted to a review of the uses of the term *adaptation*. These vernacular
uses range from a general, descriptive use (Meaning 1), usually based on a
priori inference, to a quantifiable, operational definition based on reproductive success (Meaning 4). The level at which adaptation has been
applied in past studies of behavioral development, including studies of
learning, usually has been its general and least rigorous meaning. I hasten
to add that this was not "wrong"; it merely leaves a large margin for
increased precision and depth of analysis. I therefore look forward to
further applications of the concept of ontogenetic adaptation to studies of
behavioral development. Our understanding of early learning, in particular, could benefit enormously from such efforts. We should, I believe,
attempt to move away from the psychological tradition in which learning
is regarded as entity, separable from the organism and develop an alternative view in which learning is seen as a *property of the organism*. That
is, learning is not an entity or capacity that emerges de novo or in
stages of increasing power or complexity. Instead, learning is viewed
as one dimension of organismic adaptation. Our quest is for a conceptual and procedural means by which learning can be placed in an
adaptive/evolutionary framework so that we might see learning as
an adaptive dimension of early behavior and subsequent behavioral
development.

The emergent perspective that I anticipate is one in which learning is
predicted to change during development. In contrast to other conceptualizations, the critical determinants of this ontogenetic change are not neural
development (although this may be a correlative occurrence) or a "necessary" series of stages through which an adultlike capacity is attained.
Instead, we expect changes in learning during development because the
niche inhibited by the organism changes. Thus, emphasis is not on the
development of learning per se, but the development of different niche-
appropriate learning *strategies*. These strategies should appear in sequence and in concert with the appearance of different requirements of
each niche encountered during ontogenesis.

## 1. Behavior Genetics

One way that we could strengthen our adaptive interpretations of early
learning is to conduct empirical tests that invoke assumptions and predictions of genetically based breeding outcomes. That is, if our hypothesis is
that the blockade is adaptive, in the (rigorous) sense that it has resulted
from the action of natural selection, then it should be possible to show
that the degree or frequency of this learning strategy phenotype is heritable. It should therefore be possible to breed selectively animals that var-

ied in the degree to which they displayed the blockade as pups. In order for this presumed, adaptive phenotype of learning strategy to be available as an evolutionary adaptation, it must be available to (and malleable by) selective breeding.

Derivation of two more homogenous groups from such artificial selection is a necessary, but not a sufficient, result for positing a biotic, or genetic, adaptation. Additional, more rigorous tests can be run with the methods of behavior genetics. It would be predicted, for instance, that if a particular genotype (e.g., related to a blockade strategy of learning) was operating as a selected trait, it should show *dominance* rather than mere additivity in subsequent generations. Moreover, if a trait has been established by a positive selection pressure, inbreeding should result in an overall decrease of the trait (N. D. Henderson, personal communication, 1985). That is, if the blockade faded with inbreeding (sibling matings), this would constitute evidence that its presence had been an actively selected adaptation.

### 2. Comparative-Developmental Studies

Another traditional means of fortifying our use of adaptive evolutionary concepts is to apply comparative methods, one of the most powerful tools in biology. Behavioral biology, including developmental psychobiology, would benefit from more frequent use of comparative methodologies. Our perspective on the blockade of toxiphobia posits that the dissolution of the blockade is linked both causally and adaptively to the transition from the suckling niche to the weaning niche. Within this framework, we should be able to make several predictions, including (a) The blockade of toxiphobia should be present in the suckling young of other species, most likely those with ingestive niches similar to that of *Rattus norvegicus;* and (b) dissolution of the blockade should covary with niche transition (from suckling to weaning) despite age/maturational variables.

Precocious species, that is, those born at an advanced stage of maturation, could be used as a comparative tool in tests of the blockade hypotheses. Species such as the Egyptian spiny mouse (*Acomys cahirinus*) produce offspring that are highly developed. The newborns nurse from their mother, but they also begin to eat (i.e., depart the suckling niche) within the first postnatal week. We would predict, therefore, that the suckling spiny mouse pup would demonstrate the blockade because they are challenged with the same no-choice dilemma of monophagy characteristic of the infant rat. We would further predict dissolution of the blockade to be coincident with their weaning, early in postnatal life.

### 3. Manipulating a System of Ingestive Adaptation

Throughout this chapter, the manner in which I characterized the development of ingestion in the rat was intended to convey a perspective in which the anatomy and physiology of the pup's mouth, stomach, intestine, brain, and behavior were synchronized to serve as a unified, adaptive *system* for ingestion. I use the term *system* to refer to a multileveled assembly of coordinated changes that together serve a function of lawfully related inputs and outputs.

Previous workers have shown that the development of gastrointestinal function is, to some degree, controlled by singular commands that serve to initiate or regulate multiple changes, such as shifts in enzyme levels (Yeh & Moog, 1974). I would predict that factors such as thyroid secretion, which have been shown to regulate gastrointestinal factors related to ingestive adaptation, will *also* be linked to the maturation of related learning strategies. Analyses of common controllers will be a helpful step in the accurate formulation of behavioral dimensions of complex ontogenetic adaptations.

The future of such studies will require creative, synthetic approaches to both behavior and physiology. This is characteristic of the field of developmental psychobiology, and it portends well for the future of integrative knowledge in the life sciences.

### Acknowledgments

Original research described in this chapter was supported by grants from the National Institute of Mental Health (MH28355), NIMH Research Scientist Development Award (MH00222) to J.R.A., and National Science Foundation (BNS 79-15116) to J.R.A. and D.G. Gubernick.

### References

Adolph, E. F. (1968). *Origins of physiological regulations*. New York: Academic Press.
Alberts, J. R. (1981). Ontogeny of olfaction: Reciprocal roles of sensation and behavior in the development of perception. In R. N. Aslin, J. R. Alberts, & M. R. Petersen (Eds.), *Development of perception: Psychobiological perspectives* (Vol. 1, pp. 321–357). New York: Academic Press.
Alberts, J. R. (1985). Ontogeny of social recognition: An essay on mechanism and metaphor in behavioral development. In E. S. Golin (Ed.), *Comparative development of adaptive skills: Evolutionary implications* (pp. 65–101). Hillsdale, NJ: Erlbaum.
Alberts, J. R. (1986). New views of parent–offspring relationships. In W. T. Greenough & J. M. Juraska (Eds.), *Developmental neuropsychobiology* (pp. 451–480). Orlando: Academic Press.

Alberts, J. R., & Cramer, C. P. (1986). Ecology and experience: Sources of means and meaning in developmental change. In E. M. Blass (Ed.), *Handbook of behavioral neurobiology, Vol. 9, Behavioral ecology and developmental psychobiology*. New York: Plenum.

Alberts, J. R., and Gubernick, D. J. (1984). Early learning as ontogenetic adaptation for ingestion by rats. *Learning and Motivation, 15,* 334–359.

Amsel, A., Burdette, D. R., & Letz, R. (1976). Appetitive learning, patterned alternation, and extinction in 10-day-old rats with non-lactating suckling as reward. *Nature, 262,* 816–818.

Anokhin, P. K. (1964). Systemogenesis as a general regulator of brain development. *Progress in Brain Research, 90,* 54–86.

Arnold, S. J. (1980). The microevolution of feeding behvior. In A. Kamil & T. Sargent (Eds.), *Foraging behavior: Ecological, ethological and psychological approaches* (pp. 409–453). New York: Garland.

Aslin, R. N. (1984). Sensory and perceptual constraints on memory in human infants. In R. Kail & N. E. Spear (Eds.), *Comparative perspectives on the development of memory* (pp. 39–64). Hillsdale, NJ: Erlbaum.

Brake, S. C. (1981). Suckling rats learn a preference for a novel olfactory stimulus paired with milk delivery. *Science, 211,* 506–507.

Brake, S. C., Sullivan, R., Sager, D. J., & Hofer, A. M. (1982). Short- and long-term effects of various milk-delivery contingencies on suckling and nipple attachment in rat pups. *Developmental Psychobiology, 15,* 543–556.

Bronstein, P. M., & Crockett, D. P. (1976). Maternal rations affect the food preference of weanling rats: II. *Bulletin of the Psychonomic Society, 8,* 227–229.

Campbell, B. A. (1967). Developmental studies of learning and motivation in infraprimate mammals. In H. W. Stevenson, E. H. Hess, & H. L. Rheingold (Eds.), *Early behavior: Comparative and evolutionary approaches* (pp. 43–71). New York: Wiley.

Campbell, B. A. (1984). Reflections on the ontogeny of learning and memory. In R. Kail & N. E. Spear (Eds.), *Comparative perspectives on the development of memory* (pp. 23–35). Hillsdale, NJ: Erlbaum.

Campbell, B. A., & Coulter, X. (1976). The ontogenesis of learning and memory. In M. R. Rosenzweig & E. L. Bennett (Eds.), *Neural mechanisms of learning and memory* (pp. 209–235). Cambridge: MIT Press.

Cornwall, A. C., & Fuller, J. L. (1961). Conditioned responses in young puppies. *Journal of Comparative and Physiological Psychology, 54,* 13–15.

Darwin, C. R. (1871). *The descent of man in relation to sex.* London: Murray.

Galef, B. G., Jr. (1971). Social effects in the weaning of domestic rat pups. *Journal of Comparative and Physiological Psychology, 75,* 358–362.

Galef, B. G., Jr. (1981a). Development of flavor preferences in man and animals: The role of social and nonsocial factors. In R. N. Aslin, J. R. Alberts, & M. R. Petersen (Eds.), *Development of perception: Psychological perspectives* (Vol. 1, pp. 411–431). New York: Academic Press.

Galef, B. G., Jr. (1981b). The ecology of weaning: Parasitism and the achievement of the independence of altricial mammals. In D. J. Gubernick & P. H. Klopfer (Eds.), *Parental care in mammals* (pp. 211–241). New York: Plenum.

Galef, B. G., Jr., & Henderson, P. (1972). Mother's milk: A determinant of the feeding preferences of weanling rat pups. *Journal of Comparative and Physiological Psychology, 78,* 213–219.

Gould, S. J. (1977). *Ontogeny and phylogeny.* Cambridge: Belknap Press of Harvard University Press.

Gould, S. J., & Lewontin, R. (1978). The spandrels of San Marcos and the Panglossian paradigm: A critique of the adaptationist programme. *Proceedings of the Royal Society of London, 205*, 581–588.

Gubernick, D. J., & Alberts, J. R. (1984). A specialization of taste aversion learning during suckling and its weaning-associated transformation. *Developmental Psychobiology, 17*, 613–628.

Henning, S. J. (1981). Postnatal development: Coordination of feeding, digestion, and metabolism. *American Journal of Physiology, 241*, G199–214.

James, W. T., & Cannon, D. J. (1952). Conditioned avoidance responses in puppies. *American Journal of Physiology, 168*, 251–253.

Johanson, I. B., & Hall, W. G. (1979). Appetitive learning in 1-day-old rat pups. *Science, 205*, 419–421.

Johanson, I. B., & Teicher, M. H. (1980). Classical conditioning of an odor preference in 3-day-old rat pups. *Behavioral and Neural Biology, 29*, 132–136.

Johnston, T. D. (1985). Conceptual issues in the ecological study of learning. In T. D. Johnston & A. T. Pietrewicz (Eds.), *Issues in the ecological study of learning* (pp. 1–24). Hillsdale, NJ: Erlbaum.

Kehoe, P., & Blass, E. M. (1986). Conditioned aversions and their memories in 5-day-old rats during suckling. *Journal of Experimental Psychology: Animal Behavior Processes, 12*, 40–47.

Kenny, J. T., & Blass, E. M. (1977). Suckling as incentive to instrumental learning in preweanling rats. *Science, 196*, 898–899.

Lieberman, M., & Lieberman, D. (1978). Lactose deficiency: A genetic mechanism which regulates the time of weaning. *American Naturalist, 112*, 625–627.

Lincoln, D. W., Hill, A., & Wakerly, J. B. (1973). The milk-ejection reflex of the rat: An intermittent function not abolished by surgical anesthesia. *Journal of Endocrinology, 57*, 459–476.

Lipsitt, L. P. (1971). Infant learning: The blooming, buzzing confusion revisited. In M. E. Meyer (Ed.), *Second Western Symposium on Learning: Early Learning* (pp. 5–19). Bellingham: Western Washington State College.

Martin, L. T., & Alberts, J. R. (1979). Taste aversions to mother's milk: The age-related role of nursing in acquisition and expression of a learned association. *Journal of Comparative and Physiological Psychology, 93*, 430–455.

Martin, L. T., & Alberts, J. R. (1982). Associative learning in neonatal rats revealed by heartrate response patterns. *Journal of Comparative and Physiological Psychology, 96*, 668–675.

Melcer, T., & Alberts, J. R. (1985). *Recognition of food by "food-naive," weanling-age rat pups.* Paper presented at the meeting of the International Society for Developmental Psychobiology, Dallas.

Melcer, T., Alberts, J. R., & Gubernick, D. J. (1985). Early weaning does not accelerate the expression of nursing-related taste aversions. *Developmental Psychobiology, 18*, 375–382.

Oppenheim, R. W. (1980). Metamorphosis and adaptation in the behavior of developing organisms. *Developmental Psychobiology, 13*, 353–356.

Oppenheim, R. W. (1981). Ontogenetic adaptations and retrogressive processes in the development of the nervous system and behavior. In K. Connolly & H. Prechtl (Eds.), *Maturation and behavior development* (pp. 73–109). London: Spastics Society Publications.

Pedersen, P. E., & Blass, E. M. (1982). Prenatal and postnatal determinants of the 1st suckling episode in albino rats. *Developmental Psychobiology, 15*, 349–355.

Pedersen, P. E., Williams, C. L., & Blass, E. M. (1982). Activation and odor conditioning of suckling behavior in 3-day-old albino rats. *Journal of Experimental Psychology: Animal Behavior Processes, 8,* 329–341.

Pittendrigh, C. S. (1958). Adaptation, natural selection, and behavior. In A. Roe and G. G. Simpson (Eds.), *Behavior and evolution* (pp. 390–425). New Haven, CT: Yale University Press.

Romanes, G. J. (1884). *Mental evolution in animals.* East Norwalk, CT: Appleton-Century-Crofts.

Roth, L. L., & Rosenblatt, J. S. (1967). Changes in self-licking during pregnancy in the rat. *Journal of Comparative and Physiological Psychology, 63,* 397–400.

Rovee-Collier, C. (1984). The ontogeny of learning and memory in human infancy. In R. Kail & N. E. Spear (Eds.), *Comparative perspectives on the development of memory* (pp. 103–134). Hillsdale, NJ: Erlbaum.

Rozin, P. (1976). The selection of foods by rats, humans, and other animals. In J. S. Rosenblatt, R. A. Hinde, E. Shaw, & C. G. Beer (Eds.), *Advances in the study of behavior* (Vol. 6., pp. 21–76). New York: Academic Press.

Rudy, J. W., & Cheatle, M. D. (1977). Odor-aversion learning in neonatal rats. *Science, 198,* 845–846.

Rudy, J. W., & Hyson, R. L. (1982). Consummatory response conditioning to an auditory stimulus in neonatal rats. *Behavioral and Neural Biology, 34,* 209–214.

Scott, J. P., & Marston, M. V. (1950). Critical periods affecting the development of normal and maladjusted social behavior in puppies. *Journal of Genetic Psychology, 77,* 25–60.

Smith, G. J., & Spear, N. E. (1978). Effects of the home environment on withholding behaviors and conditioning in infant and neonatal rats. *Science,* 327–329.

Stone, C. P. (1929). The age factor in animal learning: I. Rats in the problem box and the maze. *Genetic Psychology Monographs, 5,* 1–130.

Teicher, M. H., & Blass, E. M. (1976). Suckling in newborn rats: Eliminated by nipple lavage, reinstated by pup saliva. *Science, 193,* 422–424.

Teicher, M. H., & Blass, E. M. (1977). First suckling response of the newborn albino rat: The roles of olfaction and amniotic fluid. *Science, 198,* 635–636.

Thiels, E., & Alberts, J. R. (1985). Role of milk availability in weaning by the Norway rat. *Journal of Comparative Psychology, 99,* 447–456.

West, M. J., & King, J. A. (1987). Settling nature and nurture into an ontogenetic niche. *Developmental Psychobiology,* in press.

Williams, G. C. (1966). *Adaptation and natural selection.* Princeton, NJ: Princeton University Press.

Yeh, K-Y., & Moog, F. (1974). Intestinal lactose activity in the suckling rat: Influences of hypophysectomy and thyroidectomy. *Science, 183,* 77–79.

Zimmerman, R. R., & Torrey, C. C. (1965). Ontogeny of learning. In A. M. Schrier, H. F. Harlow, & F. Stollnitz (Eds.), *Behavior of nonhuman primates: Modern research trends* (Vol. 2, pp. 405–447). New York: Academic Press.

# 2

# Psychobiology of Fetal Experience in the Rat

WILLIAM P. SMOTHERMAN and SCOTT R. ROBINSON
*Laboratory for Psychobiological Research*
*Departments of Psychology and Zoology*
*Oregon State University*
*Corvallis, Oregon 97331*

## I. Introduction

In the 1920s and 1930s there was considerable scientific interest in the prenatal development of behavior (Hooker, 1952). Perhaps because the extant technical knowledge was inadequate, this early research lay fallow for nearly 40 years until the importance of prenatal influences on the physiology and behavior of offspring was rediscovered. Researchers in many fields are now becoming increasingly aware that changes in the uterine environment in which a fetus develops can have profound effects on the physical condition and behavior of offspring.

Because interest in prenatal experience has roots in so many different disciplines, the methodologies used to study continuities between prenatal and postnatal life have been equally diverse. Direct observation of surgically exteriorized animal fetuses or aborted human fetuses was one of the earliest strategies for studying fetal behavior, but technological difficulties and ethical considerations have, until recently, limited the usefulness of this strategy for understanding the role of experience during the prenatal period. Similarly, technological advances for noninvasive visualization of human fetuses have appeared only in the last decade (Reinold, 1976). For most of the history of fetal research, a more informative approach to understanding prenatal experience has involved indirect manipulation of the fetus and inference from subsequent developmental

consequences. In fact, this is the characteristic strategy employed in tera-
tological research (Landesman-Dwyer, 1982; Ward, 1984). Typically,
a pregnant female subject is exposed to various experimental conditions (drugs, other chemical substances, stress, etc.), and the effects
on the fetus are inferred from postnatal anatomic or behavioral outcomes, such as growth retardation, malformation or absence of body
parts, abnormal activity, learning impairment, or atypical behavioral
development.

Although the postnatal approach may be useful in the study of chronic
prenatal exposure to teratogens or drugs, it ignores the "black box" and
its inhabitant—the fetus in utero—which is altered by indirect manipulation of the pregnant female. Methodology is important, not just in the
conduct of individual experiments, but also in shaping the kinds of questions that are asked and the consequent biases brought to a field of study.
By placing emphasis on postnatal development, attention is directed away
from the fetus itself. In order to build a detailed understanding of the role
of experience during prenatal life, it is necessary to apply the same techniques used in studying postnatal behavioral development (as in learning)
to the fetus. Only in the last few years have we seen progress toward the
ultimate goal of directly observing the response of the fetus to immediate
changes in its intrauterine environment.

## II.  First Generation: External Stimulation

Prior to 1980, attempts to directly study the responsiveness of fetuses
to novel and conditioned stimuli were necessarily simple and employed
unsophisticated methods of manipulating the fetal environment and monitoring fetal activity. For example, the human fetus exhibits a startle response to sudden, loud noise that is detectable on the external surface of
the mother's abdomen. This fact was exploited in the first experiments
designed to assess the learning ability of the fetus (Ray, 1932; Spelt,
1948). A vibrotactile stimulus first was demonstrated to produce no fetal
response when applied to the abdomen of a pregnant woman during the
last trimester of pregnancy. This neutral stimulus was then paired with a
sudden, loud noise in a series of trials. Following a period of conditioning,
the vibrotactile stimulus was again applied without the associated noise
and was found effective in eliciting gross fetal movements. While Ray was
unsuccessful (with data from a single subject), Spelt claimed success with
these procedures in demonstrating classical conditioning of fetal movements, extinction, spontaneous recovery, and retention over a 3-week

interval during the last 2 months of pregnancy. These experiments, though innovative for the time, have since been criticized on methodological grounds, including their reliance on a small number of subjects and lack of procedural rigor.

Although new technologies have improved methods of detecting movement by the fetus in utero, the indirect approach pioneered by Ray and Spelt for manipulating the environment of the fetus has remained in use, with remarkably little change, to the present day (Leader, Baillie, Martin, & Vermeulen, 1982). Recently, external fetal monitoring has been employed successfully to describe patterns of activity in the human fetus during late gestation (Patrick, Campbell, Carmichael, & Probert, 1982). More detailed information on the behavioral repertoire of human fetuses has been obtained through the use of real-time ultrasonography (Birnholz & Benacerraf, 1983; de Vries, Visser, & Prechtl, 1982).

Perhaps the most sophisticated application of external stimulus manipulation in the study of fetal behavior is represented by the work of DeCasper and his colleagues. The intrauterine environment comprises a rich assortment of acoustic stimuli originating in the mother and the external world (Walker, Grimwade, & Wood, 1971), and the fetus is capable of auditory perception by late in the second or early in the third trimester of gestation (Birnholz & Benacerraf, 1983). DeCasper discovered that a human newborn will increase its rate of nonnutritive sucking to gain access to tape recordings of its mother's voice and that the mother's voice is preferred over the voice of an unfamiliar female (DeCasper & Fifer, 1980). Subsequent studies have similarly demonstrated that newborns exhibit a preference for the sound of maternal heartbeat (DeCasper & Sigafoos, 1983) and can discriminate between paternal and unfamiliar male voices (DeCasper & Prescott, 1984). Most recently, these neonatal acoustic preferences have been shown to be influenced by prenatal experience, as, for instance, by the mother repeatedly reading aloud a passage from a children's story during the third trimester of pregnancy (see the review by Fifer in chap. 5).

The pattern of these findings suggests several conclusions regarding fetal experience. Some form of auditory perceptual learning appears to occur when fetuses are exposed to a normal acoustic environment in utero. Viewed in a broader context, these experiences influence not only the behavior of the newborn but also the nature of parent–infant interactions. The process of voice recognition by the human newborn is thus remarkably similar to the development of individual and species recognition in birds (Gottleib, 1985) and may perform an analogous function in humans.

## III.  Second Generation: Direct Manipulation

Manipulation of the fetal environment through external stimulation can
be precise when acoustic stimuli are employed but lacks control with
other stimuli that must be transmitted or transported to the fetus by
circuitous routes. Uncertainty about the effects of stimulation is especially true of experiments that expose fetuses to teratogenic or behaviorally active chemicals. In order for these substances to reach the fetus,
they must be introduced to the mother, transported by maternal circulation, diffused across the placenta, and delivered to the fetus in sufficient
concentrations to alter fetal physiology and/or behavior. Every link in this
chain is unpredictable and lacks the measurable precision necessary to
establish causal connections between changes in the intrauterine environment and fetal behavior.

A more fruitful approach to studying the control and development of
fetal behavior has proved possible through technical procedures for directly manipulating the intrauterine environment of the fetus. Of course,
for ethical reasons this approach is only practical with nonhuman animal
subjects, such as laboratory rats. Many features of the rat fetus's environment change over the course of gestation (Smotherman & Robinson, in
press). One of the environmental features that is amenable to direct
manipulation is the fluid medium that immediately surrounds the fetus.
Amniotic fluid varies in volume, viscosity, lubricant quality, and chemical
composition during gestation and provides physical protection, promotes
osmotic stability, facilitates fetal movement, and contributes nutritional
and immunologic factors in the development of the fetus. The fluid is
ingested by the fetus and replenished by secretions of the amnion and
products of the fetal pulmonary, alimentary, and renal systems. These
dynamic processes result in turnover of the water content of amniotic
fluid, and presumably other constitutents, every 3 hr (Wirtschafter &
Williams, 1957).

Because the fluid is actively ingested and circulated, it can provide a
vehicle for presentation of chemosensory stimuli to the fetus. New prode-
dures have been described recently (Blass & Pedersen, 1980; Stickrod,
1981) by which a pregnant rat is anesthetized late in gestation, her uterus
externalized through a midventral incision, and various chemical solutions injected through the uterine wall into the amniotic fluid. The uterus
is then replaced inside the peritoneum of the mother, and the incision
closed by sutures. At term, the pups are delivered by normal vaginal
delivery or taken by cesarean section and cross-fostered to recently parturient mothers. Behavioral assessment of the effects of prenatal exposure can be conducted immediately after birth or at any subsequent time

during the postnatal period. Physical growth of pups manipulated in utero in this fashion is identical to that of untreated pups, suggesting that the procedure is benign (Smotherman, Robinson, & Miller, 1986).

The ability to manipulate the sensory characteristics of amniotic fluid has proven to be especially valuable in understanding the ontogeny of suckling in infant rats. Suckling consists of a complex sequence of activities initiated by location and attachment to the nipple. Numerous experiments have now established that olfactory cues are important in the control of nipple attachment. Pups that are rendered anosmic fail to attach to the nipple and do not suckle (Hofer, Shair, & Singh, 1976). Gentle lavage of the nipples, which removes any odor cues, similarly eliminates attachment, but application of pup saliva to washed nipples reinstates attachment (Teicher & Blass, 1977). The principal olfactory cue in pup saliva is dimethyl disulfide (DMDS), which is nearly as effective at reinstating attachment to washed nipples as fresh pup saliva (Pedersen & Blass, 1981). These findings, by elucidating the role of pup saliva in normal nipple attachment, also raised a question about the mechanisms involved in the first nipple attachment, in which pup saliva logically cannot play a role. Subsequent experiments revealed that amniotic fluid, which is normally placed on the nipples by maternal licking during parturition, directs the first nipple attachment of newborn pups (Blass & Teicher, 1980). This discovery was extended by manipulation of the prenatal experience of fetuses (Pedersen & Blass, 1982). On Day 20 of gestation, citral, a tasteless lemon scent, was injected into the amniotic fluid of fetuses in utero, then presented again immediatley after birth. Pups that receive both prenatal and postnatal exposure to citral attach to nipples painted with citral, but pups that receive only prenatal or postnatal exposure, or neither, fail to attach to citral-painted nipples. Further, citral-exposed pups fail to attach to nipples painted with normal amniotic fluid. This experiment clearly demonstrates how prenatal experience confers upon amniotic fluid its ability to regulate an important postnatal behavior such as nipple attachment and suckling.

Current evidence suggests that prenatal experience with chemicals in amniotic fluid is mediated by olfaction. Pedersen and Blass (1982) suggested at least two routes by which chemosensory stimuli could be detected by the rat fetus. First, chemical cues within the liquid medium of amniotic fluid could enter and directly stimulate the vomeronasal organ. Alternatively, amniotic fluid could stimulate the main olfactory system through contact with olfactory epithelia within the internal nares. This possiblity seems unlikely, however, in view of the fact that the accessory olfactory bulb (associated with vomeronasal reception), but not the main olfactory bulb, is functional by Day 22 of gestation (Pedersen, Stewart,

Greer, & Shepherd, 1983). Involvement of the vomeronasal system thus appears the most likely method of fetal olfaction, with subsequent generalization of fetal experience to the main olfactory system and other media of chemical exposure (i.e., gaseous) during the transition to postnatal life.

It is also noteworthy that the findings of Pedersen and Blass indicate a form of fetal learning that occurs in the absence of obvious reinforcers in the fetal environment. A similar effect has been reported for the drinking preferences of adult rats. Adults that have been exposed to apple juice in utero prefer to drink apple juice over tap water (Smotherman, 1982a). In contrast, other studies have shown that fetal learning is promoted by association of olfactory cues with aversive stimulation. Presentation of a taste or odor cue that is paired with an aversive stimulus, such as the intraperitoneal (IP) injection of LiCl, will cause the rat to avoid the taste or odor upon subsequent presentation (Garcia, Lasiter, Bermudez-Rattoni, & Deems, 1985). This learning paradigm has recently been applied to the study of prenatal experience by delivering a chemosensory stimulus (such as apple juice) to rat fetuses on Day 20 of gestation through amniotic injection, followed after a brief delay by IP injection of each fetus with LiCl (Stickrod, Kimble, & Smotherman, 1982a). Postnatal behavior of rat pups that receive the apple-LiCl pairing in utero (conditioned pups) differs from the behavior of pups that receive apple paired with an injection of saline or saline exposure paired with LiCl injection. When allowed to suckle from their anesthetized mother, pups exhibit preferential attachment to nipples as a function of prenatal experience; conditioned pups attach to apple-painted nipples less often than any control pups (Stickrod et al., 1982a). Conditioned pups also exhibit longer delays to traverse a runway suffused with the odor of apple to gain access to their mother (Smotherman, 1982b) and prefer the low-concentration end of a chamber containing a gradient of apple odor (Stickrod, Kimble, & Smotherman, 1982b).

We have recently reviewed the evidence that the rat fetus is responsive to changes that normally occur within its intrauterine environment (Smotherman & Robinson, in press). We have speculated that these behavioral alterations represent ontogenetic adaptations (Oppenheim, 1981) which have important implications for subsequent behavioral and morphological development. Second-generation studies of fetal experience confirm that manipulations of the fetal environment during the prenatal period can produce long-lasting changes in the behavior of offspring that contribute to their survival and development. The rat fetus exhibits a form of olfactory sensitization or imprinting that is important in postnatal suckling and consummatory behavior. It is also capable of olfactory associative learning in utero which can be retained into postnatal life. These experiments illustrate how the use of nonhuman animal subjects and controlled manipulations of the fetal environment permit experimental designs that incorporate the control groups necessary for testing competing hypotheses. For this reason alone, methods for directly manipulating the sensory environment of the fetus offer a significant advance over imprecise maternal exposure and indirect inference.

## IV. Third Generation: Prenatal Observation

The second-generation approach to studying the capacity of fetuses to learn has proved successful in establishing associations in utero but is still limited by the necessity of assessing the effects of learning postnatally. Either all fetuses within a female must receive the same treatment, eliminating the possibility of within-litter comparisons, or fetuses from known uterine positions must be taken by cesarean section and cross-fostered, with some consequent mortality of pups (Smotherman, Robinson, La Vallee, & Hennessy, in press). Further, when all fetuses within a female are treated, the prolonged surgical procedure necessitates the use of a long-lasting maternal anesthetic, exposing fetuses for longer periods to the effects of general anesthesia. The actual conditioning trial occurs when the mother is completely anesthetized, after the fetuses have been exposed to the general anesthetic for 15–20 min, and the mother may not fully recover until several hours after surgery. Finally, the need to anesthetize the mother precludes the assessment in utero of both the immediate effects of conditioning and the later expression of a learned aversion by the fetus; all behavioral effects must be judged postnatally. This is a notable limitation, not only because the behavior of fetuses is interesting in its own right, but also because changes in the patterns of behavior exhibited by fetuses in utero may be retained into postnatal life. For example, in utero exposure to drugs such as morphine (Kirby, 1981) or alcohol (Smotherman, Woodruff, Robinson, del Real, Barron, & Riley, 1986) produces a general suppression of fetal activity, and long-term suppression could retard the offspring's normal development of coordinated and complex movements. We know that fetuses behave and learn in utero, but the relative influence of altered fetal behavior on subsequent behavioral development is almost unexplored.

The methods employed in our laboratory for studying learning by the fetus combine the advantages of prenatal manipulation of the fetal environment with procedures for directly observing the behavior of fetuses in utero (Narayanan, Fox, & Hamburger, 1971; Smotherman, Richards, & Robinson, 1984; Smotherman, Robinson, & Miller, 1986). Briefly, fetuses are observed late in gestation (Days 19–21) following spinal preparation of the mother with one of two procedures: chemomyelotomy or reversible lidocaine anesthesia. Under brief ether anesthesia, a small volume of either 100% ethyl alcohol (for chemomyelotomy) or lidocaine containing 1% epinephrine is injected into the spinal cord of the pregnant female between the first and second lumbar vertebrae. Both procedures are effective in eliminating afferent stimuli from the lower abdomen of the female without the global effects of general anesthesia. Following spinal preparation, the female is placed in a plexiglas holding device, her uterus externalized through a midventral incision, and the female's hindquarters and uterus immersed in a warm bath of isotonic saline. Following a delay of 15–20 min, during which the effects of initial ether administration completely disappear, a fetus from the ovarian end of each uterine horn is selected as the subject of observation and gently delivered through a uterine incision, taking care to maintain the amniotic membranes and umbilical/placental connection with the uterus intact.

Fetuses prepared in this way can be viewed with extreme clarity and manipulated with precision, providing detailed information on spontaneous and evoked fetal movements. For quantitative analysis, the simple movements of the rat fetus can be classified into discrete categories based on the region of the body moved (e.g., forelimb, hindlimb, head, mouth, body trunk). These categories can occur singly (simple movements) or in any combination (complex). In addition, the sum of movements in each basic category provides a measure of overall fetal activity. We have found these observation methods provide a replicable continuous, sequential record of all fetal movements during an observation session, permitting detailed analysis of spontaneous behavior and responsiveness to controlled stimulation (see Smotherman & Robinson, 1986a, for a more detailed discussion of observation procedures and behavioral categories).

In a systematic survey of the behavior of rat fetuses observed with this methodology (Smotherman & Robinson, 1986a), we found that spontaneous activity begins to appear on Day 16 of gestation, quickly rises to a peak on Days 17–18, and remains at high levels through term. Forelimb and curl (lateral or ventral flexion of the trunk) movements are the most common behaviors of young (Day 16) fetuses, head and hindlimb movements become more common on Days 17–18, mouth movements peak on Day 19, stretch (straightening or extension of the trunk) movements occur rarely until Day 20, and twitch (thoracic spasm) movements remain rare throughout gestation. As the fetus grows older, its behavioral repertoire expands with the addition of new movement patterns (such as eye-blink and ear-wiggle) and coordinated combinations of old patterns (such as wiping, a synchronous forelimb-and-mouth movement). Uncommon patterns also become more common, leading to a general increase in behavioral diversity. By Day 18, fetuses begin to exhibit temporal patterning and behavioral organization, with movements tending to cluster in bouts and simultaneous bursts. By Day 20, interlimb coordination is evident (A. Bekoff & Lau, 1980; Smotherman & Robinson, 1986a). We believe these normative data on the spontaneous behavior of rat fetuses to be generally valid. Recently, we have begun to employ a new procedure that enables direct visualization of fetuses while circumventing the need to externalize the uterus into a water bath. This technique, which employs a slender endoscope designed for use in arthroscopic surgery, has shown that fetuses viewed within the maternal abdomen exhibit a behavioral repertoire apparently as diverse as that of externalized fetuses (Smotherman & Robinson, 1986b).

By applying this same methodology to the study of fetal experience, it has proven possible to both condition and assess the effects of conditioning within the prenatal period (Smotherman & Robinson, 1985b). As in earlier experiments, fetuses are conditioned by delivery of a chemosensory stimulus (a mint solution) into the amniotic fluid and IP injection of LiCl. Unlike previous experiments, conditioning occurs at an earlier age (Day 17), and the behavior of fetuses in response to mint, LiCl and their pairing is measured both at the time of conditioning and at a later time (Day 19) when the effects of conditioning are assessed. Quantitative data on fetal behavior collected in these situations have provided valuable information pertaining to questions about the ability of fetuses to acquire and express conditioned responses in utero.

Rat fetuses exhibit little change in behavior to the taste/odor of mint presented in utero. Two patterns of behavior—twitch and complex movements—increase slightly in frequency following exposure to mint on Day 19, but no other patterns of fetal behavior are influenced by mint presentation. There is no evidence of long-lasting effects of exposure to mint, nor of any influence of familiarity to the mint stimulus. It appears that the taste/odor of mint is behaviorally neutral, relative to isotonic saline, when presented to fetuses within the amnion; and in the few cases where it does influence fetal behavior, it serves to activate or increase the frequency of movement. Therefore, there is no evidence that the fetus becomes sensitized to the CS (mint) through prior experience.

Studies of learning in adult animals implicitly assume that the behavior of experimental subjects will not undergo a spontaneous change in repertoire during the period of conditioning and testing (Garcia et al., 1985). This cannot be assumed in studying the behavior of young animals, which exhibit a rapidly changing repertoire. Ideally, learning in the fetus could be assessed by comparing its behavior in response to the pairing of CS

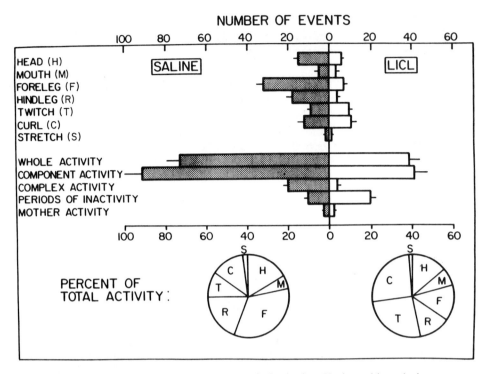

**Fig. 1.** Response of fetuses to LiCl on Day 19 of gestation. Horizontal bars depict mean frequency plus SEM for eleven categories of fetal behavior and one category of maternal movement. The sections within each circle graph represent the mean percentage of total activity for the seven basic patterns of fetal movement following saline or LiCl injection. From Smotherman & Robinson (1985b). Copyright 1985 by the American Psychological Association.

(mint) and US (LiCl) on Day 17 (the day of conditioning) to its behavior upon representation of the CS on Day 19. However, the behavioral repertoires of different-aged fetuses are not directly comparable. Therefore the response of the fetus to LiCl at both ages is important for meaningful interpretation of the fetus's behavior following exposure to the CS alone (the critical test for an effect of conditioning).

In fact, the rat fetus reponds to IP injection of LiCl with a suppression of overall activity on both Days 17 and 19 of gestation. Because a smaller repertoire of behavior is exhibited on Day 17, fewer patterns of behavior are affected by LiCl at this age. On both days, however, nearly all categories of fetal movement that are common are affected, including foreleg, hindleg, head, overall activity, and complex movements (Fig. 1). Conversely, the number of 15-s periods in which no movement occurs (periods of inactivity) increases following LiCl injection. A similar pattern of effect is apparent on Day 17 when fetuses are first exposed to mint and then injected with LiCl, the experimental circumstance presented when fetuses are actually conditioned. Further, the similarity of fetal response to LiCl alone and to the pairing of mint and LiCl speaks to the benign nature of mint as a CS.

Following the pairing of mint and LiCl on Day 17, rat fetuses respond to reexposure to mint on Day 19 with a marked suppression of overall activity. This behavioral suppression contrasts sharply with the behavior of fetuses exposed to mint on Day 19 following the pairing of saline and LiCl on Day 17. The conditioned suppression is similar—in both magnitude and range of behaviors affected—to the unconditioned suppression produced by LiCl alone. Exceptions to the overall pattern of suppression accentuate the similarity of the conditioned and unconditioned response of the fetus. Two patterns of behavior, curl and twitch, show an increase in relative frequency (when expressed as a percentage of total activity) following injection of LiCl, and both patterns also increase in relative frequency upon representation of the conditioned mint stimulus (see Figs. 1 and 2). The alterations in spontaneous fetal activity observed in this experiment cannot be ascribed to effects of novelty or familiarity with the mint CS, nor to long-term effects of the LiCl US. Therefore, these data provide convincing evidence that rat fetuses can acquire a conditioned aversion to mint as early as Day 17 of gestation (the earliest age yet found) and can express this learned aversion in utero through altered spontaneous behavior on Day 19.

In a subsequent series of experiments, this general conditioning effect in the rat fetus has been replicated and extended (Smotherman & Robinson, 1985a). As earlier, fetuses are conditioned by exposure to mint (100%) and injection of LiCl on Day 17 of gestation. Two days later, these conditioned fetuses are again exposed to a chemosensory stimulus consisting of one of several concentrations of mint (consisting of 100%, 200%, 50%, 10%, or 1% of the concentration presented during conditioning), to a novel taste/odor of lemon, or to a control saline solution. Fetuses exposed to the 100% mint CS again exhibit a conditioned suppression of behavior paralleling the original finding. Fetuses presented with 200% mint also show suppressed activity, suggesting that they do not discriminate between 200% mint and the original 100% mint CS. Mint solutions of 50% and 10% of the concentration of the original CS continue to suppress fetal behavior upon presentation on Day 19, but the overall level of activity remains higher than for fetuses exposed to 100% mint. Fetuses exposed to 1% mint exhibit little, if any, behavioral suppression; their behavior does not differ measurably from that of saline-exposed controls. The novel

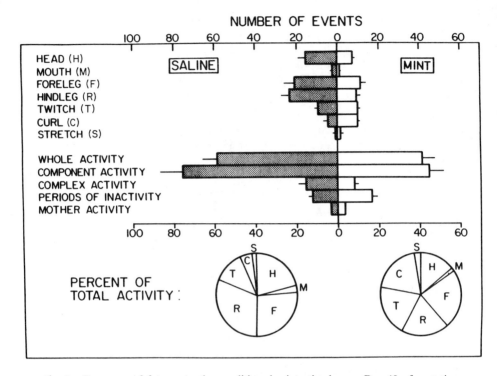

**Fig. 2.** Response of fetuses to the conditioned mint stimulus on Day 19 of gestation. Fetuses were exposed to either saline or mint, then injected with LiCl on Day 17, and were reexposed to mint before observation on Day 19. Bars represent mean frequencies plus SEM. Sections of each circle show the percentage of total activity associated with the seven basic movement patterns of fetuses exposed to saline or mint. From Smotherman & Robinson (1985b). Copyright 1985 by the American Psychological Association.

lemon stimulus also fails to influence fetal activity when compared to controls, suggesting that there is no generalization of the conditioning effect to other novel chemosensory stimuli (Fig. 3). The pattern of these experimental results argues that fetuses exhibit a conditioned aversion that is specific to the chemosensory cue experienced at the time of conditioning. Response to this cue, upon representation, falls off as a function of the discrepancy between the training and test stimuli. The existence of this apparent threshold in response suggests that the rat fetus is capable of discriminating among subtle characteristics of chemosensory stimuli experienced within its uterine environment.

The third-generation methodology for investigating the role of fetal experience has provided insights into the prenatal development of behavior that are unobtainable by other methods. In the first series of condition-

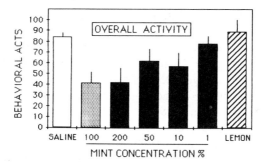

**Fig. 3.** Overall activity of conditioned fetuses exposed to different concentrations of mint, lemon, or saline on Day 19 of gestation. All fetuses were conditioned to 100% mint on Day 17. Bars represent mean frequency plus SEM. From Smotherman & Robinson (1985a).

ing experiments alone (Smotherman and Robinson, 1985a, 1985b), we have learned that (a) The rat fetus can detect and respond to chemical changes in its uterine environment. (b) It can form associations between environmental and internal stimuli as early as Day 17 of gestation. (c) Associations formed in utero can influence the form and frequency of subsequent prenatal behavior. (d) The fetus is capable of discriminating among chemosensory stimuli that it experiences in utero. This last finding is noteworthy in itself, as it suggests that conditioning and observing the fetus in utero may provide a tool with which to investigate sensory thresholds and acuity during prenatal development.

## V. Fourth Generation: Controlled Stimulus Exposure

Direct manipulation of the fetus's intrauterine environment through amniotic injection is still a relatively new tool; the full range of its potential applications has not been realized. Nevertheless, certain methodological limitations are becoming apparent with this approach to investigating fetal responsiveness to sensory stimuli. An implicit assumption in presenting chemosensory stimuli by amniotic injection is that different fetuses are equally exposed to chemicals within the amniotic fluid. However, fetuses can regulate their intake of amniotic fluid through alterations in their behavior, so variable activity may cause differential exposure to test stimuli. A single amniotic presentation of a chemosensory cue therefore does not provide sufficiently precise control over stimulus exposure, and repeated presentation is not possible without handling or otherwise disturbing the subject fetus.

Further experimental limitations arise from the presence of the chorionic and amniotic membranes that surround the fetus. Intact membranes can reduce the effectiveness of other modes of stimulus presentation, such as tactile stimulation, by physically shielding or buffering the fetus. The amniotic sac also physically restrains the fetus, thereby altering the amount and kinds of spontaneous movement exhibited by the fetus (Smotherman & Robinson, 1986a). Observation of the fetus within the amnion (but outside the uterus) is further complicated by the extreme fragility of the amniotic membranes and paucity of amniotic fluid near term (Days 21–22). For these reasons, investigation of prenatal–postnatal behavioral continuities may be hampered by observation of the fetus within the amnion.

Some of the limitations imposed by observation of the fetus in amnion can be eliminated by removing the amniotic membranes and allowing the fetus to float freely within the warm saline bath. The fetus can be delivered from the uterus and amnion without compromising the umbilical/placental connection with the uterus at any fetal age after Day 16 (Smotherman & Robinson, 1986a). Fetuses observed in bath (out of the amnion) on Day 19 are more active than fetuses in amnion (with mothers prepared by chemomyelotomy, mean overall activity per 10-min period: in amnion = $72.5 \pm 7.6$; in bath = $101.3 \pm 10.0$) and distribute this activity differently among various categories of movement. The behavioral activation of fetuses in bath may reflect a general effect of reduced fetal restraint (Smotherman & Robinson, 1986a).

Because a chemosensory stimulus delivered into the amniotic fluid quickly dissipates after removal of the amniotic membrane, an alternative method for controlled presentation of stimulus solutions is desirable. Ideally, chemical stimuli should be presented to the sense organs of the fetus in a manner that is both repeatable and nondisruptive, thereby providing precise control over stimulus exposure. We have approximated this ideal by adapting a procedure for implanting an intraoral cannula and delivering fixed volumes of chemosensory solutions directly into the fetus's mouth. The cannula is installed following procedures described by Hall (1979) for the rat pup, with additional care to remove the amniotic membranes while maintaining the fetus underwater with a healthy umbilical/placental attachment to the uterus. With the cannula in place and connected to a micrometer syringe, fetuses can be repeatedly exposed to precise volumes (20 $\mu$l) of chemosensory solutions. In the experiments described below, this cannula system was used to deliver pulses of mint, saline, and various other chemosensory solutions at 2-min intervals over the course of each 10-min observation session.

Experiments designed to assess the effects of the cannulation procedure have demonstrated no qualitative or quantitative differences in the

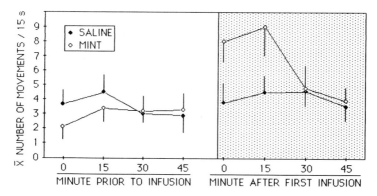

Fig. 4. Number of fetal movements during the 1-min periods preceding and following a single intraoral infusion of mint or saline. Points represent mean frequency per 15-s interval; vertical lines depict SEM.

behavior of fetuses with a cannula in place versus fetuses with no cannula. Further, fetuses that receive an infusion of saline through the cannula do not behave differently than fetuses that receive no infusion. These findings argue that intraoral cannulation is innocuous and does not disrupt spontaneous fetal behavior.

When unconditioned fetuses are presented with mint on Day 19 in amnion, few behavioral effects are noted (Smotherman & Robinson, 1985b). However, a single 20 $\mu$l infusion of mint to fetuses in bath produces marked activation of fetal behavior relative to saline controls (Fig. 4). The disparate responses of fetuses to different methods of mint presentation may be due to the environmental context in which behavior is observed (in amnion versus in bath) or, alternatively, to the more direct application of the chemosensory stimulus through the cannula to the fetal sensory receptors.

Fetal responsiveness to mint is not unusual; fetal behavior is also strongly activated by intraoral infusion of other chemosensory stimuli, such as solutions of lemon, orange, and almond extracts. On Day 19 of gestation, this behavioral response characteristically takes the form of a sharp rise in activity within 15 s of the infusion, which quickly dissipates over the next 60 s. Following infusion of lemon or orange, the level of fetal activity is over threefold greater than during the 60 s preceding the infusion. With successive infusions of the same stimulus, delivered at 2-min intervals, the magnitude of this peak response gradually diminishes, suggesting a waning responsiveness to repeated exposure.

Not all chemosensory stimuli are effective in activating fetal behavior. Intraoral infusions of 10% w/v sucrose. 0.003 $M$ quinine hydrochloride

(QHCl), or milk (commercially available light cream) to Day 19 fetuses fail to elicit the characteristic spike in activity seen following infusions of mint, lemon, orange, or almond. At least to a human observer, sucrose, QHCl, and milk lack the strong odor characteristic of lemon, orange, mint, and almond oils.

In an effort to further specify the mechanism of fetal responsiveness to certain chemosensory cues, we have also delivered intraoral infusions of aldehyde solutions, such as citral and benzaldehyde, which are widely represented as tasteless odors. Day 19 rat fetuses respond to infusions of citral, a lemon scent, with a typical spike pattern of activity indistinguishable from their response to lemon, which contains both olfactory and gustatory components. Fetal responses to benzaldehyde, which resembles almond odor, are similar to their responses to almond infusions. These findings provide further support that the chemosensory responsiveness of fetuses is mediated by olfaction, although they do not conclusively exclude a possible role for lingual, palatine, or pharyngeal chemical receptors (Mistretta & Bradley, 1986).

Each of the examples of fetal activation to chemosensory infusions described above involved the first time the fetus was exposed to the test stimulus (lemon, citral, etc.). Prior experience with the stimulus in utero, however, can alter the pattern of fetal response to infusions. Employing second-generation procedures for delivering a chemosensory cue by intra-amniotic injection, fetuses were exposed to mint on Day 17 and later tested by repeated infusion of mint on Day 19. Close inspection of the behavior of fetuses during infusion suggested that the novelty or familiarity of the mint stimulus influenced the pattern of fetal response (Fig. 5). Fetal activity scores were examined during the 5-s interval in which the infusion occurred and the three subsequent 5-s intervals. These data were compared to the baseline rate of fetal movement during the 60 s preceding each infusion.

Two general patterns of fetal response were apparent in this analysis. Fetuses that experienced mint for the first time showed an initial suppression in activity during the infusion interval. In contrast, fetuses that had experienced mint earlier in gestation exhibited a slight increase in activity during each infusion. The findings from postinfusion intervals, however, replicated for both novel and familiar mint the general activational effect found in earlier experiments. These data provide evidence that rat fetuses can discriminate between novel and familiar chemosensory stimuli and further support the view that fetuses are sensitive to changes in their intrauterine environment and can modify their behavior as a result of prior experience in utero. Moreover, the delayed responsiveness of fetuses exposed to novel mint is remarkably similar to the typical orienting

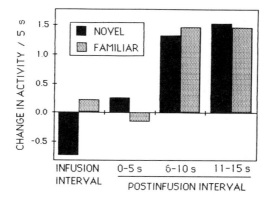

**Fig. 5.** Differential response of rat fetuses to intraoral infusions of novel or familiar mint solutions. Responses are plotted relative to baseline activity per 5 s, which is derived from the mean number of fetal movements during the 1-min period preceding each infusion. Response scores reflect the mean change from baseline in fetal activity during the 5-s interval in which the infusion was delivered (left) and three 5-s intervals subsequent to infusion (right).

reflex to novelty exhibited by many adult animals (Rohrbaugh, 1984; Sokolov, 1960).

Other aspects of fetal sensory responsiveness also can be influenced by prenatal experience. By combining techniques for conditioning fetuses (second generation), reexposing fetuses to the CS (third generation), and subsequently delivering infusions of a novel stimulus (fourth generation), we have begun to investigate the role of olfactory context on fetal chemosensory responsiveness. Olfactory context was manipulated prior to observation on Day 19 by exposing conditioned fetuses in uterus to either mint (which had been presented with LiCl on Day 17) or saline. After a delay of 2 min, each fetus was removed from the uterus and amnion, fitted with a cannula, and repeatedly infused with either lemon or saline. These experiments have demonstrated that the normal response of rat fetuses to a chemosensory stimulus (novel lemon) is altered by the presence of a salient contextual stimulus (mint CS) (Fig. 6). Fetuses in a saline context behaved much like unmanipulated fetuses exposed to lemon: fetal activity increased substantially (relative to saline-infused fetuses) following the first infusion of lemon, but the magnitude of behavioral activation waned with subsequent infusions. Fetuses in a mint context also were activated by infusions of lemon, but to a lesser degree. Further, their responsiveness to lemon showed little or no change with repeated exposure. Overall, saline-exposed fetuses were more active than mint-exposed fetuses following the first infusion of lemon but were less active than mint-exposed fetuses after the fourth infusion.

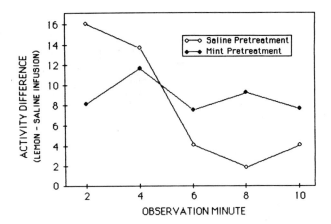

**Fig. 6.** Differential response of rat fetuses to intraoral infusions of lemon in the presence of saline or conditioned mint. Each point represents the mean activity difference between lemon-infused and saline-infused fetuses. Infusions were delivered immediately prior to the second, fourth, sixth, eighth, and tenth minute of each observation session. Activity scores are the total number of fetal movements during the 1-min interval subsequent to infusion.

The implication of this experiment is that fetal responsiveness to lemon infusion is context dependent and subject to influence by prior experience. Analogous findings have been identified in the responsiveness of rat fetuses to tactile stroking. This kind of contingent responsiveness is consistent with criteria for identifying behavior states in the fetus (Nijhuis, Prechtl, Martin, & Bots, 1982): The change in response is centrally coordinated, as evidenced by the cross-modal effect on sensory stimulation, and is expressed simultaneously in more than one behavioral variable (response to mint, response to lemon, response to stroking). It therefore appears that reexposure to the CS induces a change of behavioral state in the rat fetus.

The numerous infusion experiments we have conducted demonstrate the utility of intraoral cannulation in the study of behavioral control and development in the rat fetus: (a) The cannula does not alter spontaneous fetal behavior. (b) Fetuses in bath do not respond to infusions of saline, sucrose, or QHCl but (c) are dramatically activated by infusions of mint, lemon, orange, almond, citral, or benzaldehyde. (d) Fetal responsiveness to mint is modified by prior experience, with distinctive behavioral alterations appearing upon exposure to novel or familiar mint. (e) Fetal responsiveness to lemon is also influenced by prior experience and by the olfactory context present at the time of testing. (f) The ability of rat fetuses to modify their behavior through experience in utero therefore appears to be a robust, general phenomenon, although specific behavioral effects of learning vary across different testing procedures and fetal microenviron-ments. Moreover, the fourth generation of methods for investigating fetal learning has provided insights into the CNS control of fetal behavior unanticipated by earlier studies, such as evidence suggesting the exis-tence of behavioral state phenomena and orienting reflex to novelty in the fetus.

Controlled infusion of chemosensory cues to the fetus may provide a powerful tool for investigating other aspects of learning and perception in utero. Fine control over stimulus presentation is essential in studying the processes of habituation to and extinction of repeated stimuli. It will also be possible to vary stimulus characteristics and measure the capability of the fetus to discriminate among chemosensory cues presented in succes-sion. In this way, perceptual abilities of the fetus may be delineated, thereby improving our understanding of the relationship between fetal behavior and the intrauterine environment. Finally, by conditioning and testing the fetus in the same session, it will be possible to study the effects of different reinforcing stimuli, including the use of both negative and positive reinforcers, and to extend the experimental analysis of fetal be-havior to other forms of learning, such as appetitive conditioning.

## VI. Implications of Fetal Learning: Competence, Continuity, and Consequences

Accumulating from many sources is evidence that the mammalian fetus is responsive to sensory stimuli encountered during gestation and that behavioral modifications during the prenatal period can be retained into postnatal life. The list of competencies of human and animal fetuses is impressive: perception of tactile, acoustic, and chemosensory cues in utero; olfactory discrimination, olfactory sensitization, and habituation to neutral stimuli; orientation to novel stimuli; aversive conditioning; and behavioral adaptation to variations in the uterine environment. Parallel to these emerging abilities is the increasing organization of spontaneous fetal behavior late in gestation, as evidenced by the expansion of the behav-ioral repertoire; development of interlimb coordination and synchronous movement of body parts; appearance of temporal patterning and cyclicity of fetal activity; and the existence of behavioral states (see review by Smotherman & Robinson, in press). These discoveries portray the fetus as substantially different than once thought. The fetus bears more than the potential for future behavioral and cognitive complexity; it *is* behav-iorally sophisticated in utero.

There is also a growing recognition that behavioral abilities which emerge during the prenatal period contribute to the formation and development of postnatal behavior. Associations formed in utero can be retained and expressed after birth as odor, taste, or auditory preferences or aversions. Many of the perceptual, associative, and motor skills originally identified in infant rats and humans now appear to have their roots in the fetus. Motor practice that occurs in utero may be critically important in the normal development of coordinated movement and neuromuscular control (M. Bekoff, Byers, & A. Bekoff, 1980). Moreover, prolonged reduction or absence of fetal movement has been linked with morphological consequences, such as abnormal limb development and growth retardation (Moessinger, 1983). Although still relatively unexplored, these and other postnatal consequences of prenatal behavior may be common in the course of normal ontogeny.

## Acknowledgments

W.P.S. is supported by a grant from the National Institute of Child Health and Human Development, HD16102-04 and Research Career Development Award HD00719-01. The authors wish to thank Patricia La Vallee for her assistance in the preparation of this chapter.

## References

Bekoff, A., & Lau, B. (1980). Interlimb coordination in 20-day-old rat fetuses. *Journal of Experimental Zoology, 214*, 173–175.

Bekoff, M., Byers, J. A., & Bekoff, A. (1980). Prenatal motility and postnatal play: Functional continuity? *Developmental Psychobiology, 13*, 225–228.

Birnholz, J. C., & Benecerraf, B. R. (1983). The development of human fetal hearing. *Science, 222*, 516–518.

Blass, E. M., & Pedersen, P. E. (1980). Surgical manipulation of the uterine environment of rat fetuses. *Physiology and Behavior, 25*, 993–995.

Blass, E. M., & Teicher, M. H. (1980). Suckling. *Science, 210*, 15–22.

DeCasper, A. J., & Fifer, W. P. (1980). Of human bonding: Newborns prefer their mothers' voices. *Science, 208*, 1174–1176.

DeCasper, A. J., & Prescott, P. A. (1984). Human newborns' perception of male voices: Preference, discrimination, and reinforcing value. *Developmental Psychobiology, 17*, 481–491.

DeCasper, A. J., & Sigafoos, A. D. (1983). The intrauterine heartbeat: A potent reinforcer for newborns. *Infant Behavior and Development, 6*, 19–25.

DeVries, J. I. P., Visser, G. H. A., & Prechtl, H. F. R. (1982). The emergence of fetal behavior: I. Qualitative aspects. *Early Human Development, 7*, 301–322.

Fifer, W. P. (1987). Neonatal preference for mother's voice. In N. A. Krasnegor, E. M. Blass, M. A. Hofer, & W. P. Smotherman (Eds.), *Perinatal development: A psychobiological perspective*. Orlando: Academic Press.

Garcia, J., Lasiter, P. A., Bermudez-Rattoni, F., & Deems, D. A. (1985). A general theory of aversion learning. In N. S. Braveman & P. Bronstein (Eds.), *Experimental assessments and clinical applications of conditioned food aversions. Annals of the New York Academy of Sciences, 443,* 8–21.

Gottlieb, G. (1985). On discovering significant acoustic dimensions of auditory stimulation for infants. In G. Gottlieb & N. A. Krasnegor (Eds.), *Measurement of audition and vision in the first year of postnatal life: A methodological overview.* (pp. 3–29). Norwood, NJ: Ablex.

Hall, W. G. (1979). Feeding and behavioral activation in infant rats. *Science, 205,* 206–209.

Hofer, M. A., Shair, H., & Singh, P. (1976). Evidence that maternal ventral skin substances promote suckling in infant rats. *Physiology & Behavior, 17,* 131–136.

Hooker, D. (1952). *The prenatal origin of behavior* (18th Porter Lecture Series). Lawrence: University of Kansas Press.

Kirby, M. L. (1981). Effects of morphine and naloxone on spontaneous activity of fetal rats. *Experimental Neurology, 73,* 430–439.

Landesman-Dwyer, S. (1982). The relationship of children's behavior to maternal alcohol consumption. In E. L. Abel (Ed.), *Fetal alcohol syndrome: Vol. 2. Human studies* (pp. 127–148). Boca Raton, FL: CRC.

Leader, L. R., Baillie, P., Martin, B., & Vermeulen, E. (1982). The assessment and significance of habituation to a repeated stimulus by the human fetus. *Early Human Development, 7,* 211–219.

Mistretta, C. M., & Bradley, R. M. (1986). Development of the sense of taste. In E. M. Blass (Ed.), *Handbook of behavioral neurobiology: Vol. 8. Developmental psychobiology and developmental neurobiology* (pp. 205–236). New York: Plenum.

Moessinger, A. C. (1983). Fetal akinesia deformation sequence: An animal model. *Pediatrics, 72,* 857–863.

Narayanan, C. H., Fox, M. W., & Hamburger, V. (1971). Prenatal development of spontaneous and evoked activity in the rat. *Behaviour, 40,* 100–134.

Nijhuis, J. G., Prechtl, H. F. R., Martin, C. B., Jr., Bots, R., S. G. M. (1982). Are there behavioural states in the human fetus? *Early Human Development, 6,* 177–195.

Oppenheim, R. W. (1981). Ontogenetic adaptations and retrogressive processes in the development of the nervous system and behaviour: A neuroembryological perspective. In K. J. Connolly & H. F. R. Prechtl (Eds.), *Maturation and development: Biological and psychological perspectives* (pp. 73–109). Philadelphia: Lippincott.

Patrick, J., Campbell, K., Carmichael, L., & Probert, C. (1982). Patterns of gross fetal body movements over 24-hour observation intervals during the last 10 weeks of pregnancy. *American Journal of Obstetrics and Gynecology, 142,* 363.

Pedersen, P. E., & Blass, E. M. (1981). Olfactory control over suckling in albino rats. In R. N. Aslin, J. R. Alberts, & M. R. Peterson (Eds.), *The development of perception: Psychobiological processes* (pp. 359–381). Hillsdale, NJ: Erlbaum.

Pedersen, P. E., & Blass, E. M. (1982). Prenatal and postnatal determinants of the 1st suckling episode in albino rats. *Developmental Psychobiology, 15,* 349–355.

Pedersen, P. E., Stewart, W. B., Greer, C. A., & Shepherd, G. M. (1983). Evidence for olfactory function in utero. *Science, 221,* 478–480.

Ray, W. S. (1932). A preliminary study of fetal conditioning. *Child Development, 3,* 173–177.

Reinold, E. (1976). Ultrasonics in early pregnancy: Diagnostic scanning and fetal motor activity. *Contributions to Gynecology and Obstetrics, 1,* 148.

Rohrbaugh, J. W. (1984). The orienting reflex: Performance and central nervous system manifestations. In R. Parasuramam & D. R. Davies (Eds.), *Varieties of attention* (pp. 323–373). New York: Academic Press.

Smotherman, W. P. (1982a). In-utero chemosensory experience alters taste preferences and corticosterone responsiveness. *Behavioral and Neural Biology, 36,* 61–68.

Smotherman, W. P. (1982b). Odor aversion learning by the rat fetus. *Physiology and Behavior, 29,* 769–771.

Smotherman, W. P., Richards, L. S., & Robinson, S. R. (1984). Techniques for observing fetal behavior in utero: A comparison of chemomyelotomy and spinal transection. *Developmental Psychobiology, 17,* 661–674.

Smotherman, W. P., & Robinson, S. R. (1985a). Novel and aversive chemosensory stimuli: Discrimination by the rat fetus in utero. *Society for Neuroscience Abstracts, 11,* 837.

Smotherman, W. P., & Robinson, S. R. (1985b). The rat fetus in its environment: Behavioral adjustments to novel, familiar, aversive and conditioned stimuli presented in utero. *Behavioral Neuroscience, 99,* 521–530.

Smotherman, W. P., & Robinson, S. R. (1986a). Environmental determinants of behaviour in the rat fetus. *Animal Behaviour, 34,* 1859–1873.

Smotherman, W. P., & Robinson, S. R. (1986b). A method for endoscopic visualization of rat fetuses in situ. *Physiology and Behavior, 37,* 663–665.

Smotherman, W. P., & Robinson, S. R. (1986c). The uterus as environment: The ecology of fetal behavior. In E. M. Blass (Ed.), *Handbook of behavioral neurobiology: Vol. 9. Developmental psychobiology and behavioral ecology.* New York: Plenum.

Smotherman, W. P., Robinson, S. R., La Vallee, P. A., & Hennessy, M. B. (in press). Influences of early olfactory environment on the survival, behavior and pituitary-adrenal activity of caesarean delivered preterm rat pups. *Developmental Psychobiology.*

Smotherman, W. P., Robinson, S. R., & Miller, B. J. (1986). A reversible preparation for observing the behavior of rat fetuses in utero: Spinal anesthesia with lidocaine. *Physiology and Behavior, 37,* 57–60.

Smotherman, W. P., Woodruff, K. S., Robinson, S. R., del Real, C., Barron, S., & Riley, E. P. (1986). Spontaneous fetal behavior after maternal exposure to ethanol. *Pharmacology, Biochemistry and Behavior, 24,* 165–170.

Sokolov, E. N. (1960). Neuronal models and the orienting reflex. In M. A. B. Brazier (Ed.), *The central nervous system and behavior* (pp. 187–276). Madison, NJ: Madison Printing.

Spelt, D. K. (1948). The conditioning of the human fetus in utero. *Journal of Experimental Psychology, 38,* 338–344.

Stickrod, G. (1981). In utero injection of rat fetuses. *Physiology and Behavior, 27,* 557–558.

Stickrod, G., Kimble, D. P., & Smotherman, W. P. (1982a). In utero taste/odor aversion conditioning in the rat. *Physiology and Behavior, 28,* 5–7.

Stickrod, G., Kimble, D. P., & Smotherman, W. P. (1982b). Met-5-enkephalin effects on associations formed in-utero. *Peptides, 3,* 881–883.

Teicher, M. H., & Blass, E. M. (1977). First suckling response of the newborn albino rat: The roles of olfaction and amniotic fluid. *Science, 198,* 635–636.

Walker, D., Grimwade, J., & Wood, C. (1971). Intrauterine noise: A component of the fetal environment. *American Journal of Obstetrics and Gynecology, 109,* 91–95.

Ward, I. L. (1984). The prenatal stress syndrome: Current status. *Psychoneuroendocrinology, 9,* 3–11.

Wirtschafter, Z. T., & Williams, D. W. (1957). Dynamics of the amniotic fluid as measured by changes in protein patterns. *American Journal of Obstretrics and Gynecology, 74,* 309–313.

# 3

# Behavioral Characteristics of Emerging Opioid Systems in Newborn Rats

ELLIOTT M. BLASS
*Department of Psychology*
*Johns Hopkins University*
*Baltimore, Maryland 21218*


PRISCILLA KEHOE
*Department of Psychology*
*Trinity College*
*Hartford, Connecticut 06106*

## I. Introduction

Altricial mammals—laboratory rats as examples—have been classically and instrumentally conditioned even at birth. Extreme excitation caused experimentally by manipulations as diverse as anogenital stimulation (Pedersen, Williams, & Blass, 1982), oral injections of liquid diet in food-deprived rats (Hall, 1979), or electrical stimulation of the medial forebrain bundle (Moran, Schwartz, & Blass, 1983) has typically been required for conditioning to occur. This stimulation always produced an affective state characterized by extremely high levels of activity and a variety of integrated postural adjustments. Moreover, 1–3-day-old rats, provided with the opportunity to create this state, did so by pushing a paddle to deliver liquid diet to the mouth (Johanson & Hall, 1982) or electrical current to the brain (Moran, Lew, & Blass, 1981).

Extreme excitation also supports classical conditioning: Animals so stimulated in the presence of an odor later prefer that odor (Johanson & Teicher, 1980). Moreover, presenting the conditioned olfactory stimulus elicits behaviors that had previously been elicited by the US of intraoral milk infusions (Johanson & Hall, 1982). These studies have significantly advanced our understanding of natural conditions under which learning might occur (Johanson & Terry, in press; Rosenblatt, 1983), their underlying neurology (Coopersmith & Leon, 1984; Greer, Stewart, Teicher, & Shepherd, 1982; Pedersen, Stewart, Greer, & Shepherd, 1983), and the properties of emerging motivational systems during development (Moran, 1986; Rosenblatt, 1983).

In contrast, there have not been any studies in rodents younger than 10 days of age aimed at identifying and analyzing the motivational properties of calming stimuli. This is readily understood because the excitatory qualities of the nest are easy to identify, as are maternal and sibling stimulation. It seems to us, however, based on the human infant literature, our own parenting experiences, and the subhuman primate and kitten literatures, that "calming" stimuli are powerful motivators in neonates.

Our approach to understanding reinforcement of calming in infants was to explore the developing opioid systems. This decision was based on the theoretical implications of calming for the development of reward and motivational systems, for identifying natural circumstances of conditioning, and for its obvious clinical importance. We chose to study, therefore, the development of behaviorally functional opioid systems. There are now a significant number of pharmacological (Coyle & Pert, 1976) and immunohistological studies that point to the development of opioid systems in rats by fetal Day 16 (Bayon, Shoemaker, Bloom, Mauss, & Guillemin, 1979). All of the components of functional opioid systems appear to be in place at birth, although in an extremely immature form (Khachaturian, Alessi, Munfakh, & Watson, 1983). It is not known whether these nascent opioid systems were behaviorally functional at birth or shortly thereafter and how they might contribute behaviorally during development. One study by Stickrod, Kimble, and Smotherman (1982) suggests a functional system prenatally. An extensive series of studies by Panksepp (1981) and his colleagues (Panksepp, Herman, Conner, Bishop, & Scott, 1978) have shown that by 2 weeks of age opioid systems appear behaviorally functional in albino rats (Panksepp & DeEskinazi, 1980) and other animals (Panksepp, Siviy, Normansell, White, & Bishop, 1982). Accordingly, we herein summarize our studies on the properties of this developing system, provide evidence that it mediates stress in isolated rats, and establish continuity in the behavioral system from birth to weaning in rats.

## II. Experimental Findings

Our initial strategy was to capitalize on the ability of very young rats to become classically conditioned and to remember the relationship between conditioned and unconditioned stimuli. This information is expressed, for example, in changed intakes of fluids that have served as the conditioning stimulus (Gemberling & Domjan, 1981). Accordingly, 5-day-old rats were conditioned by allowing them to ingest, while suckling over the course of 30 min, a 0.5% Na saccharin solution, through an indwelling tongue cannula (Hall & Rosenblatt, 1977). They were then injected intraperitoneally with either isotonic saline or 0.50, 0.75, 1.0, or 2.0 mg of morphine/kg of body weight (BW). The cannulae were then removed, and the rats returned to their mother and littermates, where they remained undisturbed for the next five days. On Day 10, they once again had the tongue cannula implanted. The cannula was connected to a reservoir suspended above the test cage so that by exerting suction while suckling, the pup could control the amount of fluid ingested during the 30-min test period (Brake, 1981).

Figure 1 demonstrates that saccharin intake in Day 10 rats that had earlier received the morphine dose of 0.5 mg/kg BW increased markedly. The linearly declining dose–response relationship demonstrates morphine aversiveness at high doses. This finding accords well with the adult literature of positive reinforcement at low doses and discomfort and malaise at high doses of morphine (Hunter & Reid, 1983; Mucha, Van der Kooy, O'Shaughnessy, & Buceniems, 1982). These data clearly demonstrate that learning in rats 5 days of old can occur while they are engaged in suckling from the nipple. These associations were both negative (with elevated doses) and positive (with low doses of morphine). Learning about negative events that shortly follow suckling extends our earlier findings concerning aversion to flavors paired with LiCl toxicosis (Kehoe & Blass, 1986). The suckling act per se does *not* protect the infant from forming aversions.

To establish an opioid basis for the positive association at 0.50 mg morphine/kg, we pretreated rats with the morphine antagonist naloxone before initiating conditioning. Such rats ingested as much saccharin as control animals during conditioning and then received morphine as above. If morphine is acting on opioid receptors during conditioning, then naloxone should block its pharmacological and, therefore, reinforcing qualities. This should impair conditioning in naloxone treated rats on Day 5, and these rats should *not* show enhanced saccharin intake on Day 10.

Figure 2 bears out this prediction. Rats pretreated with naloxone on Day 5 did not on ingest more saccharin on Day 10 than control animals

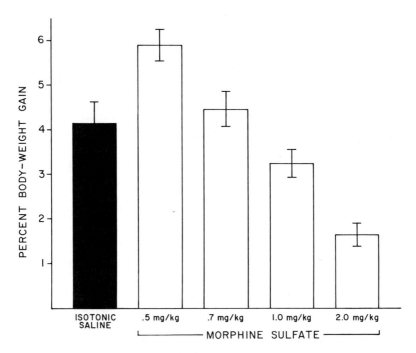

**Fig. 1.**  Each histogram represents the mean percentage body-weight gain at the Day 10 suckling intake test of pups given either saline, or morphine 0.5 mg/kg, 0.7 mg/kg, 1.0 mg/kg, or 2.0 mg/kg subsequent to saccharin infusion on Day 5.

receiving saline, pre- and postsaccharin ingestion. This cannot be attributed to a lingering malaise caused by naloxone injections because rats treated with naloxone grew normally and drank normal amounts of saccharin solution on Day 10. We suggest specificity of blockade and, furthermore, that morphine was acting on endogenous opioid receptors. A series of control experiments established that Day 10 enhanced saccharin intake could be attributed only to saccharin predicting morphine delivery on Day 5. That is, enhanced intake reflected conditioning and was not due to a general property of the experimental treatment (Kehoe & Blass, 1986a).

   This initial set of findings supports the following conclusions concerning the behavioral properties of opioid systems in 5-day-old albino rats: (a) Opiatelike receptors are available to 5-day-old albino rats, (b) they interact with systems that participate in classical conditioning, (c) these receptors are available to oropharangeal afferents that detect saccharin, and (d) this system is available to long-term memory processes.

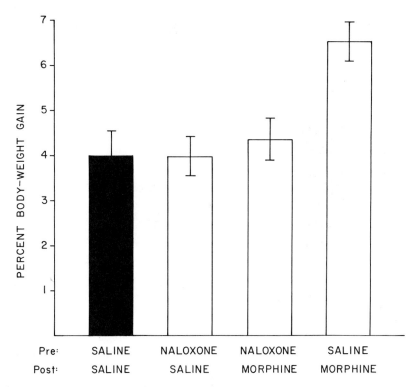

**Fig. 2.** Percentage body-weight gain at the Day 10 test of pups that had received saline or naloxone subcutaneously (SC) prior to and saline or morphine IP after a saccharin oral infusion on Day 5.

In an effort to better establish the validity of this finding, and to allow for comparisons between this reward system and that normally engaged by excitation, we paired morphine with an odor. Preference for that odor against one normally preferred was determined 5 days later. Specifically, in a standard classical conditioning paradigm, animals 5 days of age were placed in a container for 30 min that contained orange-scented chips; they were then injected IP with either isotonic saline or 0.5 mg/kg BW morphine. They were returned to the dam and studied 5 days later for odor preference.

Figure 3 demonstrates that an odor, orange in this case, that predicted the receipt of morphine (0.5 mg/kg BW) became preferred to the normally preferred odor of plain bedding (pine chips). Specifically, control rats spent only 27% of their test time over the orange odor. In contrast, rats for which orange predicted morphine spent twice as much time over

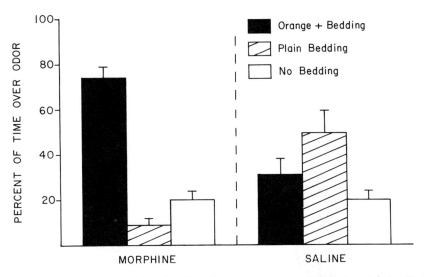

**Fig. 3.** Mean percentage of time that Day 10 pups spent over each area in a chamber that contained three areas: orange, plain, or no bedding. Pups on Day 5 had received morphine or saline (IP) subsequent to experiencing orange-scented bedding.

orange than over pine. Thus, the memory of morphine paired with the orange was sufficient to override the preference behavior otherwise determined by the sensory qualities of the orange and pine chips (Kehoe & Blass, 1986a).

Conditioning was specific: Morphine in conjunction with orange did not cause a generalized change in behavior; conditioned rats did not prefer the smell of cloves over that of pine at 10 days of age. The reverse also held, of course; that is, rats conditioned with cloves did not prefer orange. Rats pretreated with a different antagonist, naltrexone, on Day 5 did not prefer the orange odor (Fig. 4) when tested on Day 10. They reacted to the orange in a manner that was indistinguishable from that of control rats that had received isotonic saline both prior to and following orange exposure. This was in marked contrast to littermates that had received morphine IP following isotonic saline injection and exposure to orange odor.

Thus, concerning the properties and potentials of the motivational systems that involve endogenous opioids, we conclude that (a) Odors, like tastes, can gain access to the opioid motivational system; (b) these odors can be used as conditioned stimuli; (c) there is at least a 5-day memory for the conditioning event; and (d) the opioid motivational system can gain access to the processes involved in decision making that are expressed in preference.

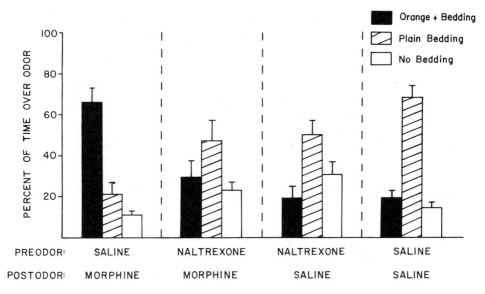

**Fig. 4.** Percentage of time that Day 10 pups spent over each area of a chamber that contained orange, plain, or no bedding. Pups on Day 5 had received either saline or naltrexone SC before orange odor exposure and morphine or saline IP after.

These processes are central in nature. Specifically, we induced preferences for orange in 10-day-old rats by pairing orange on Day 5 with intracerebroventricular injections of morphine in doses ranging from 0.15 μg up to 0.35 μg. Amount of time spent over the orange on Day 10 was linearly related to morphine dose. Moreover, the peripheral morphine effect demonstrated in Fig. 3 could be completely abolished as in Fig. 4 by intracerebroventricular pretreatment with 0.25 μg naltrexone. It appears, therefore, that the phenomena we have described in detail above can be fully explicated by central opioid receptor systems that have access to central motivational systems concerning classical conditioning, its memory, and choice behavior in rats that are 10 days of age (Kehoe & Blass, 1986c).

## A. The Stimulus Control of Affect in Classical Conditioning

A defining property of classical conditioning is that the CS comes to elicit the conditioned response; that is, the CS gains control over autonomic and muscular functions. In the case of infants excited by the stimulation, the presentation of the CS elicits complex motor patterns (Johanson & Hall, 1982) and controls preference (Johanson & Teicher, 1980).

The CS therefore, has at least two properties: affective and informational. The paradigms that we have just described present the opportunity to separate cognitive from affective aspects of performance under classical conditioning. If presentation of the CS (orange) on Day 10 to previously conditioned rats elicits an effective state (i.e., in parallel with the motor patterns elicited by stimuli associated with excitation) that sustains preference for the otherwise nonpreferred odor, then blocking that affective state should cause preference to be determined by the sensory qualities of the odor. That is, conditioned rats injected with naltrexone *at testing* should prefer pine to orange because the orange no longer elicited the opioidlike state. Stated differently, orange may cause and sustain the release of endogenous opioids to cause the marked preference seen above.

Rats were trained as before by pairing orange and morphine treatment on Day 5. On Day 10, 30 min prior to preference testing, they received an IP injection of naltrexone. They were then allowed to express their preference for orange or for pine chips. Naltrexone treatment, on Day 10, eliminated orange preference (Fig. 5). Naltrexone administration did not incapacitate the animals as ambulation appeared normal. Moreover, naltrexone did not impair their ability either to make olfactory discriminations or to choose between the two sides of the test arena. This is demon-

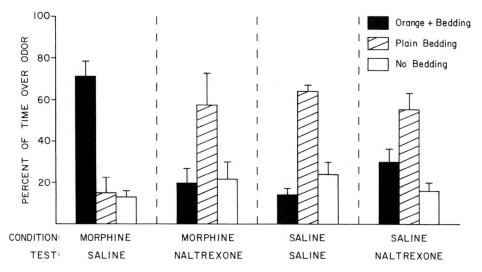

**Fig. 5.** Percentage of time spent over orange scent by rats that received saline or morphine treatments at 5 days of age and saline or naltrexone injections 30 min prior to testing on Day 10.

strated in Fig. 6. Animals that had been injected with naltrexone exhibited a preference for home-cage odors identical to that of control siblings that either were not injected or received isotonic saline 30 min prior to testing.

To more fully validate the conclusion that the conditional stimulus caused a rise in endogenous opioid levels, we sought confirming evidence from a different source. There is now a substantial psychopharamacological literature on the effects of morphine and other opioidlike substances on pain mediation. The most reliable measure utilized in behavioral psychopharmacology for assessing opioidlike effects on the pain system is the hot-plate test. A rat is placed on a plate warmed to 46–48°C and the latency either to lift all four paws off the substrate or to lick a forepaw is recorded. This behavior is very sensitive in adults to a variety of exogenous opiate substances and also reflects changes in endogenous opioid levels. In short, this behavioral bioassay is valid and reliable (Sherman & Liebeskind, 1980). We modified this assay for 10-day-old rats and established its sensitivity to morphine in a series of experiments that we will address shortly. For the moment, accept this as a reliable and valid test sensitive to the influence of morphine and naloxone administrations and to stress.

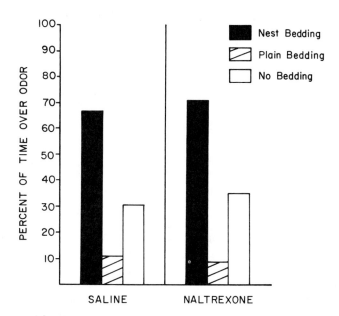

**Fig. 6.** Percentage of time that pups spent over each area of a chamber that contained nest, plain, or no bedding. Each pup was injected 30 min prior to the preference test, with either naltrexone or saline SC.

Animals that had associated orange with the onset of a morphinelike state should show elevated paw-lift latencies (PLLs) when tested in orange. Figure 7 bears out this prediction. Specifically, rats that had been exposed on Day 5 to orange scent followed by 0.5 mg/kg BW morphine had elevated PLLs (by 50%) when exposed to orange scent prior to testing on Day 10. Exposure to orange alone did not cause this enhancement: Control litter mates that received isotonic saline injections on Day 5 following orange exposure did not respond with enhanced PLL on Day 10. This study provides converging evidence that the conditioned olfactory stimulus gains control over the endogenous opioid system to functionally increase either circulating levels of opioids or the rate at which endogenous opioids are detected and integrated by the receptors and the behavioral systems they influence.

## B.   The Opioid System and Stress in Developing Rats

While establishing the validity of the hot-plate technique in indirectly assessing endogenous opioid activity, we revealed a number of properties concerning stress and its opioid mediation in development. The paw-lick hot-plate test in adults has been demonstrated to be sensitive to (a) morphine administration, (b) its antagonist blockade, and (c) stress. Specifically, morphine increases PLL in adults in a dose-related fashion; naloxone blocks such elevations, and stress induces increased PLL, or *stress-induced analgesia*. If our metric is valid, then rats 10 days of age should also demonstrate the same changes in the latencies with which they remove their paws from a hot plate set at 46°C.

We devised an easy-to-use, highly reliable system. The test arena was a stainless steel disk that was completely covered with insulating tape except for a 1 cm by 3 cm opening through which contact was established between the rat's left paw and the hot plate. This was achieved by the experimenter slowly lowering the rat to the hot-plate surface. Lowering the animal caused a digital splay, ensuring good contact. Contact activated a timer, and paw removal terminated its advance.

The initial experiment consisted of two housing conditions. In one, rats remained with the mother until test initiation; in the second, they were isolated from her at 34°C, nest temperature. This might be considered a relatively mild social stress. One half of the animals in each group was injected with naloxone, while the other half was injected with isotonic saline. All rats received a second injection: 50%, morphine; the rest, saline. Accordingly, animals were catagorized by living conditions—dam versus nondam; by initial injection of naloxone versus saline; and by a

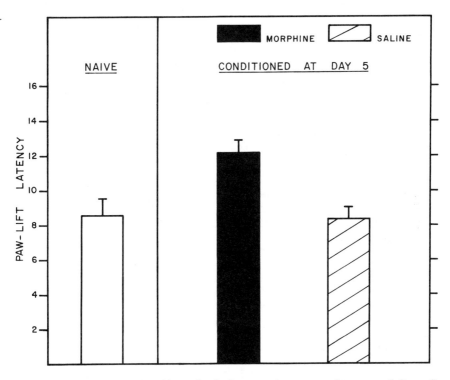

**Fig. 7.** Mean PLL of 10-day-old rats that had not ever been exposed to orange (left panel) and of rats that had been exposed to orange on Day 5 followed by morphine or saline. The latter two groups of rats were exposed to orange at the time of the hot-plate test.

second injection of morphine versus saline. Thus eight groups of animals were derived from a 2 × 2× 2 design.

The left portion of Fig. 8 reveals that rats in the S-M group living with their mother displayed markedly elevated PLL for 30 min postinjection. This is consistent with the reports on adults rats tested under analogous conditions. Naloxone administered prior to morpine normalized PLL. As expected, naloxone did not reduce PLL of control animals (Kehoe & Blass, 1986b). This is also in keeping with the findings in adult experiments in which naloxone administration is essentially without effect (Lester & Fanselow, 1985).

The right-hand portion of Fig. 8 demonstrates how maternal separation affected PLL and interacts with morphine administration and naloxone blockade. First, rats receiving morphine during the group-isolation period maintained markedly elevated PLL throughout the 1.5-hr duration of the experiment. Second, this elevated response was eliminated during the

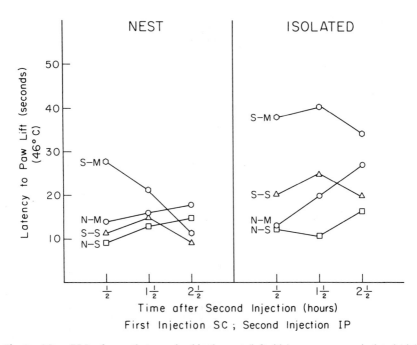

**Fig. 8.** Mean PLL of pups that remained in the nest (left side) or were group-isolated (right side) and received saline-morphine (S-M), naloxone-morphine (N-M), saline-saline (S-S), or naloxone-saline (N-S) combinations. Pups were tested 1/2, 1 1/2, and 2 1/2 hr after the second injections.

first half hour by naloxone injection. Third, naloxone apparently lost its efficacy as the PLL of animals treated with both naloxone and morphine increased linearly during the course of separation. Fourth, saline-treated, group-isolated rats showed an elevated and prolonged PLL throughout the test; a response that was completely normalized by the naloxone pretreatment. Thus, concerning opioid involvement in adult pain responsivity, morphine responsiveness, naloxone blockade, and stress-induced analgesia, infant rats appear similar to adults qualitatively, although the quantitative comparisons cannot be readily made. These findings validate the technique for use in further behavioral-pharmacological explorations.

That relatively mild stress-elevated PLL led us to determine whether the more severe stress of individual isolation would enhance latencies further yet. Thus, 10-day-old rats were individually isolated for 5 min in styrofoam cups containing pine bedding and tested for PLL. Littermate rats were injected with either isotonic saline or naltrexone. There were two additional groups. In one, individually isolated rats had their bedding

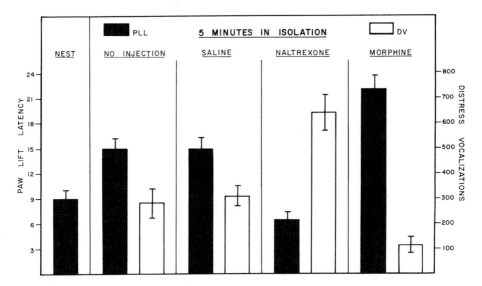

**Fig. 9.** Black bars represent the mean PLL to a hot plate at 48°C for pups either removed directly from the nest or isolated for 5 min after pretreatment with nothing, saline, naltrexone, or morphine IP injections. White bars represent the mean number of distress vocalizations (DVs) during the 5-min isolation period for each group of pups.

laced with orange to determine if orange's pungency would enhance PLLs. Additional rats were deprived as a group for 5 min and received the same injection series to compare short-term effects of group versus individual isolation.

We also determined whether the natural behavioral response to isolation, ultrasonic vocalization (distress vocalization), would be responsive to manipulations of the opioid system in neonatal rats. If such a system is opioid mediated, then morphine should reduce the numer of distress vocalizations while enhancing PLL, and naloxone should enhance distress vocalizations while normalizing PLLs. These predictions were born out (Fig. 9). The left panel presents PLL of animals taken from the nest (there are no DVs in the nest). The right panel demonstrates the effects of 5 min isolation; there was a significant increase in PLL *and* in the number of DVs in 5-min isolated rats. This profile was not altered by injections of isotonic saline (right panel, second section).

The effects of morphine and naltrexone administration were remarkable and, as predicted, operated in opposite directions. Morphine enhanced PLL while markedly attenuating ultrasonic vocalizations. Naltrexone had the opposite effect: It attentuated PLL and enhanced distress vocalizations. These data very strongly support the

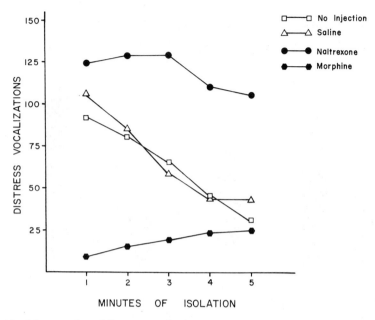

**Fig. 10.** Mean number of distress vocalization emitted by the pups in each treatment group for each minute of the 5-min isolation period.

conclusion that the endogenous opioid system in 10-day-old rats partici- pates in coping with the distress of total isolation (Kehoe & Blass, 1986b).

A more detailed analysis of the ultrasonic data provides additional in- sights into one mechanism through which the endogenous opioid system may function naturally. Figure 10 presents the minute-by-minute DVs of noninjected control rats and of rats that received isotonic saline, mor- phine, and/or naltrexone injections. In regard to control rats, DVs started very high and decreased monotonically with time. Naltrexone-injected rats maintained a relatively steady rate of distress calls throughout the entire 5-min test at about 110 ultrasonic vocalizations per minute. In contrast, morphine-treated rats barely emitted any ultrasonic calls. The extremes, as bounded by naltrexone and morphine, demonstrate that iso- lated rats are capable of both sustained vocalizations for protracted peri- ods of time and relative silence. This very wide latitude of behavioral expression presumably reflects opioid availability. Nondrugged rats pre- sented a specific and interesting behavior pattern: They vocalized during the first minutes of isolation and relatively infrequently thereafter despite their capacity of additional vocalization.

One can speculate upon the adaptiveness of this behavioral pattern. According to Rosenblatt and Lehrman (1963), rat mothers closely attend their Day 10 infants and retrieve them quickly. Thus for infants that have been displaced individually from the nest by sudden maternal departure or have been inadvertently dropped by her during litter transport from location to location (Woodside & Leon, 1980), the strategy of emitting frequent vocalizations in her immediate vicinity should capture her attention. To the extent that the dam has not responded during the first minute or two of isolation, the strategy of a continuous vocalization might serve to alert potential predators, such as other rats or small rodents that live in the vicinity, to the plight of the isolated individual and perhaps even its siblings. Thus a continued and profound level of calling could possibly be inimical. This hypothesis is currently being tested.

If separation distresses, then does maternal return alleviate? If it does, then rats returned to the mother after separation should show normalized PLL and diminished distress vocalizations. Accordingly, animals were removed from the nest, their distress vocalizations recorded, and PLL determined at 1, 3, or 5 min in separate groups of rats. Other rats were individually isolated for 5 min and then returned to an anesthetized mother and tested either at 1, 3, or 5 min postisolation.

The calming effect of the mother is unmistakable (Fig. 11). As shown in the left panel, PLL was enhanced by isolation, even after 1 min, and remained elevated. Distress vocalizations increased monotonically throughout the isolation period. These profiles were abruptly reversed within the first minute of return to the mother (right panel): Distress vocalizations were completely arrested; PLLs were normalized within the first minute and remained so for the duration of the 5-min reunion. This is a potentially important finding, as it provides us with the means for identifying which maternal aspects comfort the isolated infant and allows for an analysis of the sensory properties of the dam and the experiential contributions to what reflects a calming set of stimuli (see Hofer & Shair, 1978, for an important start on this issue).

Rats were isolated individually for 5 min and then returned either to an anesthetized dam, an anesthetized virgin female, a container bearing home shavings, or a container with pine shavings (i.e., the isolation condition). Paw-lift latency was recorded at various intervals. Figure 12 demonstrates the abrupt drop in PLL in animals presented with an anesthetized dam or an anesthetized virgin. The female does not have to be suckled to return PLL to normal levels (Kehoe & Blass, 1986d).

Returning isolated Day 10 rats to a familiar odor also reduced distress vocalization and PLL, but after a 5-min interval. Clearly, the richness of a warm body was more effective, although the olfactory stimulus, despite

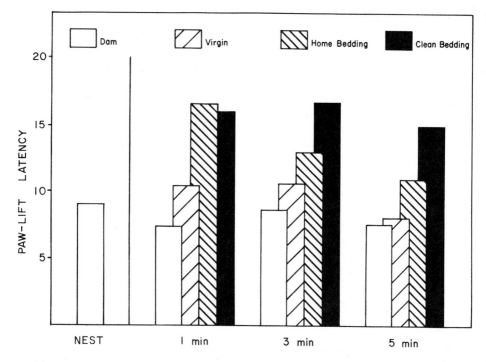

**Fig. 11.** Mean cumulative paw-lift latencies and distress vocalizations of rats isolated from their dams for 1, 3, or 5 min and the effects of return to the dam. Note the rapidity with which both DVs and PLL were normalized.

the absence of any thermotactile change, was able to normalize PLL. We do not yet know how this manipulation affected DVs. Finally, PLL, as expected, remained markedly elevated in those animals that remained isolated in fresh pine shavings for the duration of the test.

In summary, this aspect of our experimental analysis has identified a naturally occurring behavioral circumstance, isolation, and the behavioral response to this stress as being mediated, at least in part, by the endogenous opioid system. We have identified circumstances of activating the opioid system in a graded manner and have also identified stimuli sufficient for inhibiting the already-activated system, again in a graded manner.

## III. General Discussion

These studies have presented pharmacological and behavioral evidence that behaviorally functional opioid systems are available in rats as early as Day 5 for learning and reinforcement, both appetitive and aversive. More-

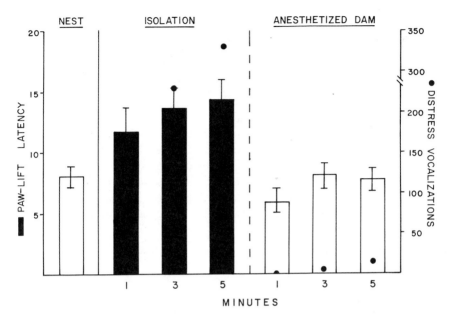

**Fig. 12.** Mean paw-lift latency of pups taken directly from the nest (left panel) or isolated for 5 min and then placed (right panel) for 1, 3, or 5 min on either clean bedding, home bedding, anesthetized virgin, or anesthetized dam.

over, a naturally occurring behavior, stress-induced vocalization, may be mediated by endogenous opioids. The opioid systems appear to be controlled and modulated by some of the sensory qualities of the mother as well as acquired properties of the nest, olfaction in particular. The following discussion revolves around the pharmacological and biologic evidence for opioid-based influence of behavior, an analysis of reinforcement, and the potential contribution of endogenous opiods to learning and memory processes.

## A. Pharmacological Evidence

First, injections of morphine, especially at the dose of 0.5 mg/kg BW, is an effective reinforcer for classically conditioning taste or olfactory stimuli. Second, opioid antagonists effectively block the formulation of classical conditioning when they precede morphine administration. Third, relatively high doses of morphine cause sustained aversions in neonatal rats, as judged by reduced saccharin intake. Fourth, microgram intracerebroventricular injections of morphine cause positive conditioning, and microgram injections of naltrexone intraventricularly block the formation of classical conditioning in animals that received morphine paired with

orange scent. This suggests behaviorally functional central opioid receptors that engage motivational and conditioning systems in 5-day-old rats.
Naloxone and naltrexone administration indicate opioid specificity.

The stress experiments speak to endogenous opioid involvement in
pain and stress mediation. Specifically, morphine caused a marked rise in
PLL that was prevented by naltrexone or naloxone pretreatment. Moreover, morphine administration interacted with the stress produced by
long-term group isolation or short-term individual isolation. Latencies for
individually isolated rats were considerably higher than for group-isolated
rats. Thus the endogenous systems involved in stress mediation are sensitive, even in 10-day-old rats, to graded biologic stress. In this regard, the
neonatal and adult systems are similar, for adult rats show graded responses to social stimuli (Fanselow, 1985; Lester & Fanselow, 1985).

## B.  Biological Evidence

The ultrasonic vocalization studies suggest opiate modulation of stress
in isolated rats. Naloxone elevated and sustained levels of ultrasonic
vocalizations; morphine exerted the opposite effect. We are impressed by
the linear reduction over time in the levels of DVs by isolated 10-day-old
rats and suggest that selection may have worked against those animals
that advertised their position by continuously calling and against those
that were silent (i.e., the latter would not have alerted their mother to
their isolation).

Our studies have also started to identify characteristics of the mother
that ameliorate stress. Specifically, contact alone with a warm, furry body
appears to be sufficient for the 10-day-old rat to normalize PLL and
essentially eliminate DVs. This is reminiscent of the Hofer and Shair
(1978) findings in 14-day-old rats. Distress vocalizations were reduced in
an additive fashion by tactile, thermal, and olfactory attributes of Day 14
pups. In the present study, we identified characteristics of the mother and
the nest that reduced DVs. The latter characteristic, nest odors, is of
significance because the capacity of nest odors to reduce distress vocalization was probably acquired. This is similar to Albert's (1981) finding
that contact with an attentive thelectomized dam was sufficient to establish a preference for huddling with objects bearing her odor. Identifying
whether processes involved in quieting distressed pups are homologous
with those supporting olfactory huddling in 15–20-day-old pups represents an important step in identifying the nexus of events that support
social development and differentiation and later fillial behaviors.

Reinforcing qualities of morphine share certain characteristics of other
more conventional reinforcers such as food or mates. Specifically, rats

conditioned to orange odor, when provided the opportunity, spent more time over the orange odor than control rats receiving isotonic saline injections or those for whom morphine was preceded by naltrexone. Choice shift is particularly noteworthy because the animal's disposition to stay away from the side of the arena containing orange (possibly due to orange's irritating quality) was overcome. The effect appears to be specific because the rats tracked the conditioned scent as opposed to any novel scent.

These studies' most significant contributions lie in the effects of CS reexposure on choice and escape behavior. Specifically, rats trained on Day 5 to orange did not express the preference for orange on Day 10 when naloxone preceded the preference test. Moreover, conditioned rats' PLLs were elevated by 50% by CS reexposure at test. Together these data suggest that the conditioned stimulus causes a release of endogenous opioids that become available to pain systems and to mechanisms determining and sustaining choice.

## C. Classes of Infantile Reinforcement Systems

We can now identify at least four states that appear to be reinforcing to infant rats. First are states of overt, sustained activation. This has been most clearly demonstrated empirically in the studies of Hall (1979) and his collaborators (Hall & Bryan, 1980; Johanson & Hall, 1982) which showed that warm, deprived infant rats, even on the day of birth, would become highly excited by infusions of warm liquid diet into the mouth. This excitement was marked by the expression of complex, integrated motor behaviors including lordosis and by the ability of rats to learn certain contingencies conerning operant as well as classical conditioning. The same holds for 3-day-old rats that received electrical stimulation to the medial forebrain bundle (Moran *et al.*, 1981). Such animals showed essentially the same behavioral patterns as those in the Johanson and Hall studies, although nondeprived. These animals also learned to push a paddle for brain reinforcement and to discriminate "effective" from "ineffective" paddles.

A second class of reinforcement systems, opioid-mediated, has been described in the present studies. We have not identified spontaneous natural occasions for "pleasurable" opioid mediation during the nesting period. Negative affective circumstances, like distress of separation, might be naturally buffered by the endogenous opioid systems, however.

A third class of reinforcing events is also of a calming nature but probably not opioid mediated: calming by maternal or sibling stimulation. Contact comfort is probably not mediated through endogenous opioids because PLLs were normalized from their exaggerated form in isolates. Further work is necessary to more exactly classify the mediators of the calming effects. If anything, the opioid system is activated by the removal of these standard contact stimuli.

A fourth class of rewarding stimuli are acquired by predicting one or more of the "primary" reinforcers. We tentatively suggest that each of the classes of secondary reinforcers may be mediated in part by the states associated with its predicted primary reinforcer. This is supported by our own studies and by those of Johanson and Hall (1982) in which exposure to an odor associated with stimulation caused the animals to exhibit some of the behavioral patterns associated with the infusion of milk into the oropharynx.

Finally, we have provided a link between the report of Stickrod *et al.* (1982) and those of Panksepp (Panksepp, 1981; Panksepp & DeEskinazi, 1980; Panksepp, Herman *et al.*, 1978; Panksepp, Siviy *et al.*, 1982) and his colleagues. Stickrod *et al.* demonstrated that fetal rats exposed to morphine in the presence of apple juice preferred the odor and taste of apple juice relative to control rats, suggesting that the components of the endogenous opioid systems may be behaviorally functional in the fetus. Panksepp and his colleagues have identified circumstances under which endogenous opioids may contribute to weaning and social process. The current studies extend Panksepp's reports to demonstrate the subtlety and characteristics of the opioid sytems in younger animals. This field of research offers considerable promise for understanding developing behavioral mechanisms and their central underlying processes.

### Acknowledgments

These studies were supported by Grant in Aid of Research AM28560 to E. M. B. from the National Institute of Arthritis Metabolism and Digestive Diseases. The studies were conducted during P. K.'s tenure as National Institute of Mental Health predoctoral fellow (MH09211) and E. M. B.'s as a research scientist (MH00925).

### References

Alberts, J. R. (1981). Ontogeny of olfaction: Reciprocal roles of sensation and behavior in the development of perception. In R. N. Aslin, J. R. Alberts, & M. R. Peterson (Eds.), *The development of perception: Psychobiological perspectives* (pp. 321–357). New York: Academic Press.
Bayon, A., Shoemaker, W. J., Bloom, F. E., Mauss, A., & Guillemin, R. (1979). Perinatal development of the endorphin- and enkephalin-containing systems in the rat brain. *Brain Research, 179,* 93–101.

Brake, S. C. (1981). Suckling infant rats learn a preference for a novel olfactory stimulus paired with milk delivery. *Science, 211,* 506–508.

Coopersmith, R., & Leon, M. (1984). Enhanced neural response to familiar olfactory cues. *Science, 225,* 849–851.

Coyle, J. T., & Pert, C. B. (1976). Ontogenetic development of (H)-naloxone binding in rat brain. *Neuropharmacology, 15,* 550–555.

Fanselow, M. (1985). Odors released by stressed rats produce opioid analgesia in unstressed rats. *Behavioral Neuroscience, 99,* 589–592.

Gemberling, G. A., & Domjan, M. (1981). Selective associations in one-day-old rats: Taste-toxicosis and texture-shock aversion learning. *Journal of Comparative and Physiological Psychology, 96,* 105–113.

Greer, C. A., Stewart, W. B., Teicher, M. H., & Shepherd, G. M. (1982). Functional localization of the olfactory bulb and a unique glomerular complex in the neonatal rat. *Journal of Neurosciences, 2,* 1744–1759.

Hall, W. G. (1979). The ontogeny of feeding in rats: I. Ingestive and behavioral responses to oral infusions. *Journal of Comparative and Physiological Psychology, 93,* 977–1000.

Hall, W. G., & Bryan, T. E. (1980). The ontogeny of feeding in rats: II. Independent ingestive behavior. *Journal of Comparative and Physiological Psychology, 94,* 746–756.

Hall, W. G., & Rosenblatt, J. S. (1977). Suckling behavior and intake control in the developing rat pup. *Journal of Comparative and Physiological Psychology, 91,* 1232–1247.

Hofer, M. A., & Shair, H. (1978). Ultrasonic vocalization during social interaction and isolation in 2-week-old rats. *Developmental Psychobiology, 11,* 495–504.

Hunter, G. A., Jr., & Reid L. D. (1983). Assaying addiction liability of opioids. *Life Sciences, 33,* 393–396.

Johanson, I. B., & Hall, W. G. (1982). Appetitive conditioning in neonatal rats: Conditioned orientation to a novel odor. *Developmental Psychobiology, 15,* 379–397.

Johanson, I. B., & Teicher, M. H. (1980). Classical conditioning of an odor preference in 3-day-old rats. *Behavioral and Neural Biology, 29,* 132–136.

Johanson, I. B., & Terry, L. M. (in press). Learning in infancy: A mechanism for adaptive change in behavioral development. In E. M. Blass (Ed.), *Developmental psychobiology and behavioral ecology.* New York: Plenum.

Kehoe, P., & Blass, E. M. (1986). Conditioned aversions and their memories in 5-day-old rats during suckling. *Journal of Experimental Psychology: Animal Behaivor Processes, 12,* 40–47.

Kehoe, P., & Blass, E. M. (1986a). Behaviorally functional opioid systems in infant rats: I. Evidence for olfactory and gustatory classical conditioning. *Behavioral Neuroscience, 100,* 359–367.

Kehoe, P., & Blass, E. M. (1986b). Behaviorally functional opioid systems in infant rats: II. Evidence for pharmacological, physiological and psychological mediation of pain and stress. *Behavioral Neuroscience, 100,* 624–630.

Kehoe, P., & Blass, E. M. (1986c). Central nervous system mediation of positive and negative reinforcement in neonatal albino rats. *Developmental Brain Research, 27,* 69–75.

Kehoe, P., & Blass, E. M. (1986d). Opioid-mediation of separation distress in 10-day-old rats: Reversal of stress with maternal stimuli. *Developmental Psychobiology, 19,* 385–398.

Khachaturian, H., Alessi, N. E., Munfakh, N., & Watson, S. J. (1983). Ontogeny of opioid and related peptides in the rat CNS and pituitary: An immunocytochemical study. *Life Sciences, 33,* 61–64.

Lester, L. S., & Fanselow, M. S. (1985). Exposure to a cat produces opioid analgesia in rats. *Behavioral Neuroscience, 99,* 756–759.

Moran, T. H. (1986). Environmental and neural determinants of behavior in development. In E. M. Blass (Ed.), *Handbook of behavioral neurobiology: Vol. 8. Developmental psychobiology and developmental neurobiology* (pp. 96–128). New York: Plenum.

Moran, T. H., Lew, M. F., & Blass, E. M. (1981). Intracranial self-stimulation in 3-day-old rats. *Science, 214,* 1366–1368.

Moran, T. H., Schwartz, G. J., & Blass, E. M. (1983). Organized behavioral responses to lateral hypothalamic electrical stimulation in infant rats. *Journal of Neuroscience, 3,* 10–19.

Mucha, R. F., Van der Kooy, D., O'Shaughnessy, M., & Buceniems, P. (1982). *Brain Research, 243,* 91–105.

Panksepp, J. (1981). Brain opioids—a neurochemical substrate for narcotic and social dependence. In S. J. Cooper (Ed.), *Theory in psychopharmacology (Vol. 1,* pp. 149–175). New York: Academic Press.

Panksepp, J., & DeEskinazi, F. G. (1980). Opiates and homing. *Journal of Comparative and Physiological Psychology, 94,* 650–663.

Panksepp, J., Herman, B., Conner, R., Bishop, P., & Scott, J. P. (1978). The biology of social attachments: Opiates alleviate separation distress. *Biological Psychiatry, 13,* 607–618.

Panksepp, J., Siviy, S., Normansell, L., White, K., & Bishop, P. (1982). Effects of B-chlornaltrexamine on separation distress in chicks. *Life Sciences, 31,* 2387–2390.

Pedersen, P. E., Stewart, W. B., Greer, C. A., & Shepherd, G. M. (1983). Evidence for olfactory function in utero. *Science, 221,* 478–480.

Pedersen, P. E., Williams, C. L., & Blass, E. M. (1982). Activation and odor conditioning of suckling behavior in 3-day-old albino rats. *Journal of Experimental Psychology: Animal Behavior Processes, 8,* 329–341.

Rosenblatt, J. S. (1983). Olfaction mediates developmental transition in the altricial newborn of selected species of mammals. *Developmental Psychobiology, 16,* 347–375.

Rosenblatt, J. S., & Lehrman, D. S. (1963). Maternal behavior of the laboratory rat. In H. L. Rheingold (Ed.), *Maternal behavior in mammals.* New York: Wiley.

Sherman, J. E., & Liebeskind, J. D. (1980). An endorphinergic, centrifugal substrate of pain modulation: Recent findings, current concepts, and complexities. In Bonica (Ed.), *Pain.* New York: Raven.

Stickrod, G., Kimble, D. P., & Smotherman, W. P. (1982). Met-5-enkephalin effects on associations formed in-utero. *Peptides, 3,* 881–883.

Woodside, B., & Leon, M. (1980). Thermoendocrine influences on maternal nesting behavior in rats. *Journal of Comparative and Physiological Psychology, 94,* 41–60.

# 4

# The Role of Sensory Modality in the Ontogeny of Stimulus Selection

NORMAN E. SPEAR and JUAN C. MOLINA
*Center for Developmental Psychobiology*
*University Center at Binghamton*
*State University of New York*
*Binghamton, New York 13901*

This chapter contains two major sections. In the first we consider evidence that the sensory modalities themselves might not be well differentiated in infancy. In doing so we discover that transfer of conditioning between sensory modalities (*intermodal transfer*) occurs quite readily in the rat prior to the age of weaning and as young as 4 days postnatal—earlier than many theorists would expect—and tends to decline in adulthood. In the second section we test some hypothetical means by which encoding and conditioning might proceed in infant rats without regard to sensory modality (*amodal processing*). This information is relevant to the general issue of how ontogenetic change in stimulus selection might promote "infantile amnesia," the more rapid forgetting observed for infants than for adults (Spear, 1979).

Stimulus selection determines which of all of the events in a conditioning episode are in fact learned. The emphasis here is on how selection of stimuli changes ontogenetically in terms of sensory modality; specifically, we suggest that, early in life, relatively little use may be made of sensory modality differences in the animals' representations of events to be learned.

While the term *stimulus selection* has not always been used, it seems applicable even to general theories of infantile amnesia emphasizing that human infants do not linguistically encode learned events and yet ostensibly attempt to remember these events in linguistic terms (e.g., Neisser,

1962). Any ontogenetic change in how the world is represented by an individual would seem to lead to difficulty in the retrieval of infantile memories. The general reasoning for this language-based theory has been that retrieval of infantile memories fails due to too little contact between what is to be retrieved and the adult's linguistically mediated devices for retrieval. This may or may not be an accurate assessment, but it helps illustrate that our use of the term *stimulus selection* incorporates the nature of the individual's encoding as well as which particular events are encoded for memory.

An elementary source of ontogenetic differences in nonlinguistic stimulus selection would be in the particular sensory modality used by the animal. For example, the neonatal rat seems fairly proficient in processing information from thermal or tactile events. It is also quite adept with olfactory events and can discriminate taste differences. Audition and vision are not used until the latter part of the second postnatal week (see Alberts, 1984, for a review). We might expect that during this period of early infancy, the rat's options for stimulus selection within the typical, multiple-event conditioning episode are fairly well set in terms of its sensory capabilities. We could predict that thermal and tactile events probably would be detected and learned by the neonatal rat, olfactory events somewhat less so, gustatory events even less, and auditory and visual events not at all. We would expect remembering of that neonatal episode later as an adult to be impeded both by the change in the animal's disposition to notice and encode auditory and visual events rather than tactile ones and by the animal's enhanced olfactory and gustatory abilities, which would lead it to notice quite different aspects of these sensory modalities than before.

If stimulus selection by the infant rat were indeed based on sensory modality in this way, it could explain infantile amnesia. Our evidence, however, casts doubt on the presumed importance of sensory modality as a basis for stimulus selection. We will also give reason to doubt that differences in sensory modality applied by the animal do serve even as a basis for differentiation of stimuli in general during the period of infancy (prior to postnatal Day 21). Our basic hypothesis is that, when faced with the same conditioning episode and circumstances, what is learned by infant animals is different from what is learned by adults.

Even controlled experimental circumstances permit differences in what might be learned. This is perhaps most obvious with instrumental learning. A rat that successfully learns to obtain food by following a route in a maze or by pressing a lever at the correct amount can do so by learning any of a number of cues or response patterns. Pavlovian conditioning is somewhat more useful for studying differences in what is learned because it allows us to know more precisely what stimulus the animal is responding to. This learning paradigm also permits more precise control over the temporal and stochastic relationship between that stimulus, the CS, and the critical predicted consequence, the US. Yet, even with Pavlovian conditioning, neither the CS, US, nor context need be perceived by the animal as unitary. The separable elements of each permit considerable differences in what is learned, even in a conditioning situation as simple as this. And even if we consider only a CS as simple as a pure tone, we must still allow the possibility that the animal might not perceive this event as a fundamentally acoustic one, processing it instead in terms of one of its amodal properties common to other sensory events, such as intensity.

Our research has indicated that infant animals encode an episode differently from adults in three respects: (1) in their processing or "integration" of multielement stimuli (Spear, 1984b; Spear & Kucharski, 1984a, 1984b); (2) in their differentiation of single-element stimuli according to sensory modality; and (3) in their use of memory attributes that are orthogonal to conventional physical definitions of stimuli. In this chapter we focus on respects (2) and (3).

The experiments we wish to discuss have dealt with ontogenetic differences in what is learned about relatively unitary stimuli, that is, single odors, tastes, or textures that are discriminated from alternative odors, tastes, or textures. There is general difference in the potential for stimulus selection with single-element stimuli compared to that with compound stimuli. For the latter, animals may differ in which element or elements are selected for learning. With single-element stimuli, however, stimulus selection may instead be more a question of how the subject chooses to represent that particular stimulus.

## I. Transfer between Sensory Modalities

### A. Intermodal Equivalence and Intermodal Transfer

Our first indications that different sensory modalities might not be differentiated early in life came from a series of experiments indicating that infants (but not adults) may treat the odor and taste of alcohol as equivalent (Molina, Hoffmann, & Spear, 1985; Molina, Serwatka, & Spear, 1984; Molina, Serwatka, Spear, & Spear, 1985; Serwatka, Molina, & Spear, 1986). If preweanling rats were merely exposed to the odor of ethanol, they were subsequently more inclined to consume ethanol. We also found that if the ambient odor of ethanol (in the absence of any

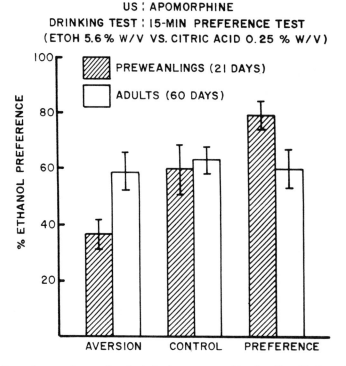

**US : APOMORPHINE**
**DRINKING TEST : 15-MIN PREFERENCE TEST**
**(ETOH 5.6 % W/V VS. CITRIC ACID 0.25 % W/V)**

**Fig. 1.** Percentage preference for alcohol odor as assessed in a locational test as a function of age and treatment. Aversion: Alcohol odor (1.5 cc) paired with onset of apomorphine intoxication. Control: Alcohol odor explicitly unpaired with the onset or offset of apomorphine intoxication. Preference: Alcohol odor paired with recovery from apomorphine toxicosis.

drinking) were paired with LiCl or apomorphine and consequent internal discomfort, subsequent *ingestion* of ethanol was significantly reduced, together with preference for the spatial location of the ethanol odorant; if that odor was paired with the offset of apomorphine-induced discomfort, ethanol *ingestion* increased (see Fig. 1). This was particularly interesting to us because our preliminary tests indicated that ethanol ingestion by adult rats was unaffected in this situation, even though these adults readily acquired an aversion to the location of the odor. When we paired ethanol odor with footshock rather than a drug, infants *increased* their ingestion of ethanol, an effect previously observed among adults given pairings of footshock and the ingestion of ethanol. Finally, we tested transfer of conditioning from alcohol olfaction to alcohol ingestion with much younger preweanlings—rats 5 and 10 days postpartum—given an injection of LiCl preceded by either alcohol odor, alcohol taste, or both the ambient odor and the taste presented simultaneously. Similar to our other results, we found that, relative to control conditions, an equivalent degree of aversion to alcohol consumption was conditioned whether the CS had been only the alcohol odor, only the taste, or both the odor and the taste. It was again as if the ambient odor and discrete taste of alcohol were treated alike by these preweanling rats, a tendency not found in our tests with adults.

Information from different sensory modalities might be treated as equivalent for either of two reasons. The animal might learn, or perceive directly, that these different sensory events apply to the same object or predict the same object. Alternatively, the animal might merely fail to differentiate input from different sensory modalities. In other words, (a) the odor of alcohol and the taste of alcohol might be attributed to the same object (alcohol solution), or (b) the odor might be mistaken for the taste. With regard to the first explanation, there is a long history to the issue of ontogenetic differences in the realization that the touch of a ball and the sight of a ball can apply to the same ball (Friedes, 1974; E. J. Gibson, 1969, 1983; Marks, 1978; Werner, 1940). Aside from the general philosophical and psychological significance of this issue, however, it has special importance for the study of conditioning and for approaches to developmental psychobiology. With regard to the second explanation, stimuli in studies of conditioning conventionally are selected for their sensory purity. We have expected that when an odor is paired with milk or a taste with an illness, the animal learns that a particular kind of smell predicts nutrients and a particular flavor predicts internal discomfort. That the animal might learn about something other than these physical properties of the odor or taste is not usually considered.

Within developmental psychobiology, the regular ontogeny of sensory capabilities and the influence of Anohkin's (1964) functional systems approach has led to the consideration of separate ontogenies of memory capacity for each sensory system. This consideration has been applied most thoroughly in the important series of experiments by Rudy and his colleagues (e.g., Rudy, Vogt, & Hyson, 1984) and also accepted implicitly by the first author (Spear, 1984a). But suppose that some invariant characteristic of objects other than sensory quality is learned, or that an odor is somehow interpreted by the rat pup as a sound. In that event, conditioning of an olfactory stimulus may tell us nothing about olfactory conditioning per se, response to an acoustic CS may not necessarily indicate auditory learning, and so forth.

Our results clearly indicated that transfer between the smell and the taste of alcohol is especially likely in younger rats. But the results did not indicate the generality of such ontogenetic differences. For example, the preweanlings' transfer of conditioning across sensory modalities might apply only to the special case of olfaction and gustation. There was precedent in the literature, however, for the notion that transfer of conditioning across sensory modalities—conventionally, *cross-modal* or *intersensory transfer*—might be a general feature of infantile behavior (E. J. Gibson, 1969, 1984). On this basis we were encouraged to view our effects as not necessarily restricted to transfer from olfaction to ingestion, nor constrained to substances such as ethanol.

The cross-modal transfer effect itself may involve virtually any combination of sensory modalities, although different species may be disposed to certain sensory combinations, such as sound and color in the case of humans; it does not require language; it has a potential basis in neuroanatomic action; and it could be a consequence, if only in small part, of synesthesia, which itself seems to decrease with ontogeny (for reviews, see Friedes, 1974; Marks, 1975, 1978).

## B.  Tests of Intermodal Transfer

Our experiments with ethanol indicate that preweanling rats may show cross-modal or intermodel transfer analogous to that observed in tests of human infants or adult chimps and primates (e.g., Friedes, 1974; Marks, 1975, 1978). In these tests, the animal first learns with Sensory Modality A, then is tested for expression of this conditioning in terms of Sensory Modality B. The stimulus item to be conditioned has been the same for the two sensory modalities. In our case it was alcohol solution, smelled during conditioning and tasted during the test.

We also tested transfer of learning between two sensory modalities that did not represent the same stimulus item but had as a common feature the US paired with those sensory modalities. Two CSs were derived from different physical objects, and their detection was mediated by different sensory receptors. We were interested in whether the animal's response to one of these CSs would be affected by learning about the alternative CS.

Our approach involved conditioning within Sensory Modality A, followed by a subthreshold level of conditioning within Stimulus Modality B such that its conditioning would not ordinarily be expressed. The question was whether the prior conditioning to A would promote this expression. Our first experiment required a moderate amount of conditioning to an odorant, methyl salicylate, and a subthreshold level of conditioning to a black, as opposed to white, compartment. We had determined that six pairings of methyl salicylate with the US, footshock, would condition a moderate but significant aversion to it but that a single pairing of the black compartment with this US would induce no measurable aversion. To assess conditioning to methyl salicylate we measured the rat's preference for the location of this odorant relative to that of a novel odorant, lemon. To assess conditioning to the black compartment we measured the rat's preference for a black compartment relative to a white compartment of the same dimensions.

### 1. Transfer between Olfaction and Vision at 16 or 60 Days Postpartum

We compared the cross-modal transfer of rats 16 days old (infants) and 60 days old (adults). The question was whether conditioning to the black compartment would be facilitated by prior conditioning to the methyl salicylate. A trio of conditions exemplifies the experimental paradigm used throughout this series. The paradigm includes these three conditions in each of our studies: (1) the basic transfer condition in which moderate conditioning within sensory modality A precedes subthreshold conditioning to sensory modality B; (2) subthreshold conditioning to B only, with prior unpaired presentations of A and the US; (3) conditioning to A only, with unpaired presentations of B and the US.

Figure 2 shows the results of the first experiment. It is clear that, for the infants, conditioning to the black compartment occurred only when preceded by conditioning to the odorant methyl salicylate. In contrast, the adults exhibited no transfer from olfactory conditioning to visual conditioning. Prior olfactory conditioning promoted visual conditioning for preweanlings but not for adults. Did the visual conditioning reciprocally strengthen the olfactory conditioning? If potentiation of conditioning to the black compartment were due to its treatment as somehow similar to the odor, conditioning of the odor may be further strengthened by conditioning its "equivalent," the black compartment.

To test this, another experiment was conducted with exactly the same procedures as the first except that odor aversion rather than visual aversion was assessed. Results are shown in Fig. 3. As expected from our previous experiments, olfactory conditioning was significant for both the infants and the adults, as assessed by the difference between subjects given pairings of the odorant and footshock (O+) and those given unpaired presentations of the odorant and footshock (O−). The conditioned aversion to methyl was further strengthened by the subsequent conditioning to the black compartment (V+), but this effect, too, occurred only for the preweanlings. For the adults, visual conditioning did not strengthen olfactory conditioning.

For preweanlings, olfactory conditioning facilitated visual conditioning and vice versa. This mutual strengthening of conditioning with two differ-

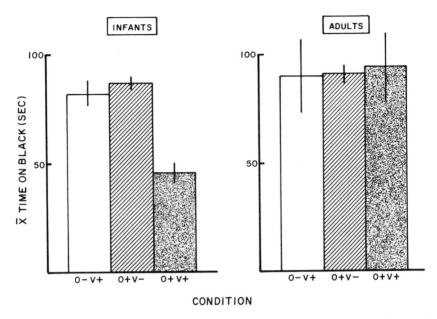

**Fig. 2.** Time spent in the black compartment of a visual discrimination test as a function of treatment and age. Abbreviations: O, olfactory CS (methyl salicylate, 2.0 cc); V, visual CS (black compartment); −, unpaired presentations between olfactory or visual stimuli and footshock; +, paired presentations between olfactory or visual stimuli. Conditioned aversion to black is in terms of the mean number of seconds that the rats spent in the black compartment; their alternative was to spend time in the adjacent white compartment. Each test lasted a total of 180 s.

ent sensory modalities implies that the olfactory and visual stimuli were in some sense treated as equivalent by the rat. But still another test of this hypothesis is possible. One should expect that for rats conditioned with both the olfactory (O+) and visual (V+) CSs, weakening of conditioning to the odor, methyl, should weaken conditioning to the particular brightness, black. Four groups of 16-day-old rats were given the basic transfer conditions, olfactory conditioning followed by visual conditioning. Prior to testing for visual conditioning, however, half the rats in each experiment were given a 20 min nonreinforced exposure to methyl salicylate. This extinction treatment of olfactory conditioning was given either before or after the visual conditioning. In each case, the expected result occurred: Visual conditioning was weakened by a weakening of the olfactory conditioning.

Generally speaking, the infants seemed to be treating a transparent compartment scented with methyl salicylate as if it were the same as a black unscented compartment. As far as we could tell, the only major

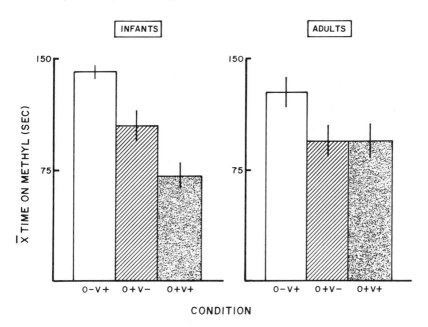

**Fig. 3.** Time spent over location scented with methyl (2.0 cc) as a function of treatment and age. Abbreviations: O, olfactory CS (methyl); V, visual CS (black compartment); −, unpaired presentations between olfactory or visual stimuli and footshock; +, paired presentations between olfactory or visual stimuli and footshock.

factor common to the two compartments was the mildly punishing foot-shocks administered in each. And furthermore, whatever other feature or features these two stimulus events may have had in common was undetected not only by us but also by the adult rats.

The age difference also suggested that this effect was more than general learning-to-learn (why should the adults show less?). Yet we were frankly surprised at the strength of this transfer effect and a little surprised that it had occurred at all. With no precedent for such an effect and certainly none with our procedures, we had not been optimistic about its occurrence when we first set out to test it. Moreover, some of our pilot experiments indicated that this "odor–brightness" transfer might not occur under some parametric variations, and we did not have a firm grasp on which particular parameters were critical. These gaps in our understanding of the basic effect suggested that our next step should be a test of its generality, with quite different procedures that engaged different sensory modalities. This course was also suggested by other considerations, discussed next.

### 2.  Intersensory Transfer with Various Sensory Modalities

In the previous experiments we found intermodal transfer of conditioning for 16-day-old rats but not for adults. This finding could indicate an ontogenetic decrease in intersensory transfer, or it could indicate something peculiar about the 16-day-old rat with regard to the special circumstances of transfer between olfactory and visual learning. For instance, the 16-day-old rat has only recently opened its eyes; perhaps it is especially disposed to transfer information from a familiar sensory modality such as olfaction to this relatively unfamiliar sensory modality of vision. As a first step toward reconciling these alternatives, we tested intermodal transfer of conditioning with a variety of sensory modalities and for rats in their first and third postnatal weeks.

Given limited space, we present here only samples of these tests to make the point that intersensory transfer is reasonably widespread for the infant rat. In the first example, transfer between olfactory and tactile conditioning was observed for the 4-day-old rat; the second observation was transfer between visual and gustatory conditioning for the 16-day-old rat; and the third observation was tactile and gustatory conditioning for the 4-day-old.

***a.  Olfactory-Tactile Transfer, 4 Days Old.***   The standard three conditions were tested. For the basic transfer condition, pairings of the odor of methyl salicylate and lateral shock (a mild electrical current applied to the rat's lateral portions, just behind the front legs) preceded pairings of exposure to the soft piling of a rug and lateral shock. For one control group, the odor–lateral shock pairings preceded unpaired presentations of texture and lateral shock. For the other control group, unpaired presentations of odor and lateral shock preceded the texture–lateral shock pairings.

The basic phenomenon of intersensory transfer of conditioning was again quite clear. The open bars in Fig. 4 show that, relative to the control conditions, prior olfactory conditioning enhanced the conditioning of aversion to texture. The tactile aversion was tested by allowing the rat pup a choice between being on the soft pile or being on a rough surface (the back side of the same type of carpeting). Also in Fig. 4 (darker bars) are shown the results of a subsequent experiment in which olfactory extinction, analogous to that in the previous series with 16-day-olds and adults, was given. Specifically, nonreinforced presentations of the methyl odor were given to each animal for 20 min following the paired, or unpaired, presentations of texture and lateral shock. This olfactory extinction significantly decreased the texture aversion, reducing it to a level equivalent to that of the control conditions.

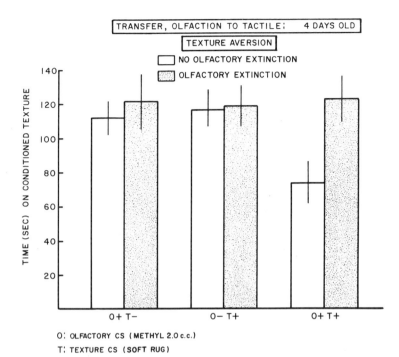

**Fig. 4.** Time spent on the conditioned texture (soft piling of a rug) as a function of conditioning and olfactory extinction treatments. +, Paired presentation; −, unpaired presentation.

### b. Visual-Gustatory Transfer, 16 Days Old.

If adult rats are given pairings of a distinctive taste with footshock, a conditioned aversion to the tasted substance is either unlikely to occur (for reviews, see Domjan, 1985) or very difficult to achieve (e.g., Pelchat, Grill, Rozin, & Jacobs, 1983). We asked whether such conditioning would be promoted in the preweanling rat by prior visual conditioning. Rat pups 16 days of age were cannulated with the procedures of Hall and Rosenblatt (1977) and water-deprived 6 hr before conditioning. Each pup in the experimental condition was then given six pairings of the black compartment and footshock. In the basic transfer condition, this was followed by six intraoral infusions of 15% sucrose solution, each 20 s in duration, accompanied by footshock during seconds 8–10 and 18–20 of each infusion. In the two control conditions, only the black-footshock pairings or the sucrose-footshock pairings were received, together with unpaired presentations of the alternative combinations.

Conditioning of aversion to the sucrose solution was promoted by prior conditioning of the visual stimulus. This result is shown in Fig. 5 in terms of each of two measures of conditioned aversion. Infusion of the sucrose solution was the same for all three conditions, and placement of the cannula was such that the rat pup could reject the sucrose solution, that is, could spit it out or allow it to spill out of its mouth. Since greater aversion to sucrose solution would be accompanied by less ingestion of it, the greater the conditioned aversion, the less the weight gain. Spillage was made readily detectable by coloring the sucrose solution red and placing a piece of white paper beneath the testing apparatus. The time of the first appearance of red on the white paper was taken as the time of rejection; the shorter the time of rejection, the greater the aversion.

These measures agreed in showing conditioned aversion to the taste of sucrose solution if and only if conditioning of the visual stimulus—black compartment paired with footshock—had preceded conditioning of the taste stimulus—sucrose solution paired with footshock. Not only did

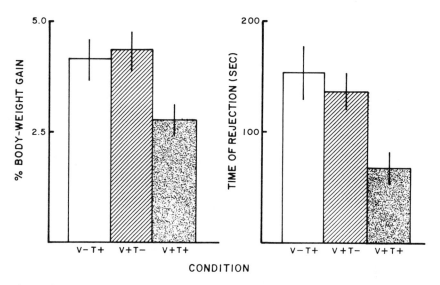

**Fig. 5.** Percentage body-weight gain—(postinfusion weight − preinfusion weight) × 100/ preinfusion weight—and latency to reject a sucrose solution (15% w/v) during the ingestional test. Abbreviations: V, visual CS (black compartment); T, taste CS (15% w/v sucrose solution); −, unpaired presentations between visual or taste stimuli and footshock; +, paired presentations between visual and taste stimuli. The left panel of this figure represents a conventional index of taste aversion with infant rats: percentage body-weight gain as a consequence of ingesting the conditioned substance during testing. Represented in the right panel is latency between onset of the infusion of sucrose solution and the first indication of rejection by the pup: actual spillage from the mouth.

prior visual conditioning potentiate taste conditioning, but the visual conditioning was itself further strengthened as a consequence of the subsequent taste conditioning.

*c. Tactile-Gustatory Transfer, 4 Days Old.* The final set of our experiments usefully mentioned here also tested intermodal transfer involving conditioning of a taste US to a footshock US, but with 4- rather than 16-day-old rats.

Tactile aversion was conditioned and tested as in the previous experiment, with 4-day-olds. Conditioning of the taste aversion included six pairings of the infused sucrose solution and shock delivered with the same procedures and schedule as had been used for the 16-day-old rats, except that lateral shock rather than footshock was used for the 4-day-olds and total volume and rate of infusion were less, scaled to the sizes of the pups.

In the first experiment, the pups in the critical transfer condition were given pairings of the texture and lateral shock followed 20 min later by pairings of the taste and lateral shock. The pups in the control conditions were given pairings with lateral shock for only one of the two CSs and explicitly unpaired presentations of the alternative CS and lateral shock. Conditioned aversion to the sucrose solution that had been paired with lateral shock is shown in Fig. 6; the two response measures used are the same as those used for the 16-day-old rats. It was found that conditioning of taste aversion was enhanced by prior conditioning of texture aversion. Animals given conditioning to texture prior to conditioning to taste gained less BW as a consequence of the sucrose infusion and more readily rejected as the solution than did either of the two control groups.

A surprising, but possibly important, result was that pairings of taste and shock were sufficient in themselves to induce a significant taste aversion. This aversion is assessed relative to the sucrose intake of rats given explicitly unpaired presentations of the taste and shock preceded by conditioning of the texture aversion. Such conditioning of a taste aversion to peripheral shock with relatively few pairings suggests that the neonatal rat may be less subject to biologic constraints on CS-to-US compatibility than are adults. This would indicate still another instance of ontogenetic change in stimulus selection. This taste aversion occurred in special circumstances, and caution about its generality is reasonable. Yet, this effect has been replicated by Heather Hoffmann in our laboratory with 5-day-old rats, with comparison against conventional control conditions; notably, taste-footshock conditioning did not occur when 15-day-olds were tested with the same procedures.

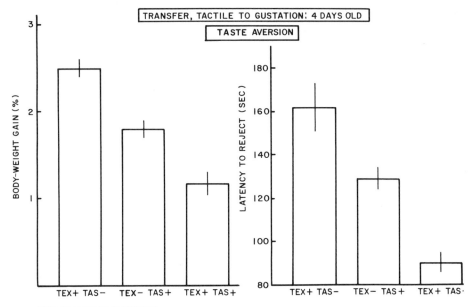

**Fig. 6.** Percentage body-weight gain—(postinfusion weight − preinfusion weight) × 100/preinfusion weight—and latency to reject a sucrose solution (15% w/v) as a function of treatment. +, Paired presentation; −, unpaired presentation.

### 3. Summary and Comment

We may now summarize the results of these initial tests of intermodal transfer. We found that transfer of conditioning occurred between an olfactory CS and a visual CS, but only for 16-day-old rats, not for adults. This was a mutually facilitatory transfer, such that olfactory conditioning facilitated visual conditioning and the visual conditioning strengthened still further the olfactory conditioning. It was as if successive conditioning trials had been given the same CS rather than the different CSs actually presented. Following conditioning of both CSs, extinction of either CS weakened the conditioning strength of the alternative. This further indicated that intermodal equivalence was established, that is, that the preweanlings (but not the adults) were somehow treating information gathered through one sensory modality as equal to that gathered through a different modality.

We observed similar intermodal transfer among infant rats in a variety of circumstances: 4-day-old rat pups transferred conditioning from olfactory to tactile stimuli; 16-day-old rats transferred conditioning between visual and taste stimuli, even though the nocioceptive US was peripheral (footshock) and conditioning of taste aversion with such a US is known to be impossible or very difficult among adult rats; and 4-day-olds also readily conditioned an aversion to a taste paired with shock when that episode was preceded by tactile conditioning. Our study of these effects is still in its early stages, however. Not all of these variations have included explicit comparisons between infant and older rats. Also, not all of the several phenomena indicating intersensory equivalence with infants given olfactory-visual transfer have been observed with all the varieties of transfer we have tested. For instance, with 4-day-olds given olfactory-tactile transfer, a tendency for the mutual strengthening of olfactory conditioning by subsequent tactile conditioning, analogous to the strengthening of olfactory conditioning by subsequent visual conditioning among the older preweanlings, was not significant. Generally speaking, however, the nature of these intersensory transfer effects has been similar for all of the combinations of sensory modalities we have tested among infants, and we have seen none of these effects as yet with older rats.

It is difficult not to take an incredulous view of these results. Generalization across sensory modalities seems even less adaptive than that within sensory modalities. Moreover, unlike intrasensory generalization, the advantage of capitalizing on an ever-changing world would seem to be lost: Why should it be adaptive that a particular odor, when revisited in slightly different circumstances, would be treated the same as a particular visual event? Unlike our initial experiments that tested transfer between olfactory learning about ethanol and subsequent ingestion of ethanol, however, these subsequent transfer experiments were not conventional tests for assessment of generalization. Instead, a common US was paired with each of the two CSs presented sequentially.

That this common US could provide the mediation link for learned equivalence has been confirmed by a recent test in our laboratory. Briefly, a requirement of such a test is two different USs that yield equivalent reinforcement. We established a concentration of infused citric acid which, when paired with an odor, yielded the same degree of conditioning as that found with a specified intensity and duration of footshock. We then observed that transfer to a visual CS occurred only when both stimuli were accompanied by the same US (citric acid or footshock) and not if the odor CS was paired with one US and the visual CS with another. The intersensory transfer apparently was mediated by the common "affordance" (the US).

This does not, however, exclude other means by which intersensory equivalence might be achieved. An equally likely explanation is in terms of amodal characteristics that are held in common by the stimuli for which we observed intersensory transfer. The implication here is that, in some circumstances, the rat may not learn strictly in accord with sensory modality.

## II. Intersensory Equivalence and Amodal Learning

Thus far we have provided evidence that preweanlings appear not to differentiate events according to the different sensory modalities used to detect these events. To say this another way, preweanlings may treat as equivalent, stimuli detected on separate occasions by different sensory modalities. Indifference to sensory modality is consistent with Gibsonian thinking in general (e.g., J. J. Gibson, 1966) and with the ontogeny of stimulus differentiation and perceptual learning as well (E. J. Gibson, 1969). In the Gibsonian view of perception, there is no need to be concerned with sensory systems per se; the concept of *perceptual systems* is used instead. This view is based on a strict realism that considers perception as direct and based on information that exists fully in the environment. This information is picked up multimodally and dynamically: To perceive a ball, one may touch it, look at it from different locations, hear it bounce.

Early in life an infant should come to expect that detection through different sensory receptors may apply to the same object. E. J. Gibson (1984) suggests that precoordinated perceptual systems are available for use from birth, at least in humans, permitting the infant to acquire "knowledge of multi-modally specified invariants" (p. 28). Within Gibsonian theory what is perceived is affordances of objects—what an individual might do with or to an object or what the object might do to the individual. E. J. Gibson (1984) suggests that "it may be that common *affordances* also provide a basis for unity" [of the senses] (p. 33). This theory of perception accounts for both failure to differentiate sensory modalities early in life and also coordination of input from different sensory modalities in such a way as to treat the different sources of sensory input as equivalent, that is, as applying to the same object.

Whatever theory of conditioning and learning one accepts, it seems necessary that events to be associated or somehow integrated must be differentiated from other events. An associative interpretation of Pavlovian conditioning applied in the present experiments therefore requires a relatively unambiguous representation of the CS by the animal. This is needed to allow the CS to be distinguished from other events that do not predict the US. If not in terms of the sensory modalities through which the CS is detected, how is such a representation achieved? One possibility is through other attributes of the memory of a CS that can lead to differentiation independent of sensory modality, a sort of *amodal conditioning* that can lead to amodal transfer.

There are a number of precedents for the consideration of amodal conditioning and transfer: in theories attempting to reconcile and understand the "unity of the senses" (Hartshorne, 1934, cited by Marks, 1978); in the investigation of perception and cognition in human children (e.g., Wagner & Sakovits, 1983; Wagner, Winner, Cicchetti, & Gardner, 1981); and in the basic conditioning and learning of adult animals (e.g., Church & Meck, in press; Holt & Kehoe, 1985; Kehoe, Morrow, & Holt, 1984). Perhaps the most thorough tests of cross-modal transfer of learning have been completed by Church and Meck (in press) in the context of timing behavior. They show quite clearly, for example, that learning based on different durations of a visual stimulus transfers readily to an auditory stimulus presented with the corresponding durations, or vice versa. They conclude that "it is now known that animals have amodal systems for the analysis of attributes such as time and number, and these attributes can be transferred across modalities" (p. 94).

The latter suggestion is consistent with the experiments discussed next. Although they do not involve the attributes of duration and number, these experiments consider other attributes that are common to events detected by different sensory modalities and that seem likely to be used by infants. The above examples of cross-modal or amodal processing with animals have tested only adults. There is good precedent for such effects with infants, however. The theory and data of Turkewitz and his colleagues (e.g., Turkewitz, Gardner, & Lewkowicz, 1984) provide a compelling argument that during the first month or so of postnatal life, human infants may primarily respond to (and perhaps learn about) the intensities of stimuli rather than their more qualitative sensory features such as the sensory modality through which a particular stimulus is detected. Our analysis, too, indicates that this tendency for amodal processing may be stronger in younger animals.

## A.  Familiarity as an Amodal Mediator of Transfer of Conditioning

Rats behave differently to an unusual odor they previously have experienced than to a completely novel odor. From their second postnatal week to adulthood, when given a mere 3 min of exposure to an ambient novel odor, the rat will prefer to be in the location of that odor rather than the location of one that it has not previously smelled. This effect supersedes even the apparently aversive consequences of the rat pup being isolated from its home while it is becoming familiar with the odor (Caza & Spear,

1984; Smith, Kucharski, & Spear, 1985; Wigal, Kucharski, & Spear, 1984). Relative familiarity of an odor is therefore an important determinant of the infant rat's behavior. In our laboratory, Nancy Lariviere tested whether an acquired aversion to an odor that is especially familiar to the developing rat would transfer to an equally familiar odor quite different in quality from the first.

The odorants used by Lariviere were commercially produced representations of those one can smell in the real world (peppermint, lemon, and garlic); but aside from the controlled familiarization experiences (2 hr per day for 5 days) and conditioning episodes, these odors were quite unique in the lives of the animals tested. For rats familiarized with two odors, the question was whether preference for a familiarized but not peviously conditioned odor would be significantly reduced if the other familiarized odor were made aversive. The full experimental design was a 2 × 2 × 2 factorial at each of the three ages; either the animals were familiarized previously with odors or they were not, given pairings of one familiarized odor and footshock or explicitly unpaired presentations of the same events, and conditioned with peppermint and tested with garlic or vice versa.

The results indicated that the younger preweanlings could learn amodally on the basis of relative familiarity. This effect was observed for both 12- and 16-day-old preweanlings but not for rats 21 days of age. The relative familiarity of a CS seemed to mediate transfer of conditioning to a CS of quite different sensory quality. Fig. 7 shows that for either 12-day-old or 16-day-old rats previously familiarized with both peppermint and garlic, significant transfer of conditioning occurred from the conditioned to the nonconditioned familiar odor. This is indicated by the differences between those given actual paired presentations of CS and US during prior conditioning and those given unpaired presentations. For animals not given prior familiarization, the paired and unpaired conditions did not differ. With 21-day-old rats, however, there was no indication that prior familiarization led to significantly greater transfer of aversion for the paired relative to the unpaired animals.

Transfer of conditioning may be mediated in 12- and 16-day-old rats by familiarity, apparently independent of similarity between the sensory aspects of the stimuli. That 21-day-olds did not show this effect is of potentially great interest, although we cannot at this point elaborate why this might be so. It is quite clear, however, that the effect occurs in younger preweanlings. Although interpretation of these results in terms of sensory preconditioning is conceivable—that is, an association between the sensory aspects of the two odors could have taken place during familiarization—our previous data indicate that the sequential exposure to the two odors make sensory preconditioning an unlikely possibility in rats of these ages (Spear & Kucharski, 1984a).

## B.  Stimulus Encoding in Terms of Affect

Familiarized novel odors might become more preferred because of a change in the affect elicited by them. We could say that because of the increased preference for an odor to which an infant rat has been exposed for several days, this odor elicits more of a positive affect, or less of a negative affect, than does a novel odor. An additional experiment in our laboratory by Lariviere (unpublished) indicated that infant rats may encode events on the basis of the affective response elicited by an odor. Briefly, the question was whether conditioning of an aversion to a highly preferred odor would be more likely to transfer to a different highly preferred odor than to a different odor of relatively low preference.

This study included three separate experiments, each with 16-day-old rats. First, a preference scale for a variety of odors was established by comparing the rat's preference for the location of each of several novel odors relative to that of clean home shavings. This produced an ordering of odors from very low preference to very high preference. Examples of less preferred odors are lemon and orange; more preferred odors include maple and butter. The next step was to condition an aversion to one of the high-preference odorants, with counterbalancing, and test whether the transfer of aversion would be greater to another high-preference odor than to a low-preference odor. The results indicated more transfer of aversion to a highly preferred odor than to a highly unpreferred odor. It was as if the infant had learned that novel odors of initially higher affect (i.e., relatively preferred) are more likely to be accompanied by foot-shock.

Yet, there existed the possibility of primary stimulus generalization between odors of equal preference. To test this, rats were given a highly preferred odor paired with footshock and a moderately preferred odor *not* paired with footshock. Lariviere then assessed their preference between a different moderately preferred odor and an odor of ordinarily very low preference. If primary generalization between the two moderately preferred odors were an important factor, then, due to the initial "safe" experience with a moderate odor, we would expect greater preference of the other moderate odor. But if the rats had learned that a more highly preferred odor is more likely to be paired with footshock, they should choose the odor of very low preference over the moderately preferred odor. The rats did the latter, indicating that relative affect determined the transfer

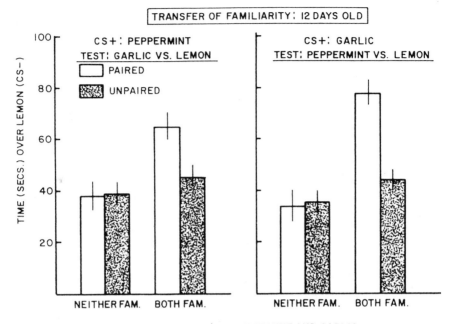

FAMILIARITY WITH PEPPERMINT AND GARLIC

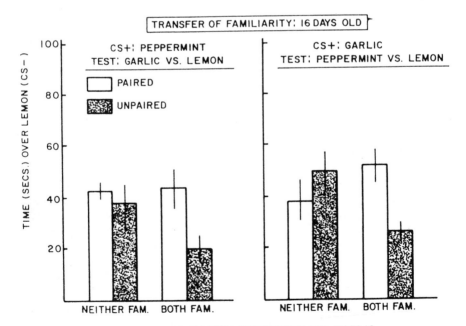

FAMILIARITY WITH PEPPERMINT AND GARLIC

between odors and that primary generalization had comparatively little influence in the previous experiment.

Finally, a study with 15-day-old preweanling rats has tested the use of affective encoding in other circumstances (Meehan & Spear, 1986). The stimuli to be encoded were visual—black versus white. These alternative levels of brightness were paired with ambient temperatures that were either preferred or not preferred. The first test was to determine the nature of the resultant preference for black (or white, counterbalanced) when the black compartment had been accompanied by an ambient temperature of 23°, 26°, 29°, 32°, or 35°C. Interspersed among the pairings of black and one of the ambient temperatures were equivalent exposures to the white compartment always at 23°C. For the test for brightness preference, room temperature in both the black and white compartments was always 23°C. Temperature regulation for 15-day-old rats is not accomplished internally with nearly the effectiveness of 25-day-olds. When a 32°C temperature was paired with the black compartment, a significant *preference* for that brightness was conditioned for 15-day-olds, but a significant aversion was conditioned for 25-day-olds (see Fig. 8).

We may now ask what the 15-day-old animals learned about the black compartment when it was accompanied by an ambient temperature of 32°C. At one extreme, the animal could learn that black predicts a specific value of temperature in absolute terms, that is, the physical properties of 32°C. Alternatively, the pup could have learned that black predicts thermal comfort or the absence of thermal discomfort, that is, the black affords positive affect. This can be tested by pairing the black compartment with 32°C when the animal is 15 days old and testing for preference of the black compartment when the animal is 25 days old. Animals 15 days old forget conditioning very rapidly. But, with a high degree of conditioning and widely distributed practice, infantile amnesia can to some extent be overcome (Spear, 1979), so conditioning in this study included extensive conditioning sessions on each of postnatal Days 15 and 16, and retention was enhanced accordingly.

Our data indicate that at 25 days of age, rats find 32°C quite aversive. Therefore, if the 15-day-old had learned that black predicts the absolute physical properties of a 32°C temperature, that memory should be ex-

**Fig. 7.** (Top) Time spent over lemon odor (1.0 cc) as a function of familiarity and conditioning treatments in 12-day-old rats. (Bottom) Time spent over lemon odor (1.0 cc) as a function of familiarity and conditioning treatments in 16-day-old rats. These results are presented in terms of time on the completely novel odor during testing: The higher the number, the greater the transfer of aversion to the alternative, familiarized-but-not-conditioned odor.

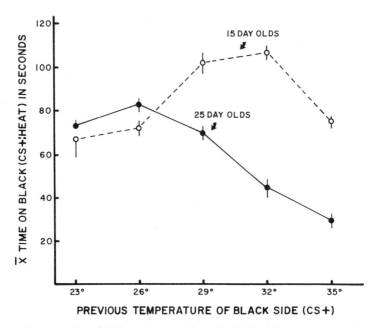

**Fig. 8.** Time spent in a black compartment in a visual discrimination test as a function of age and previous experience with different temperatures paired with the CS+ (black compartment).

pressed at 25 days of age in terms of aversion to the black compartment. Alternatively, if the rat had encoded its 15-day-old experience with black as predicting general thermal comfort or generally positive affect, the memory of that experience should be expressed in terms of a preference for the black compartment.

When the rats were tested 9 days later at 25 days of age, their preference for the black compartment was about 35% greater than that of control animals that had been given explicitly unpaired presentations of black and 32°C. Evidently what had been learned about the black compartment by the 15-day-old rat pup was that black predicted general thermal comfort—positive affect—not that it predicted a particular temperature.

## III.  Summary and Conclusions

We have found that the preweanling rat is capable of transferring the consequences of Pavlovian conditioning across sensory modalities and across different instances of a single sensory modality. This transfer is accomplished in a variety of circumstances, and with surprising efficacy.

In contrast, the adult rat shows little evidence of such transfer in these same circumstances.

We first tested transfer from conditioning of the olfactory properties of alcohol to expression in terms of alcohol's gustatory properties. During each of their first, second, and third postnatal weeks, preweanlings showed transfer of such magnitude as to suggest that they treated the smell and taste of this particular substance as equivalent. Adults, however, gave no indication of any significant transfer of this kind. We subsequently found that in terms of potentiation of conditioning involving one sensory modality by prior conditioning with another, intersensory transfer was evident in a variety of circumstances for rats during their first and third postnatal weeks. These instances included transfer between olfaction and vision, between vision and taste, between olfaction and tactile reception, and between tactile reception and taste. Adult rats gave no evidence for such intersensory transfer in comparable tests.

The final set of our studies tested whether preweanlings might encode stimuli in conditioning irrespective of the sensory modality through which detection occurred. Preweanlings during their second postnatal week readily transferred conditioning from one odorant to a discriminably different odorant, provided that these odorants had an equal degree of familiarity. It was as if the rat learned that a familiar odor predicted a particular consequence and generalized this to other equally familiar odors, without regard to the physical properties of the odor. Such transfer was also evident during the beginning of the third postnatal week but not toward the end (21 days of age). Other experiments indicated that among preweanlings, transfer between stimuli of different physical characteristics might be mediated by affect—that is, they may encode stimuli as "good" and "something to approach" on the one hand or "bad" and "something to avoid" on the other, sometimes without regard to the qualitative physical properties of that object.

We cannot assert categorically how each of these transfer effects changes ontogenetically. Clear age-related differences have been observed each time we looked for them, but it is difficult to arrange strictly comparable tests for preweanlings and adults and we have yet to do so for all of the transfer effects. It is unlikely that adults will show no intermodal transfer in each instance. The data of Church and Meck (in press) are especially clear in showing robust transfer of this kind among adult rats. The nature of the ontogenetic change, when it occurs, and the boundary conditions for intersensory transfer among animals of all ages are further questions that require answers before a great deal can be made theoretically of the effects reported in this chapter.

With these limitations in mind, we may now comment on a few implications of the intersensory transfer and amodal encoding we have observed among preweanling rats. These results are generally consistent with the ontogeny of stimulus selection in circumstances involving relatively complex multievent stimuli. In a variety of circumstances, age-related differences in overshadowing, potentiation, or blocking were tested, together with ontogenetic comparisons of contextual learning during conditioning and of sensory preconditioning. The results indicated generally less overshadowing and blocking for preweanlings than for adults, but more potentiation, more sensory preconditioning, and more processing of contextual events among the younger rats. As a whole, these results were consistent with the general notion that preweanling animals are less likely than adults to differentiate among elements of a CS or between a CS and context. It was as if the preweanling animals perceived the circumstances of conditioning as an integral unit of undifferentiated events, perhaps analogous to the integral processing of preschool children that differs from the separable processing observed at older ages (see Spear, 1984b; Spear & Kucharski, 1984a, 1984b).

This general theme of less differentiation among stimuli by immature animals is consistent with the present phenomena of intersensory transfer. In the latter case, however, reference is primarily to differentiation among sensory modalities. The idea of an ontogenetic increase in sensory differentiation is certainly not new; the possibility of such an ontogenetic change has been recognized for at least the past 100 years, and perhaps longer (Cytowic & Wood, 1982). Within the past 20 years it has been elaborated most eloquently by E. J. Gibson, together with other issues of ontogenetic change in stimulus differentiation (e.g., E. J. Gibson, 1969).

What is new in our experimental findings is that such effects can be observed quite clearly in the developing rat, which provides an opportunity to test more directly some of the general implications. We may now apply the present conditioning procedures to determine the ontogeny of differentiation among and within sensory modalities at the behavioral level. We may also reconcile a variety of basic issues: whether sensory differentiation is possible at a particular age yet not expressed or not implemented; the nature of the encoding that is employed in lieu of sensory differentiation; and what neuroanatomic and neurophysiological changes occur ontogenetically that may correspond to and perhaps directly constrain the development of sensory differentiation at the behavioral level (cf. Almli, 1984).

Some specific implications for the developmental psychobiology of learning and memory are also suggested by our evidence. Suppose that infant altricial mammals may not differentiate a touch from a sound, a smell from a sight or a taste from a smell, so that the initial stage of cognition during infancy is differentiation of the sensory modalities themselves. We would certainly be less inclined, then, to focus our experiments and theories of memory development on specific sensory systems. On the other hand, for infant animals that learned an aversion or a preference to a taste, an odor, or a texture, the learning has seemed fairly specific; aversion or preference has not been exhibited to all events nor even to all tastes, odors, or textures. Decisions regarding the boundary conditions of what is learned must now be considered before drawing any conclusions about the efficacy of learning in general at any particular age.

Many developmental psychobiologists, including ourselves, have not been inclined to consider a unitary capacity that develops to promote, in uniform fashion, all kinds of learning or memory. Instead, it has seemed that the ontogeny of learning and memory will depend on the "system" or "kind" or learning and memory in question (Spear, 1984a). One approach is to divide up kinds of learning along the lines of sensory modalities—the sensory system accordingly becomes the functional system. We mentioned earlier the astute series of studies by Rudy and his colleagues that indicates, for instance, that the capacity for acquiring an olfactory aversion emerges before that of a taste aversion, and the capacity for each of these precedes that for acquiring an auditory aversion or a visual aversion (Rudy et al., 1984). These ontogenetic changes in learning correspond to those for basic sensory detection, although mature detection is carefully shown by Rudy and his colleagues to be only a necessary case for learning and not sufficient in itself. Differences in maturational rates for memory capacity (in the sense of forgetting) seem to be similar in that they also accord with the sensory modality required to process the CS, although the facts on this matter are less well developed so far than are those for initial conditioning (Markiewicz, Kucharski, & Spear, 1986).

In conventional thinking, this relationship among the maturation rates for sensory capacity, learning, and memory seems so reasonable as to be almost unremarkable. The capacity for learning and memory about stimuli processed by a particular modality such as the "visual system" or the "olfactory system" emerges all at once for stimuli within the realm of the particular modality. But what happens before the sensory modalities are differentiated? What if learning during the perinatal or infant periods does not involve sensory modality as a means for identifying what is learned? We would then find it difficult to allude to learning within, say, the "visual system" or the "olfactory system(s)." We could not even talk about "visual learning" or "olfactory learning," only visual or olfactory detection. We would have to devise another arrangement for classifying learning and memory, at least early in development. At this time, these matters of classification may need to be postponed until we achieve a better grasp of the extent to which infant learning proceeds without regard to sensory modality and until we can identify more precisely what is learned in the absence of sensory differentiation.

## Acknowledgments

This research was supported by a grant from the National Institute of Mental Health (1 RO1 MH35219) to N.E.S. and by a fellowship awarded to J.C.M. by the National Council of Research of Argentina (CONICET). The authors express their appreciation to Norman G. Richter for his technical assistance and to Teri Tanenhaus for preparation of the manuscript. The authors are also grateful to Phil Kraemer, Heather Hoffmann, and Gail Baker for their critical reading and suggestions on an earlier draft of this manuscript.

## References

Alberts, J. R. (1984). Sensory-perceptual development in the Norway rat: A view toward comparative studies. In R. Kail & N. E. Spear (Eds.), *Comparative perspectives on the development of memory* (pp. 65–102). Hillsdale, NJ: Erlbaum.

Almli, C. R. (1984). Early brain damage and time course of behavioral dysfunction: Parallels with neural maturation. In S. Finger & C. R. Almli (Eds.), *Early brain damage: Vol. 2. Neurobiology and behavior* (pp. 99–116). Orlando: Academic Press.

Anohkin, P. K. (1964). Systemogenesis as a general regulator of brain development. *Progress in Brain Research, 90,* 54–86.

Campbell, B. A., & Spear, N. E. (1972). Ontogeny of memory. *Psychological Review, 79,* 215–236.

Caza, P. A., & Spear, N. E. (1984). Short-term exposure to an odor increases its subsequent preference in preweanling rats: A descriptive profile of the phenomenon. *Developmental Psychobiology, 17,* 407–422.

Church, R. M., & Meck, W. H. (in press). Acquisition and cross-modal transfer of classification rules for temporal intervals. In M. L. Commons, A. R. Wagner, & R. J. Herrnstein (Eds.), *Quantitative analysis of behavior: Discriminative processes* (Vol. 4, pp. 75–97). Cambridge, MA: Ballinger.

Cytowic, R. E., & Wood, F. B. (1982). Synesthesia: I. A review of major theories and their brain basis. *Brain and Cognition, 1,* 23–35.

Domjan, M. (1985). Cue-consequence specificity and long-delay learning revisited. In N. S. Braveman & P. Bronstein (Eds.), *Experimental assessments and clinical applications of conditioned food aversions. Annals of the New York Academy of Sciences, 443,* 54–66.

Freides, D. (1974). Human information processing and sensory modality: Cross-modal functions, information complexity, memory, and deficit. *Psychological Bulletin, 81,* 284–310.

Gibson, E. J. (1969). *Principles of perceptual learning and development.* New York: Appleton-Century-Crofts.

Gibson, E. J. (1984). Development of knowledge about intermodal unity: Two views. In L. Liben (Ed.), *Piaget and the foundations of knowledge* (pp. 19–41). Hillsdale, NJ: Erlbaum.

Gibson, J. J. (1966). *The senses considered as perceptual systems.* Boston: Houghton Mifflin.

Hall, W. G., & Rosenblatt, J. S. (1977). Suckling behavior and intake control in the developing rat. *Journal of Comparative and Physiological Psychology, 91,* 1232–1247.

Hartshorne, C. (1934). *The philosophy and psychology of sensation.* Chicago: University of Chicago Press.

Holt, P. E., & Kehoe, E. J. (1985). Cross-modal transfer as a function of similarities between training tasks in classical conditioning of the rabbit. *Animal Learning & Behavior, 13,* 51–59.

Kehoe, E. J., Morrow, L. D., & Holt, P. E. (1984). General transfer across sensory modalities survives reduction in the original conditioned reflex in the rabbit. *Animal Learning & Behavior, 12,* 129–136.

Markiewicz, B., Kucharski, D., & Spear, N. E. (1986). Ontogenetic comparison of memory for Pavlovian conditioned aversion in temperature, vibration, odor or brightness. *Developmental Psychobiology.*

Marks, L. E. (1975). On colored-hearing synesthesia: Cross-modal translations of sensory dimensions. *Psychological Bulletin, 82,* 303–331.

Marks, L. E. (1978). *The unity of the senses: Interrelations among the modalities.* New York: Academic Press.

Meehan, S. M. & Spear, N. E. (1986). *Learning and retention of thermal cues in 15- and 25-day-old rats: Evidence for encoding of affective attributes.* Paper presented at meetings of the Midwestern Psychological Association, Chicago.

Molina, J. C., Hoffmann, H., & Spear, N. E. (1985). Conditioning of aversion to alcohol orosensory cues in 5- and 10-day old rats: Subsequent reduction in alcohol ingestion. *Developmental Psychobiology, 19,* 175–183.

Molina, J. C., Serwatka, J., & Spear, N. E. (1984). Changes in alcohol intake resulting from prior experience with alcohol odor in young rats. *Pharmacology, Biochemistry, and Behavior, 21,* 387–391.

Molina, J. C., Serwatka, J., Spear, L. P., & Spear, N. E. (1985). Differential ethanol olfactory experiences affect ethanol ingestion in preweanlings but not in older rats. *Behavioral and Neural Biology, 44,* 90–100.

Neisser, U. (1962). Cultural and cognitive discontinuity. In T. E. Gladwin & W. Sturtevant (Eds.), *Anthropology and human behavior.* Washington DC: Anthropological Society of Washington.

Pelchat, M. L., Grill, H. J., Rozin, P., & Jacobs, J. (1983). Quality of acquired responses to taste by *Rattus norvegus* depends on type of associated discomfort. *Journal of Comparative Psychology, 97,* 140–153.

Rudy, J. W., Vogt, M. B., & Hyson, R. L. (1984). A developmental analysis of the rat's learned reaction to gustatory and auditory stimulation. In R. Kail & N. E. Spear (Eds.), *Comparative perspectives on the development of memory* (pp. 181–208). Hillsdale, NJ: Erlbaum.

Serwatka, J., Molina, J. C., & Spear, N. E. (1986). Weanlings' transfer of conditioned ethanol aversion from olfaction to ingestion depends on the unconditioned stimulus. *Behavioral and Neural Biology, 45,* 57–70.

Smith, G. J., Kucharski, D., & Spear, N. E. (1985). Ontogenetic differences in the conditioning of an odor aversion using isolation from the home nest environment as the unconditioned stimulus. *Developmental Psychobiology, 18,* 421–434.

Spear, N. E. (1979). Memory storage factors in infantile amnesia. In G. Bower (Ed.), *The psychology of learning and motivation* (Vol. 13 pp. 91–154). New York: Academic Press.

Spear, N. E. (1984a). Behaviors that indicate memory. *Canadian Journal of Psychology, 38,* 348–367.

Spear, N. E. (1984b). Ecologically determined dispositions control the ontogeny of learning and memory. In R. Kail & N. E. Spear (Eds.), *Comparative perspectives on the development of memory* (pp. 325–358). Hillsdale, NJ: Erlbaum.

Spear, N. E., & Kucharski, D. (1984a). Ontogenetic differences in stimulus selection during conditioning. In R. Kail & N. E. Spear (Eds.), *Comparative perspectives on the development of memory* (pp. 227–252). Hillsdale, NJ: Erlbaum.

Spear, N. E., & Kucharski, D. (1984b). Ontogenetic differences in the processing of multi-element stimuli: Potentiation and overshadowing. In H. Roitblat, T. Bever, & H. Terrace (Eds.). *Animal cognition* (pp. 545–567). Hillsdale, NJ: Erlbaum.

Turkewitz, G., Gardner, J. M., & Lewkowicz, D. J. (1984). Sensory/perceptual functioning during infancy: The implications of a quantitative basis for responding. In G. Greenberg & E. Tobach (Eds.), *T. C. Schneirla Conference on Levels of Integration and Evolution of Behavior* (pp. 167–195). Hillsdale, NJ: Erlbaum.

Wagner, S., & Sakovitz, L. (1983). *Cross-modal information processing: The effects of modality, age, complexity and number.* Paper presented at the meeting of the Society for Research in Child Development, Dallas.

Wagner, S., Winner, E., Cicchetti, D., & Gardner, H. (1981). "Metaphorical" mapping in human infants. *Child Development, 52,* 728–731.

Werner, H. (1940). *Comparative psychology of mental development.* New York: Harper.

Wigal, T., Kucharski, D., & Spear, N. E. (1984). Familiar contextual odors promote discrimination learning in preweanling but not in older rats. *Developmental Psychobiology, 17,* 555–570.

# 5

# Neonatal Preference for Mother's Voice

WILLIAM P. FIFER
*New York State Psychiatric Institute*
*Department of Developmental Psychobiology*
*Columbia University*
*New York, New York, 10032*

## I.  Introduction

"For behold, the moment that the sound of thy greeting came to my ears, the babe in my womb lept for joy." John the Baptist was the lone subject in this observational study referenced in Luke. Most of the evidence for such precocious fetal auditory competence in humans remains largely anecdotal. Though published empirical data directly investigating a fetal capability for auditory recognition can currently only be found in the animal literature, there is a rapidly accumulating body of evidence that supports the notion that prenatal experience plays a major role in the development of human newborn auditory preferences and capabilities. In our laboratory we are investigating what may be a direct consequence of this early fetal experience, the newborn's preferential responsiveness to voices. Examination of this capability may not only provide a window into the processes underlying early attachment, neonatal learning, and perceptual development but may also provide us with another vantage point from which to focus our investigative lenses on the fetus.

## II.  Fetal Auditory Experience

Though significant gaps remain, there is substantial evidence that voices are transmitted in utero, that the fetus is capable of responding to auditory stimulation, and that the combination of the acoustic and filtering

**111**

characteristics of the womb may provide an optimal environment for extensive experience with the maternal voice. The human fetus has an intact, well-developed auditory system by the final trimester of gestation. Thorough reviews of the development of the fetal auditory system can be found in Pujol and Hilding (1973), Lecanuet, Granier-Deferre, and Busnel (1985), and Rubel (1985). In addition to the numerous anecdotal reports by mothers describing fetal kicking to different sounds, there is a substantial body of data demonstrating fetal responsiveness to auditory stimuli dating back to Peiper (1925) and Forbes and Forbes (1927). Fetal heart rate changes, independent of maternal responses, have been observed in response to externally presented pure tones as early as 24 weeks gestational age (Bernard & Sontag, 1947; Sontag & Wallace, 1936). Johansson, Wedenberg, and Westin (1964) observed increased pulse rates following presentation of tones during the last 7 weeks of gestation. Eye blinks following vibroacoustic stimulation were recorded in a 25-week-old fetus (Birnholz & Benacceraf, 1983). Recent advances in ultrasound imaging have allowed observations of global body and limb movement to external sounds (Gelman, Wood, Spellacy, & Abrams, 1982; Leader, Baile, Martin, & Vermuelen, 1982). Jensen (1984) has demonstrated that changes in fetal cardiac response occur as early as 32 weeks and then begin to increase as a function of gestational age. Finally, recent studies have shown that, similar to the newborn, fetal responses to acoustic stimulation are modulated by states of alertness (Lacanuet, Granier-Deferre, Cohen, Busnel, & Sureau, 1984).

Though tranmission across the maternal tissues and through the amniotic fluid causes some distortion and filtering to occur, certain sounds appear to be transmitted to the fetus. Recent technological advances have allowed more direct measurement of intrauterine sounds. Although original estimates put background noises and maternal vascular and other internal sounds as high as 95 dB (Bench, 1973; Henschall, 1972; Murooka, Koie, and Suda, 1976; Walker, Grimwade, & Wood, 1971), recent access to more sophisticated equipment has allowed a reassessment of the sounds in the womb. The overall intensity of the background noises, most of which are below 300 Hz, are more in the range of 50–60 dB (Querleu, Renard, & Crepin, 1981; Versyp, 1985). The frequencies primarily associated with voices are subject to the least amount of filtering (Armitage, Baldwin, & Vince, 1980; Querleu et al., 1981; Versyp, 1985). Additionally, external voices are probably not substantially masked by the low-frequency intrauterine vascular sounds. In fact, male voices may be transmitted as clearly as female voices, that is subject to minimal masking. A greater amount of experience with the female voice, however, may occur since the maternal voice is also transmitted internally and with considerably less attenuation (Lacanuet *et al.*, 1985; Versyp, 1985). A number of researchers have suggested that the sounds transmitted to the fetus are particularly biased toward experience with the dominant frequencies found in speech sounds (Aslin, Pisoni, & Jusczyk, 1983). Rubel (1985) notes that the transmission of sounds favoring low frequencies, while attenuating high frequencies, parallels auditory neuronal development. The developing system, with low-frequency sensitivity emerging first, may be making optimal use of the available stimuli. Moreover, the experience with external sounds may serve a role of enrichment, facilitation, or fine tuning of the system (Gottlieb, 1985; Lacanuet *et al.*, 1985). Developmental changes in sound transmission resulting from changes in the shape and density of the maternal abdominal wall, relative amount of amniotic fluid, and fetal head position throughout pregnancy may play a role as well in the development of hemispheric specialization (Turkewitz, in press). Turkewitz has made the further suggestion that coupling of auditory stimulation with the sensations resulting from movement of the mother's diaphragm while talking, may not only serve to make maternal speech more salient but can provide an important source of contingent and multimodal experience for the fetus.

Though the technology needed to determine exactly what sounds eventually reach the inner ear is not yet available, both animal and human studies have provided some data on the intelligibility of sounds transmitted into the amniotic fluid. Most recent in utero recordings indicate that external speech sounds are minimally distorted, though intensity may be attenuated on the average by as much as 20 dB (Lacanuet *et al.*, 1985; Versyp, 1985). The intrauterine recordings of the maternal voice when played to adult listeners, though approximately 15 dB louder than speech sounds originating externally, are heard as more distorted and less intelligible. The intonation or melodic contour is perceived as identical and may be the critical factor underlying subsequent postnatal responsiveness to voices (Panneton, 1985).

### III.  Newborn Auditory Capabilities

The newborn immediately after birth appears to be particularly responsive to sound. For thorough reviews see Eisenberg (1976) and Aslin, Pisoni, and Jusyck (1983). The evidence for precocious postnatal auditory competency begins with studies showing both behavioral and electrophysiological responding to sound in preterm infants (Aslin *et al.*, 1983; Eisenberg, 1976; Gregg, Haffner, & Korner, 1976). Full-term newborn infants will orient toward a sound source. They will turn their eyes toward an auditory stimulus (Wertheimer, 1961) and will visually scan the location of a sound source (Mendelson & Haith, 1967). Under controlled laboratory situations, neonates will also localize sound sources by turning their heads (reviewed in Muir & Clifton, 1985).

The newborn's auditory capabilities may include a special sensitivity to the frequency and band width components of human speech. For example, infants less than 3 days old show reliable cardiac responses to a restricted band of noise, but not to pure tones, demonstrating a sensitivity to band width (Turkewitz, Birch, & Cooper, 1972). Noise bands were also more effective than pure tones in eliciting muscular movement in newborns (Hutt, Hutt, Lenard, Bernuth, & Muntjewerff, 1968). Using habituation of body movement as the dependent measure, infants as young as 21 hr were observed to discriminate between signals of 200 and 1,000 Hz (Leventhal & Lipsitt, 1964). A 150-Hz tone has more reliable soothing effects than does a 500-Hz tone (Birns, Blank, & Bridger, 1966). Whereas low-frequency sounds are better inhibitors of infant distress, high frequencies (above 400 Hz) tend to occasion distress (Eisenberg, 1976). Hutt and Hutt (1970) reported maximal changes in newborn heart rate to frequencies within the range for human speech. Newborns can also discriminate intensity differences at birth; for example, Bartoshuk (1962) showed heart rate change to four different tonal intensities. Neonates may also be especially sensitive to sound levels within the range of normal conversational intensities. Suzuki, Kamijo, and Kiuchi (1964) found the optimum intensity level for eliciting a change in respiration rate to be approximately 62 dB, the average intensity of normal speech.

Infants appear to be differentially sensitive to auditory cues associated with speech and speechlike sounds (Aslin et al., 1983; Moon, 1985). For example, cues associated with intonation and rise-and-fall time of a tone are discriminated by young infants (Morse, 1972). The capacity to discriminate the phonetic components of speech, which has been demonstrated in young infants (Eimas, 1975), also appears to lie within the newborn's range of capabilities (Bertoncinni & Mehler, 1981; Moon 1985).

These perceptual sensitivities undoubtedly subserve a number of auditory preferences displayed by newborns. For example, instrumental music can be distinguished from a wide-band noise, and the infant will actually work, that is, alter his rate of sucking, when such a change produces the music (Butterfield & Siperstein, 1972). Similar techniques show newborn preferences for vocal over instrumental music and speech over other nonspeech sounds (Eisenberg, 1976; Siperstein & Butterfield, 1973). The human newborn's auditory system appears especially useful for detecting cues potentially associated with mother.

## IV.  Newborn Response to Voices

Mills and Meluish (1979) showed that the maternal voice may be an important stimulus for older infants. They demonstrated a differential sensitivity to the maternal voice in infants 20–30 days old. Amount of time spent sucking and number of sucks per minute were greater when a brief presentation of mother's voice followed initiations of sucking bursts. In a study using 1 month-old infants (Mehler, Bertoncini, Bauriere, & Jassik-Gershenfeld, 1978), sucks were reinforced with either mother's or a stranger's intonated voice or either voice presented in monotone. A significant increase in sucking was only observed when mother's voice was properly intonated. Though these procedures clearly demonstrate that infants respond differentially to their mother's normal voice, the differences in responding do not necessarily indicate a preference for her voice; that is a differential sensitivity to a stimulus need not indicate a preference for that stimulus. Clinical observations, for example, Andre-Thomas (1966) and Hammond (1970), have suggested that newborn infants will preferentially orient to mother's voice. However, not until a more recent study by DeCasper and Fifer (1980) was there any direct experimental evidence that neonates prefer their mothers' voices.

### A.   Temporal Discrimination Procedure

In this procedure, 48–72-hr-old infants were observed for 5-min baseline periods in which sucks on a nonnutritive nipple were recorded, and the median time between sucking bursts was determined. A burst was defined by a series of sucks separated by less than 2 s. For one half of the infants, interburst intervals (IBIs) less than the baseline median were followed by a recorded presentation of their mother's voice reading a children's story. The voices, presented over stereo headphones, came on with the first suck of each burst and remained on until the burst ended. IBIs greater than the baseline median resulted in presentation of the recording of the previous subject's mother. Thus, each burst of sucking produced one voice or the other. The contingency was reversed for the remaining half of the infants, that is, IBIs greater than baseline produced mother's voice. Eight of nine infants showing a preference preferred their mother's voice; they produced their mother's voice more often and for a longer total period of time. Four of the infants who demonstrated this preference subsequently encountered a reversal of the initial contingencies. All four newborns reversed their earlier pattern of sucking and thus again heard more of their own mother's voice (Fig. 1).

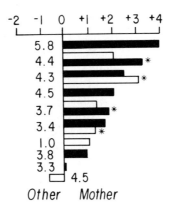

**Fig. 1.** Signed difference scores between the baseline median IBIs and the IBI during the final third of the session for each subject. Differences for the four reversal sessions are also presented (*). Positive values indicate a preference for the maternal voice, and negative values indicate a preference for the nonmaternal voice. Filled bars indicate that the mother's voice followed IBIs of less than the baseline median. Open bars indicate that her voice followed intervals greater than the median. Median IBIs of the 5-min baseline (in seconds) are shown for each subject.

B.   Signal Discrimination Procedure

Fifer (1981) replicated and further investigated the neonate's preference for the maternal voice. A new procedure was designed to enhance the measure of preferential responding in order to detect possible individual or group differences and to allow observation of infants as young as 1 day old. DeCasper and Fifer (1980) differentially reinforced interburst intervals. A preference was shown by an increased frequency of intervals that produced the mother's voice. Between-group comparisons were of limited value because of what may have been an inherent difference in the ability to learn the "greater than" versus the "less than" contingency. In addition, pilot studies using the IBI contingency indicated that the 1 day old infants were less likely to complete a no-stimulation baseline period and to sustain a full 18-min session. The need to maintain longer periods of quiet alert states in the younger infants, to minimize constraints on acquisition of a contingency based on burst duration, and to facilitate between group comparisons led to the development of a new procedure.

A discrimination procedure was developed in which the presence or absence of a tone signaled the availability of the different voices, but voices remained on for the duration of the sucking burst. Because interburst intervals are nondifferentially reinforced, the duration of each burst (the amount of time each voice is maintained) serves as an additional independent measure of responsiveness. This is also a clear departure from many auditory discrimination procedures in which a decrease in sucking, that is, habituation, is the required response. Thus, in this paradigm the likelihood of responding in the presence of each signal operationally defines one measure of preference, and the duration of sucking bursts in the presence of each voice serves as another.

Eight bottle-fed and eight breast-fed full-term female neonates served as subjects. In this study, only female infants were chosen because males were unavailable for at least 12 hours following circumcisions, and the scheduling of these operations was unpredictable. In order to maximize the probability of obtaining an alert healthy newborn, all infants had Apgar scores of at least 8 and weighed between 6 and 8.5 lb. The infants were in one of two age ranges at the time of testing, 24–48 hr or 72–96 hr. Informed consent was obtained from each mother, and she was encouraged to observe the experimental session. Following acquisition of informed consent, the mother's voice was recorded while reading a children's story. The tape was edited to omit extraneous sound and pauses longer than 1.5 s and repeatedly rerecorded on one track of a stereo tape to provide 25 min of uninterrupted prose. The recording of the mother's voice from the preceding session was placed on the other track of this tape.

Sessions began $2\frac{1}{2}$ hr after either the 6 a.m., 10 a.m., or 2 p.m. feedings in order to maximize the probability of obtaining alert infants. Newborns were moved to an adjoining nursery in their own cribs and coaxed to a state of quiet alertness (Wolff, 1966). The earphones were placed securely over both ears, and a nonnutritive nipple was placed in the infant's mouth. Any infant who could not be brought to this quiet, alert, eyes-open state was returned to the nursery and was brought back after the next feeding if time permitted. While one researcher monitored the recording equipment, the other, blind to the experimental condition, monitored the baby and held the nipple in place. The infant was allowed 2 min to adjust to the situation before presentation of the auditory stimuli. If the infant failed to reliably emit measurable sucks (approximately 20 mmHg), she was returned to the nursery.

Each experimental condition began with a 4-s presentation of a 400-Hz tone followed by a 4-s period of silence or no tone. The tone/no-tone alternation continued until a sucking burst was initiated. Depending upon which stimulus was present when the burst began, that burst produced either the mother's voice or the voice of the previous subject's mother for as long as the burst continued. A burst was defined as a series of individual sucks separated from one another by less than 2 s. The termination of each burst was followed by the tone/no-tone sequence, and each stimulus had a .50 probability of beginning the sequence.

Sessions were terminated the second time that a 1 min period of either nonresponding or crying occurred. Each session lasted at least 12 min, but not more than 20 min, and contained at least 100 presentations of tone or no-tone. Therefore, a *data baby* was one who met the selection criteria; was in an alert state at the beginning of the session; emitted measurable sucks during the adjustment period; and completed at least 12, and no more than 20 min of testing with the voices.

Both breast- and bottle-fed infants were observed in this study. The nursing infants averaged six breast feedings per day, the bottle-fed infants averaged four feedings per day with their mother. One half of each group was between 24 and 48 hr old, and the other half was between 72 and 96 hr old. For half of the infants in each group, the maternal voice was presented when a sucking burst began during the presentation of the 400-Hz tone and the voice continued for the duration of the burst. Sucks initiated during the periods of no tone resulted in the presentation of the other woman's voice. For the other half of the infants, sucking during the no-tone period produced their mother's voice and sucking while the tone was on produced the other voice.

The infants sucked significantly longer (using repeated measures analysis of variance) to presentations of the maternal voice during the final third of the session ($p < .01$) and sucked significantly more to the signal for the mother's voice ($p < .05$). There were no significant differences during the final third as a function of age or type of feeding. Analyses of individual subject data showed that during the final third of the session, 13 of 16 infants responded more often during the signal associated with their mother's voice ($p < .011$ by the binomial test). During the same period, 15 of 16 infants showed longer burst durations during presentation of mother's voice ($p < .001$). These data indicate that newborn infants as young as 1 day old can demonstrate a preference for mother's voice. They learned to respond more often to the signal associated with her voice, and further, they produced the maternal voice for longer durations. Although there was an absence of an effect of both age and feeding experience, this experiment was not designed to address the question of whether postnatal experience can influence this preference. The data, however, do indicate that a newborn with minimal postnatal experience with voices will show a preference for the maternal voice. The results are also consistent with the hypothesis that prenatal experience may play a major role in the development of this preference. Additionally, successful discrimination learning under these contingencies indicated the presence of a mechanism available during the perinatal period for acquiring associations between environmental events and further suggested that newborns are even more competent learners than is usually believed.

## C.  Syllable Discrimination Procedure

These results were replicated and extended in the first in a series of studies aimed at investigating the ability of 1- and 2-day-old infants to discriminate speech sounds at the level of the syllable (Fifer & Moon, 1986; Moon, Bever, & Fifer, 1986). The study to be reported here was also designed to facilitate individual and between-group comparisons by standardizing session length and other criteria and to explore the use of "stranger" female voices as reinforcers to decrease enormous costs of time required to prepare, record, and edit individual maternal voices.

Each infant was randomly assigned to one of these experimental conditions: mother/quiet, mother/other, and other/quiet. All were from normal vaginal deliveries with Apgar scores of 8–10 and had no pre- or perinatal medical complications. There were five female and five male babies per group. Ages ranged from 33 to 64 hr old, with a mean of 51 hr.

The infants again wore calibrated headphones and listened to recorded presentations of either their own mother's voice, another mother's voice, or periods of slience, depending upon condition. These speech sounds were presented contingent upon sucking pressure on a nonnutritive nipple. The sounds were of two types: voices—tape recordings of mothers in conversations or no-voices (periods of silence)—and signals—a computer-edited male voice repeating the syllable /pat/ or /pst/. Those in the mother/quiet group heard a recording of their own mother's voice or silence; the other/quiet group heard the previous infant's mother or silence; the mother/other group were presented with their own mother or the previous mother's voice. The speech sounds were contingent upon sucking in the following way: In the absence of a sucking burst, strings of syllables (the signals) were presented such that 4 s of one syllable alternated with 4 s of the other syllable. If the infant initiated a sucking burst, the syllables ceased and either a voice or silence was presented for as long as the sucking burst continued. For example, in the mother/other condition, if /pat/ was the signal for mother, and the infant sucked during the /pat/ string, the syllables ceased and the baby then heard mother's voice for as long as he or she continued to suck. The signal for the other voice would be /pst/, and if the baby sucked during that syllable string, the other voice would be presented for the duration of the sucking burst. At the end of a burst, the syllable strings resumed alternation. In the mother/quiet and other/quiet conditions, one syllable signaled a voice and the other signaled quiet. For five infants in each group, /pst/ signaled a voice and /pat/ signaled the alternative, whereas for the other five infants, the signal/voice pairing was reversed. The experimental sessions were 18 min long.

Infants sucked significantly more often to the signal for mother over quiet, for other female over quiet, and for mother over other female. In addition, infants in all three groups learned by the final third of the session to obtain presentations of the preferred voice for significantly longer periods of time (Fig. 2). These results demonstrate the infant's capacity to maintain an alert state for at least 18 min, to learn a differential response to two syllables shortly after birth, and to demonstrate preferences for auditory stimuli, particularly the maternal voice.

## V. Conclusion

Several researchers have suggested that such sensory competencies and stimulus preferences may play a major role in activating and reinforcing early mother–infant interactions (Ainsworth, 1979; Brazelton, Koslowski, & Main, 1974; Cairns, 1979; DeChateau, 1977; Fifer, 1981; Hofer, 1981). Though there is a gap in our understanding of the sequence of the attachment process from the infant's perspective, appreciation of a more active role for the infant has emerged from recent explorations into newborn abilities. Specifically, research on the sensory and perceptual capacities of the neonate indicates they are able to differentially respond to, interact with, and actively seek contact with a wide range of maternal stimuli.

Early discrimination of and attachment to significant others could be served if the infant was maximally and differentially sensitive to different types of maternal stimulation. Recent research findings suggest newborns are indeed sensitive to proximal cues, that is, odor, touch, nearby visual stimulation. However, since later indexes of attachment primarily consist of the infant's responses to maternal presence or absence in the auditory or visual field, a differential sensitivity in the newborn to more distal cues may more directly subserve the initial phases of the attachment process. Specifically, early discrimination and preference for mother's voice might serve to facilitate the development of the reciprocal interactions essential in the earliest stages of the attachment process.

One of a multitude of directions that continued research into these capacities can take is an exploration of prenatal influences. In fact, Spence and DeCasper (1982), Panneton (1985), and Satt (1985) have recently reported some data indicating a postnatal preference following a specific prenatal auditory experience. Another potentially fruitful direction for investigation could focus on subsequent shifts in voice preferences throughout early infancy and might shed light on the processes underlying the development of attachment, learning, and sensory integra-

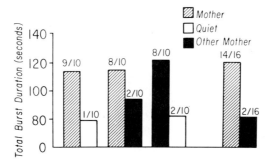

**Fig. 2.** Average total burst durations during the final third of each session for four different groups of infants in four separate experimental conditions. The number of individual infants with longer durations to the indicated sound, over the total number of subjects in that condition, is presented above each bar. The three pairs of bars on the right represent groups in the syllable discrimination procedure; mother versus quiet, mother versus other mother, and other mother versus quiet. The left pair of bars represents the results from the tone/no-tone signal discrimination procedure for mother versus other mother.

tion. For example, responsiveness to the maternal voice may change in form and intensity as maternal visual stimuli become more salient, as the constellation of other voices expands, and as the character and content of the maternal speech ("motherese") evolves. Investigation of a population of infants whose intrauterine as well as postnatal experience is markedly different, the preterm infant, could aid in our understanding of the development, limits, and adaptive value of responsiveness to voices.

We have chosen to focus our efforts on more fully characterizing the dimensions of early newborn responsiveness to voices and to develop procedures which allow us to ask more difficult questions and get stronger results. We believe this approach offers some promise for further studies of infant perceptual, learning, and memory capacities and will provide data which may guide the development of more sensitive and reliable tools for assessing individual differences during the newborn period.

### Acknowledgments

I would like to acknowledge the major contribution made by Christine Moon to much of the work reported in this chapter. I am also very grateful to Anthony DeCasper and Robin Panneton for their collaboration in the earlier studies at the University of North Carolina at Greensboro. I would like to thank Lisa Monti and Reisa Sperling for their aid in collecting the data and preparing the manuscript, and the nursery staff at both North Central Bronx Hospital and Columbia Presbyterian Medical Center for their help and cooperation. Preparation of this manuscript and much of the research was supported by the Research Foundation for Mental Hygiene, the New York State Psychiatric Institute, and a grant from the National Institute of Child Health and Human Development (HD20102).

# References

Ainsworth, M. D. S. (1979). Attachment as related to mother–infant interaction. In J. S. Rosenblatt, R. A. Hinde, C. G. Beer, & M. C. Busnel (Eds.), *Advances in the study of behavior* (Vol. 9, pp. 2–52). New York: Academic Press.

Andre-Thomas, A. S. (1966). *Locomotion from prenatal to postnatal life.* London: Spastic Society, Heinemann.

Armitage, S. E., Baldwin, B. A., & Vince, M. A. (1980). Fetal response to extrauterine sounds in sleep. *Science, 208,* 1173–1174.

Aslin, R. N., Pisoni, D. B., & Jusczyk, P. W. (1983). Auditory development and speech perception in infancy. In P. Mussen (Ed.), *Carmichael's manual of child psychology* (4th ed.): *Vol. 2. Infancy and the biology of development,* M. M. Haith & J. J. Campos (Eds.) (pp. 573–687), New York: Wiley.

Bartoshuk, A. K. (1962). Response decrement with repeated elicitation of human neonatal cardiac acceleration to sound. *Journal of Comparative and Physiological Psychology, 55,* 9–13.

Bench, J. (1973). Fetal audiometry in relation to the developing fetal nervous system. In W. Taylor (Ed.), *Disorders of auditory function* (pp. 115–119). New York: Academic Press.

Bernard, J., & Sontag, L. W. (1947). Fetal reactivity to tonal stimulation: A preliminary report. *Journal of Genetic Psychology, 70,* 205–210.

Bertoncini, J., & Mehler, J. (1981). Syllables as units in infant speech perception. *Infant Behavior and Development, 4,* 247–260.

Birnholz, J. C., & Benaceraff, B. B. (1983). The development of fetal hearing. *Science, 222,* 516–518.

Birns, B., Blank, M., & Bridger, W. H. (1966). The effectiveness of various soothing techniques on human neonates. *Psychosomatic Medicine, 28,* 316–322.

Brazelton, T. B., Koslowski, B., & Main, M. (1974). The origins of reciprocity in mother–infant interaction. In M. Lewis & L. A. Rosenbloom (Eds.), *The effect of the infant on its caregiver.* (pp. 49–76) New York: Wiley.

Butterfield, E. C., & Siperstein, G. N. (1972). Influence of contingent auditory stimulation upon non-nutritional suckle. In J. Bosma (Ed.), *Oral sensation and perception: The mouth of the infant.* (pp. 313–334) Springfield, IL: Thomas.

Cairns, R. B. (1979). *Social development: The origins and plasticity of interchanges.* San Francisco: W. H. Freeman.

DeCasper, A. J., & Fifer, W. P. (1980). Of human bonding: Newborns prefer their mothers' voices. *Science, 208,* 1174–1176.

DeChateau, P. (1977). The importance of the neonatal period for the development of synchronization in the mother–infant dyad. *Birth and the Family Journal, 10,* 41–51.

Eimas, P. D. (1975). Speech perception in infancy. In L. B. Cohen & P. Salapatek (Eds.), *Infant perception: From sensation to cognition.* (pp. 193–231) New York: Academic Press.

Eisenberg, R. B. (1976). *Auditory competence in early life: The roots of communicative behavior.* Baltimore: University Park Press.

Fifer, W. P. (1981). *Attachment in the neonate: The ontogeny of maternal voice preference.* Unpublished doctoral dissertation, University of North Carolina at Greensboro.

Fifer, W. P., & Moon, C. (1986). *Newborn discrimination learning: The value of voices.* Manuscript submitted for publication.

Forbes, H. S., & Forbes, H. B. (1927). Fetal sense reaction: hearing. *Journal of Comparative Physiological Psychology, 7,* 353–355.

Gelman, S. R., Wood, S., Spellacy, W. N., & Abrams, R. M. (1982). Fetal movements in response to sound stimulation. *American Journal of Obstetrics and Gynecology, 143,* 484–485.

Gottlieb, G. (1985). On discovering significant acoustic dimensions of auditory stimulation for infants. In G. Gottlieb & N. A. Krasnegor (Eds.), *Measurement of audition and vision in the first year of postnatal life: A methodological overview.* (pp. 3–29) Norwood, NJ: Ablex.

Gregg, C. L., Haffner, M. E., & Korner, A. F. (1976). The relative efficacy of vestibular-proprioceptive stimulation and the upright position in enhancing visual pursuit in neonates. *Child Development, 47,* 309–311.

Hammond, J. (1970). Mother's voice. *Developmental Medicine and Child Neurology, 12,* 3–5.

Henschall, W. R. (1972). Intrauterine sound levels. *Journal of Obstetrics and Gynecology, 112,* 577–579.

Hofer, M. A. (1981). *The roots of human behavior: An introduction to the psychobiology of human development.* San Francisco: W. H. Freeman.

Hutt, S. J. & Hutt, C. (1970). *Direct observation and measurement of behavior.* Springfield, IL: Thomas.

Hutt, S. J., Hutt, C., Lenard, J. G., Bernuth, H., & Muntjewerff, W. J. (1968). Auditory responsivity in the human neonate. *Nature, 218,* 888–890.

Jensen, O. H. (1984). Fetal heart rate response to controlled sound stimuli during the third trimester of normal pregnancy. *Acta Obstetricia Gynecologica Scandinavica, 63,* 193–197.

Johansson, B., Wedenberg, E., & Westin, B. (1964). Measurement of tone response by the human foetus. *Acta Oto-laryngologica, 57,* 188–192.

Leader, L. R., Baile, P., Martin, B., & Vermuelen, E. (1982). The assessment and significance of habituation to a repeated stimulus by the human fetus. *Early Human Development, 7,* 211–219.

Lecanuet, J. P., Granier-Deferre, C., Busnel, M. C. (1985). *L'audition prenatale.* Manuscript submitted for publication.

Lecanuet, J. P., Granier-Deferre C., Cohen, H., Busnel, M. C., & Sureau, C. (May 1984). *Fetal alertness and reactivity to sound stimulation.* Paper presented at the International Conference on Infant Studies, New York.

Leventhal, A. S., & Lipsitt, L. P. (1964). Adaptation, pitch, discrimination and sound localization in the neonate. *Child Development, 35,* 759–767.

Mehler, J., Bertoncini, J., Bauriere, M., & Jassik-Gershenfeld, D. (1978). Infant recognition of mother's voice. *Perception, 7,* 491–497.

Mendelson, M., & Haith, M. (1967). *The relation between audition and vision in the human newborn.* (Monograph No. 41). Society for Child Development.

Mills, M., & Meluish, E. (1979). Recognition of mother's voice in early infancy. *Nature, 252,* 123–124.

Moon, C. (1985). *Phonological universals and syllable discrimination in one- to three day-old infants.* Unpublished doctoral dissertation, Columbia University.

Moon, C., Bever, T., & Fifer, W. (1986). *Syllable discrimination by newborn infants.* Manuscript submitted for publication.

Morse, A. R. (1972). The discrimination of speech and non-speech stimuli in early infancy. *Journal of Experimental Child Psychology, 14,* 477–492.

Muir, D., & Clifton, K. C. (1985). Infant's orientation to the location of sound sources. In G. Gottlieb & N. A. Krasnegor (Eds.), *Measurement of audition and vision in the first year of postnatal life: A methodological approach* (pp. 171–194). Norwood, NJ: Ablex.

Murooka, H., Koie, I., & Suda, D. (1976). Analyse des sons intrauterines et de leurs effets tranquillisants sur le nouvea-né. *Journal de Gynecologie Obstetrique et Biologie de la Reproduction, 5*, 367–376.

Panneton, R. P. (1985). *Prenatal experience with melodies: Effect on postnatal auditory preference in human newborns*. Unpublished doctoral dissertation, University of North Carolina at Greensboro.

Peiper, A. (1925) Sinnesempfindungen des Kindes vor seiner Geburt. *Msr. Kinderheik, 29*, 236.

Pujol, R., & Hilding, D. (1973). Anatomy and physiology of the onset of auditory function. *Acta Oto-laryngologica, 76*, 1–10.

Querleu, D., Renard, X., & Crepin, G. (1981). Perception auditive et réactivite foetale aux stimulations sonores. *Journal de Gynecologie Obstetrique et Biologie de la Reproduction, 13*, 125–134.

Rubel, E. W. (1985). Auditory system development. In G. Gottlieb & N. A. Krasnegor (Eds.), *Measurement of audition and vision in the first year of postnatal life: A methodological approach* (pp. 53–90). Norwood, NJ: Ablex.

Satt, B. J. (1985). *An investigation into the acoustical induction of intra-uterine learning*. Unpublished doctoral dissertation, California School of Professional Psychology.

Siperstein, G. N., & Butterfield, E. C. (1973). *Neonates prefer vocal-instrumental music to noise and vocal music to instrumental music*. Unpublished manuscript. University of Kansas Medical Center.

Sontag, L. W., & Wallace, R. F. (1936). Changes in the rate of fetal heart in response to vibratory stimuli. *American Journal of Disabled Children, 51*, 583–589.

Spence, M. J., & DeCasper, A. J. (April 1982). *Human fetuses perceive maternal speech*. Paper presented at the International Conference on Infant Studies, Austin, Tx.

Suzuki, T., Kamijo, J., & Kiuchi S. (1964). Auditory test of newborn infants. *Annals of Otolaryngology, 73*, 914–923.

Turkewitz, G. (in press). A prenatal source for the development of hemispheric specialization. In S. Segalowitz & D. Molfese (Eds.) *Developmental implication of brain lateralization*.

Turkewitz, G., Birch, H. G., & Cooper, K. K. (1972). Responsiveness to simple and complex auditory stimuli in the human newborn. *Developmental Psychobiology, 5*, 7–19.

Versyp, F. (1985). *Transmission intra-amniotique des sons et des voix humanines*. Unpublished doctoral dissertation, University at Lille, Lille.

Walker, D., Grimwade, J., & Wood, C. (1971). Intrauterine noise: A component of the fetal environment. *American Journal of Obstetrics and Gynecology, 109*, 91–95.

Wertheimer, M. (1961). Psychomotor coordination of auditory-visual space at birth. *Science, 134*, 1962.

Wolff, P. H. (1966). The classification of states. *Psychological Issues, 5*, 23–31.

# III

## NEURAL SUBSTRATES OF BEHAVIORAL PLASTICITY

# 6

# Development of Olfactory Specificity in the Albino Rat: A Model System

GORDON M. SHEPHERD, PATRICIA E. PEDERSEN,
and CHARLES A. GREER
*Sections of Neuroanatomy and Neurosurgery*
*Yale University School of Medicine*
*New Haven, Connecticut 06510-8001*

Advances in cell biology and, more recently, molecular biology have provided common tools and a common language which have begun to bring together different disciplines concerned with the relation between the nervous system and mammalian behavior. This is especially true of the psychobiology of early mammalian development. On the one hand, behavioral studies are increasingly utilizing new tools to obtain results which not only illuminate mechanisms of early behavior but also contribute to our basic knowledge of the neural structures and physiological properties underlying those behaviors. Neuroanatomists and neurophysiologists, for their part, are increasingly searching for the behavioral correlates of their analysis of structure and function.

In analyzing the ontogeny of mammalian behavior, it is important to employ model systems wherein the properties of a part of the nervous system and their relation to specific behaviors can be elucidated. The olfactory system is particularly attractive for this purpose because it is precociously present during this period. Obviously it is an advantage in analyzing the neural mechanisms underlying the ontogeny of behavior if the system under study plays some important role in the life of the developing animal. As is well known, the sense of smell is important for most newborn mammals (Alberts, 1976, 1981; Cheal, 1975; Pedersen & Blass, 1981; Rosenblatt, 1983) and for mother–infant relationships (Leon, 1983). Recent behavioral studies are documenting the extraordinary variety of

**127**

these early functions mediated by the olfactory system, not only in most mammalian species, but also in primates and humans (Kaplan, Cubicciotti, & Redican, 1977; Macfarlane, 1975; Porter, Cernoch, & Balogh, 1985; Porter, Cernoch, & McLaughlin, 1983).

From these studies it appears that, among sensory systems, the olfactory is one of the first to differentiate and become functional in the developing mammal. It is therefore a reasonable premise that knowledge of how neural mechanisms develop in this system is important both for understanding the ontogeny of sensory function in the mammal and for understanding how this controls the emergence of behavior. This premise appears to be gaining increasing acceptance, as attested by the growing literature on experimental studies and the importance recognized by several contributors to this symposium.

Our own studies of the olfactory system have arisen from an interest in using it as a model for analyzing synaptic organization. From work in many laboratories and many different parts of the nervous system, it is becoming possible to characterize synaptic organization according to some general principles. These include recognition of several levels of organization, beginning with the single synapse, and building up through microcircuits, local circuits involving connections within a region, to pathways and systems involving several regions (see Shepherd, 1979). Parts of the olfactory system, such as the olfactory bulb, have been useful for identifying and characterizing these different levels of organization.

In pursuing these studies, we have been led earlier and earlier in ontogeny, into the neonatal and, most recently, the prenatal period. We have carried out these studies in the rat. The results thus have contributed to the growing literature establishing the albino rat as one of the most extensive models presently available for understanding the ontogeny of mammalian behavior.

In this review we will give an overview of the organization of the olfactory system in the developing mammal. We will emphasize the emerging view of the multiple subsystems into which the peripheral olfactory pathway is divided. We will summarize recent studies aimed at identifying and characterizing both cellular and functional organization of the different subsystems during early development and also the sequence in which different subsystems are expressed in order to process odor stimuli crucial for different stages of development. We will mention certain aspects of cellular organization relevant to each subsystem. These include the development and distribution of olfactory receptor neurons within the nasal cavity, the development of the olfactory glomerulus as a functional module for the processing of receptor neuron input, and the development of the dendritic microcircuits responsible for the most powerful inhibitory microcircuits within the olfactory bulb. We will show how these properties of the olfactory system reflect a general principle of multiple sequential adaptive systems which appears to characterize the early development of the mammalian nervous system.

## I. Overview of Olfactory Organization

The main elements of the developing mammalian olfactory system in the rat are shown in Fig. 1. The first level in the olfactory pathway is the receptor neurons, which are located in three main regions. The largest structure is the olfactory epithelium, which covers the medial wall of the nasal system and the convexities of the nasal turbinates. Olfactory receptor neurons are also found in a small region along the septal wall known as the septal organ, or organ of Masera. A third region is the vomeronasal organ (VNO), a separate structure ventral to the nasal cavity; this contains modified receptor neurons believed to be sensitive to volatile compounds in the liquid phase.

The second level in the olfactory pathway is the olfactory bulb. Here the receptor axons terminate in rounded regions of neuropil called glomeruli, where they make synaptic connections onto the dendrites of two types of relay neurons. The largest are the mitral cells, which convey the output of the olfactory bulb through their axons to the olfactory cortex. A smaller type of relay neuron is the tufted cell.

There are two types of interneuron. The periglomerular (pg) short-axon cell receives synaptic inputs within the glomeruli and has intrinsic connections to neighboring glomeruli. The granule cell is situated more deeply; its dendrites are studded with spines, which form a richly interconnected network of synaptic connections with secondary dendrites of mitral and tufted cells. Periglomerular cells may provide for inhibitory (Getchell & Shepherd, 1975; Shepherd, 1971) or excitatory processing of mitral or tufted cell responses to sensory input; granule cells provide for powerful inhibitory control of mitral or tufted cell output to the olfactory cortex (Rall, Shepherd, Reese, & Brightman, 1966).

In addition to these synaptic connections, olfactory bulb neurons are heavily modulated by a variety of neuropeptides and central systems (for review, see Halasz & Shepherd, 1983; Macrides & Davis, 1983). The brainstem norepinephrine and serotonin centers send a rich innervation. There is an acetylcholine (ACh) innervation by centrifugal fibers from the nucleus of the horizontal limb of the diagonal band, one of the basal

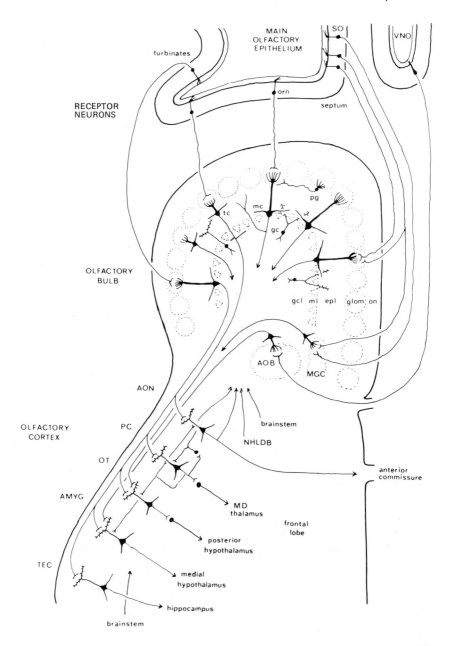

forebrain ACh regions. Other centrifugal fibers arise from olfactory cortical regions and from the median forebrain bundle. The olfactory bulb is
also rich in thyrotropin-releasing hormone. Presumably these neuroactive
substances and centrifugal pathways provide the means by which processing of olfactory information is regulated according to the developmental stage and behavioral state of the organism.

The description thus far has applied to the main olfactory bulb (MOB).
In addition, there is at least one set of modified glomeruli set apart from
the main sheet of glomeruli; this has been termed the *modified glomerular
complex* (MGC). Finally, the accessory olfactory bulb (AOB) is a distinct
structure with a cellular organization similar to that of the MOB but less
sharply differentiated into distinct cell types; it receives the terminals of
axons from receptor neurons in the VNO.

The third level of the olfactory pathway is the olfactory cortex, which is
divided into several subregions, as indicated in Fig. 1. Here the axons of
mitral and tufted cells, after coursing through the lateral olfactory tract on
the surface of the brain, terminate on the distal dendritic spines of pyramidal neurons. The pyriform cortex is usually regarded as the main olfactory
cortex; here the intrinsic organization includes local circuits for inhibition
and reexcitation (Haberly, 1985). These are analogous to corresponding
circuits in other cortical regions, such as the hippocampus. Each cortical subregion sends its output to a different target; these are indicated
in Fig. 1.

The AOB sends its output axons specifically to the corticomedial group
of the amygdaloid complex (Kevetter & Winans, 1981; Scalia & Winans,
1975) at the olfactory cortical level. This pathway is distinct from the
projection of the MOB. The projection of the MGC has not yet been
determined; preliminary data suggest that projection overlaps with that of
the MOB (Pedersen, Jastreboff, Stewart, & Shepherd, 1986).

---

**Fig. 1.**   Schematic diagram of the mammalian olfactory system. This view shows the three
levels of the system, proceeding from the receptor neurons at the top, through the olfactory
bulb, to the olfactory cortex (bottom). There is an attempt to emphasize the different
subsystems as they are seen at each level. The text discusses the emergence of the subsystems at different times during development. Abbreviations: Receptors—orn, olfactory receptor; SO, septal organ; VNO, vomeronasal organ. Bulb—tc, tufted cell; mc, mitral cell;
gc, granule cell; pg, periglomerular cell; gcl, granule cell layer; ml, mitral layer; epl, external
plexiform layer; glom, glomerular layer; on, olfactory nerve layer; AOB, accessory olfactory bulb; MGC, modified gomerular complex. Cortex—AON, anterior olfactory nucleus;
PC, piriform cortex; OT, olfactory tubercule; AMYG, amygdala; TEC, transitional entorhinal cortex; NHLDB, nucleus of the horizontal limb of the diagonal band; MD thalamus,
medial dorsal nucleus of the thalamus.

## II. Olfactory Subsystems

With this introduction to the overall organization, we will next consider each of the subsystems of the olfactory pathway. Traditionally, such an account would begin with the main olfactory pathway. However, here we will consider them in their ontogenetic sequence. Drawing on recent studies of early development, we will briefly summarize the subsystems in the order in which they appear to become functional in the developing animal.

### A. Vomeronasal Subsystem

The VNO becomes anatomically distinct at an early age, embryonic Day 11 (E11) in the fetal rat (Cuschieri & Bannister, 1975a, 1975b). It is not yet known when the receptor neurons begin to differentiate, send their axons to the AOB, and establish synaptic contacts with dendrites within the AOB glomeruli. It is generally considered that the VNO reaches its mature form by birth or soon after (Kratzing, 1976). Olfactory marker protein, the polypeptide unique to olfactory receptor neurons, cannot be demonstrated in VNO receptor neurons by immunocytochemical methods until postnatal Day 4 (P4) (Farbman & Margolis, 1980) and requires antisera at $\times$ 20 concentrations compared with olfactory receptor neurons to be visualized.

The VNO projects to the AOB; the possibility of some fibers reaching glomeruli in the MOB has begun to be tested (see below), but so far none have been found. The AOB develops early; mitral cells begin to differentiate at E13, a day or two earlier than mitral cells in the MOB (Bayer, 1983). The interneurons (pg and granule cells) have their peak generation times between E17 and E19, with granule cell generation continuing well into the first postnatal weeks (a characteristic shared with intrinsic neurons in other brain regions). The specific projections of AOB mitral cells to the medial and cortical amygdaloid nuclei begin to be laid down by E18–E19, 2–3 days before birth (Schwob & Price, 1978, 1984a, 1984b); by P3 these central connections appear mature. Together these anatomic studies indicate that each of the components of the vomeronasal–accessory bulb–corticomedial amygdala system arises early in development, and the whole system appears to have its basic relay connections in place before birth.

In view of the early anatomic maturation of the VNO system, one might suppose that this would be a prime candidate for early onset of function, but thus far there are very few data. A direct assessment of this question was undertaken by making 2-deoxyglucose (2-DG) injections into a pregnant dam 2 days before term and looking for activity patterns in the fetal olfactory bulb. These studies showed the most prominent focuses of activity over the AOB (Pedersen, Stewart, Greer, & Shepherd, 1983). This result was surprising, for several reasons: (a) It was the first suggestion of functioning of the AOB in utero; (b) it contrasted with the relative lack of 2-DG uptake in the AOB postnatally; and (c) it implied that this same region had different functions in the fetal period and in adult life, when it is known to mediate odor stimuli involved in mating (Powers & Winans, 1975; Scalia & Winans, 1975). Further studies, with the 2DG method and with other techniques, are needed to characterize the physiological properties of the neural elements in the VNO system and assess their functional roles during the fetal period.

B.  Modified Glomerular Complex Subsystem

The receptor neurons that project to the MGC have been assessed recently by making horseradish peroxidase (HRP) injections into this region in 12-day-old rats and tracing the retrograde HRP transport into the nose (Jastreboff, Pedersen, Greer, Stewart, Kauer, Benson, & Shepherd, 1984). The labeled receptor neurons are found in the main olfactory epithelium, within a circumscribed area on the septal wall, and on the convexities of several of the turbinates (Pedersen, Jastreboff et al., 1986). The receptor neurons projecting to the MGC may be presumed to be within this population. They have the morphological features commonly associated with receptor neurons in the main olfactory epithelium; thus far they have no other distinguishing features. Some labeled neurons were also found in the septal organ (Pedersen & Benson, 1986). No labeled neurons were found in the VNO. Thus far there is no specific information on the anatomic or physiological development of these receptor neurons; the closest data pertain to other receptor neurons within the main olfactory epithelium (see below).

At the olfactory bulb level, the MGC appears to differentiate early. Using the Timm stain for heavy metals, Friedman and Price (1984) showed that the MGC is prominent as early as E19, the earliest day they examined the bulb with this stain. It is clearly visualized in sections of the E21 fetus (Pedersen et al., 1983), where it is a well-defined group of glomeruli that contrasts with the less clear outlines of most of the glomeruli in the MOB.

Information about the functional properties of the MGC has come from 2-DG studies. In suckling rat pups, the MGC shows a dense focus over one or more of its constituent glomeruli (Greer, Stewart, Teicher, & Shepherd, 1982; Teicher, Stewart, Kauer, & Shepherd, 1980). Neighboring regions of the MOB also show raised activity, but not focal in nature. It has been suggested by these studies that the MGC and these neighboring glomeruli are involved in processing information about the specific odor cue that mediates suckling by the rat pup.

Studies of the projection from the MGC to olfactory cortical areas have been initiated, tracing anterograde transport of HRP from the injected MGC. In the 12-day-old, preliminary results suggest that the projection overlaps with that of the MOB. Further studies are required to determine the exact pattern and characterize its development.

## C.   Main Olfactory (Mitral) Subsystem

Receptor neurons in the main olfactory epithelium begin to differentiate from stem cells and send out axons around E10 in mouse (Cushieri & Bannister, 1975a, 1975b) and, correspondingly, 2–3 days later in rat (Farbman & Margolis, 1980). By about E14 (mouse), the axons reach the olfactory bulb and begin to establish synaptic contacts. Initially, connections are made as deep as the mitral body layer, but by birth the mature pattern of connections confined within the glomeruli has been established (Monti Graziadei, Stanley, & Graziadei, 1980). This may be taken as an example of exuberant branches found in other sensory systems (cf. Lance-Jones & Landmesser, 1980) that are later pruned back. After the axons reach the bulb, the receptor neurons differentiate their dendrites, terminal knobs, and cilia, a process that is largely completed by E17 (mouse). This has been taken to imply that maturation of these neurons is dependent on a retrograde influence from their synaptic targets in the olfactory bulb.

The functional development of receptor neurons has been studied by extracellular records in fetal rats (Gesteland, Yancey, & Farbman, 1982). Unit firing from cells in the olfactory epithelium (presumably receptor neurons) is first recorded on E16. Cells at this stage are broadly responsive to a variety of odor stimuli. Shortly before birth, the units show increased selectivity in their responses, which continues into the postnatal period. This has been interpreted as indicating that there is a progression from a mostly immature population of nonselective cells to mature, selective cells. If this progression depends on the insertion or maturation of receptor molecules in the olfactory knob or cilia, it apparently occurs after the receptor neurons have matured by the anatomic criteria cited previously. Further studies are needed to clarify this relation.

Within the olfactory bulb, embryogenesis proceeds by proliferation and migration of a series of cell types from the germinal ventricular zone. Thymidine-labeling studies have shown that mitral cells—the largest cells—are generated first, the peak occurring in the mouse at E12 (Hinds, 1968a, 1968b), and in rats at E15–E16 (Bayer, 1983). In view of the fact that the mitral cells are generated before the tufted cells, one presumes that they are the first to become functional during development. The last few days and first two postnatal weeks are a time of rapid growth in size of the mitral cells and their dendritic arbors, correlated with the proliferation of interneuronal populations (see above).

There are no reports to date of unit activity of mitral cells during the prenatal period. After birth, spontaneous activity of bulbar units (presumably mostly mitral cells) has been recorded as early as P1 (Math & Davrainville, 1980). Also beginning on P1, presumed mitral cells can be selectively excited by different odorous stimuli (Mair & Gesteland, 1982). The response patterns are simpler than the complex response patterns of the adult. It has been concluded that receptor-to-mitral synapses are functional in the neonate and that the simple response patterns reflect the lack of fully functional interneuronal local synaptic circuits, which may modulate the complex response patterns in the adult.

Among the interneuronal circuits in the bulb, the reciprocal synapses between mitral and granule cells are particularly important. These provide for self- and lateral inhibition of mitral cells and are believed to play a major role in shaping the temporal patterns of mitral cell impulse output. They also are largley responsible for generating the field potentials responsible for electroencephalogram (EEG) wave recordings. In accord with the unit response patterns, the EEG potentials do not become prominent in the developing olfactory bulb until P3–P5 (Iwahara, Oishi, Sano, Yang, & Takahashi, 1973; Salas, Guzman-Flores, & Schapiro, 1969).

These studies indicate that the development of olfactory bulb function is closely dependent on the development of the granule cells and their synaptic microcircuits. As mentioned above, their generation continues at a significant rate through at least the first 3 postnatal weeks. Although these studies have indicated the times of final differentiation of the granule cells, they do not indicate the time course of maturation of the granule cell dendrites and their synaptic circuits.

This question is presently being pursued by Greer (1984). Preliminary studies have clearly supported the presence of subpopulations of granule cells mediating local circuit interactions with mitral and tufted cells. These subpopulations were previously recognized in the adult (Mori, Kishi, & Ojima, 1983; Orona, Scott, & Rainer, 1983). These and previous studies (Brunjes, Schwark, & Greenough, 1982) have further demonstrated that the appearance of spines on dendrites is a relatively late developmental event. In general, the differentiation of spines follows the branching and elongation of parent dendritic processes. Of particular interest is evidence of overproduction of spines around 12 days postnatal. There is a significant increase in the total number of spines per cell and the density of spines per lum of dendrite, followed by a decrease by 21 days postnatal. This phenomenon is consistent with the exuberant production of neuronal elements and processes in other neural systems (see above) and may reflect a transitory developmental state which precedes the stabilization of synaptic appositions mediating the local circuit interactions. To examine this issue further, serial section Golgi electron microscopy (EM) analysis is being used (Greer, 1984). In this procedure the cytoplasmic silver deposits of the Golgi procedure are replaced with gold particles which permit ultrastructural analyses. Consequently, individual neurons may be morphologically characterized as in conventional Golgi analyses and subsequently be serially sectioned for EM assessment. With these procedures it will be possible to document the development of the reciprocal synaptic microcircuits and correlate them with morphological features of development and the developing capacity for interneuronal signal processing during the early postnatal period. This should provide further insights into the time course of sequential adaptive odor processing by parallel circuits within the perinatal olfactory system.

The overall patterns of activity in the main olfactory bulb during the early postnatal period have been analyzed using the 2-DG method. In summary, there are patterns of activity elicited in the MOB by odor stimulation already in P1, but the patterns are diffuse; the only punctate focuses are in the MGC (see above) in the suckling animal. Punctate focuses begin to be seen in the MOB at about P6. By about P15, the pattern of focuses closely resembles that seen in the adult (Greer et al., 1982). Since the 2-DG focuses are localized to the glomerular layer, their development of 2-DG focal patterns appears to reflect increasing differentiation and growth of the individual glomeruli.

Data on the anatomic and functional development of the olfactory cortical regions receiving input from the main olfactory bulb are still limited. As noted above, these connections appear to develop slightly later than those from the AOB. Several types of studies (tritiated amino acid transport, EM, horseradish peroxidase, Timm stain) have indicated that the neuronal elements of the piriform cortex show mature morphological features (Friedman & Price, 1984; Schwob & Price, 1978; Westrum, 1975) and receive synaptic connections (Schwob & Price, 1984a, 1984b) by birth. The posterior part of the olfactory bulb may mature earliest, and the parts of the piriform cortex receiving this input may correspondingly mature earliest. This may be taken as additional evidence for specificity in the developing animal; the MOB mitral subsystem may thus have subregions which mature at different rates. These subregions may well reflect coordinated schedules of gene expression in subsets of receptor neurons, mitral cells, and cortical pyramidal neurons, targeted for specific types of odor molecules at different stages of development. The nature of these subsets, and their relation to adult organization, remain to be elucidated.

## D. Main Olfactory (Tufted) Subsystem

The increasing evidence that tufted cells are distinct from mitral cells leads to the hypothesis that there is a distinct tufted cell subsystem, in addition to a mitral cell subsystem, in the olfactory pathway. The possibility that the receptor neurons projecting to tufted cells are distinct from those to mitral cells is worth considering. Thus far there is no direct evidence for this. However, indirect evidence for specificity of olfactory receptor cell axon synapses may be derived from the work of White (1973). He demonstrated that one of the types of receptor cell axon synapses found in the glomeruli, onto the pg cell dendrite, was absent in BALB/c mice. Although this is inconclusive evidence regarding the issue of subpopulations of receptor neurons projecting to specific neurons in the olfactory bulb, it does raise the issue of heterogeneity among receptor axon synapses, a question which requires much additional work.

Tufted cells are distinct from mitral cells in several properties. Their cell bodies are smaller and more peripherally located; the dendritic arbors are correpondingly smaller. In view of the *size principle*, which has been deduced for motoneurons (Henneman, 1968), it is possible that tufted cells are more excitable than mitral cells and are therefore the first to be activated at low intensities of sensory stimulation.

Tufted cells also appear to have different types of axon collaterals within the olfactory bulb and therefore must form local circuits that differ from those of mitral cells and play different functional roles (Shepherd, 1971). The dendrodendritic reciprocal synapses of tufted cells appeared to be formed with a population of granule cells different from those that interact with mitral cells (Mori *et al.,* 1983). Tufted cells are genetically distinct from mitral cells, as shown by studies of Purkinje cell degeneration–mutant mice in which mitral cells also undergo selective degeneration but tufted cells are spared (Greer & Shepherd, 1982).

Finally, tufted cells differ in their projections to the olfactory cortex. Their axons connect mainly to the olfactory tubercle (Scott, McBride, & Schneider, 1980), in contrast to mitral cells, which connect throughout the piriform cortex. On the basis of these distinct properties, it seems likely that the tufted and mitral cells form parallel subsystems within the MOB. They may be analogous in this respect to the X, Y, and W cell systems in the visual pathway (Stone & Fukuda, 1974). It is tempting to speculate that tufted cells may mediate sensory input that is less concerned with conscious discrimination and more concerned with affect and with triggering limbic system motor ouput. The tufted cell system might be adapted for transmitting pheromonal types of signals, such as the odor cue that activates the motor patterns involved in suckling in the neonatal rat.

## III.  Behavioral Plasticity and Olfactory Learning

One of the remarkable findings in developmental psychobiology during the last decade has been that pups' responsiveness to odors appears to be influenced by learning (for review, see Rosenblatt, 1983). For example, pups suckle for the first time to amniotic fluid that coats the mother's nipples at birth (Teicher & Blass, 1977). However, pups can be induced to suckle an artificial odor cue, citral, provided that they are exposed to citral during the last few days of gestation and the first hour following parturition (Pedersen & Blass, 1982). This experimental finding suggests that amniotic fluid, the normal cue for the first attachment, becomes a potent elicitor of suckling because of its presence prenatally in the amniotic-rich nest.

What are the corresponding neural changes that accompany this behavioral plasticity? Answers to this question will reveal the mechanisms by which odors become encoded to carry biologically significant information. Indeed, the prenatal period must be the starting point of the accompanying neural changes related to odor experiences. Smotherman's (see chap. 2, this volume) remarkable investigations of behavioral responses of fetuses to odors as early as E17 strongly suggest that olfactory neural structures, although few in number at that time, must support odor processing. Moreover, fetuses do not respond in a unitary manner to changes in the amniotic milieu. The characteristics of these behavioral changes, as well as the specific odor conditions under which they are expressed, may reflect the maturity of a particular subsystem and the susceptibility of the system to odor experiences. These behavioral studies must be incorporated into the neural model of how the olfactory system develops to encode odors.

One obvious strategy is to look for changes in the olfactory bulb, especially since it is undergoing dramatic neural development prenatally (for review, see Pedersen, Greer, & Shepherd, 1986) and therefore might be especially vulnerable to changes in the odor milieu. We have examined bulbar 2-DG patterns to citral odor after pups have been exposed to citral either prenatally and postnatally or not at all. Extensive areas of increased 2-DG uptake occurred in the dorsomedial regions of the bulb following exposure to citral, regardless of whether pups had prior exposure to citral (Pedersen, Greer, Stewart, & Shepherd, 1982). The overall distribution of 2-DG focuses appeared similar, but there were differences in the characteristics of the distribution between groups. The pups that received citral exposure prenatally and postnatally exhibited a higher density of 2-DG uptake in the bulbar regions that responded to citral, and their pattern of uptake appeared more localized within glomerular areas. We are currently analyzing this data further, to examine to what extent these differences exist. The differences are of interest in light of Leon's recent findings of alterations in density of 2-DG focuses following pups' experience with peppermint odor (see chap. 7, this volume). Our study supports the idea that changes may occur at the bulbar level that reflect odor experiences of pups. Moreover, Leon's findings have suggested that structural changes in the olfactory bulb accompany altered odor experiences. The elucidation of these findings will no doubt further emphasize the olfactory system as a model system for the study of the ontogeny of learning.

## IV. Conclusion

The material reviewed in this article illustrates how a system expressed early in development permits analysis of how the nervous system is assembled in order to mediate behavior. The first point is that the olfactory system is composed of several anatomic subsystems. This was first established in the adult; the anatomic distinctions between the subsystems have now been traced to the embryonic period. Second, the subsystems do not appear at the same time; there are overlapping sequences of development of the different subsystems. This sequence can be documented in terms of the anatomy, as seen in histology and electron microscopy preparations; the function, as expressed by the 2-DG mapping method; by other physiological measures (such as EEG, single units, etc.); and by behavioral analysis of odor-dependent behaviors.

The key feature of this sequence of development is that the whole system functions at a given stage of development through one or more subsystems that are specifically adapted for the particular environment at that stage. This is particularly apparent in the olfactory system. We have seen that there is a sequence of distinctly different odor milieus, and the olfactory system must be adapted appropriately for each.

The progression of development can be conceived in different ways, as illustrated in Fig. 2. Traditionally, scientists have conceived of a given system as emerging anatomically and functionally toward the adult condition in a gradual, linear fashion, either beginning at birth (A) or from before birth (B). This form of development does not apply to the olfactory

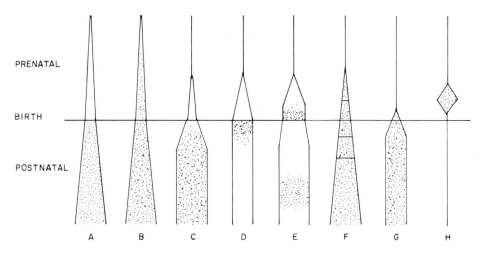

**Fig. 2.** Conceptual schema for representing the emergence of neural systems and subsystems during development. Outlines indicate anatomic growth and differentiation, while stippling indicates expression of function. (A) Gradual development after birth. (B) Gradual development beginning before birth. (C) Example of the development of the main olfactory system. (D) Example of the development of the modified glomerular complex. (E) Example of the development of the accessory olfactory bulb; note first period of function, related to suckling, and second period of function, related to reproductive activities. (F) Sequence of different functions expressed in the same system. (G) Rapid expression of a given system. (H) Transit expression of neural elements (e.g., synapses, neurons) or subsystems.

system. It is better characterized in terms of its subsystems, each of which has its own timetable for development; in the diagram, C, D, and E represent the MOB, MGC, and AOB, respectively. Note that a system, such as the AOB, may be active at two separate periods, with distinctly different functions in two periods. Other systems may express other properties; a single system may have different functions at different stages (F) or appear relatively suddenly at some particular stage (G). Finally, a subsystem or its neural elements may appear and then disappear (H); for example, neuron death or synaptic elimination are well-documented phenomena.

The result of these different timetables is that at any one time in development, one can look across the various subsystems and, as in Fig. 2, see that there is a unique combination at that time period compared with previous or subsequent time points. These observations support the general principle of ontogenetic adaptation. This has been eloquently expressed by Hofer (1981):

> Development is characterized by transformations in which certain functional patterns come into being that are not found in previous or even in subsequent

stages. Functionally as well as structurally, it is not the same creature at two different stages of its own development. The differences between stages of development in a single animal are almost as profound as those between species of vertebrates.

Finally, we add plasticity and learning to this version of development. In the olfactory system, every odor-guided behavior in the rat that has been studied in some detail has been shown to be modifiable by olfactory experience. Furthermore, olfactory learning takes place as early as the fetal period. The way that the entire system develops provides the capacity for each subsystem to be modifiable by odor experience, and for this modification to be coordinated with the subsequent development of that subsystem and the other subsystems, so that behavioral integrity of the mature organism is achieved.

## References

Alberts, J. R. (1976). Olfactory contribution to behavioral development in rodents. In R. L. Doty (Ed.), *Mammalian olfaction, reproductive processes and behavior* (pp. 67–94). New York: Academic Press.

Alberts, J. R. (1981). Ontogeny of olfaction: Reciprocal roles of sensation and behavior in the development of perception. In R. N. Aslin, J. R. Alberts, & M. R. Petersen (Eds.), *Development of perception: Psychobiological perspectives* (Vol. 1, pp. 322–357). New York: Academic Press.

Bayer, S. A. (1983). $^3$H-thymidine-radiographic studies of neurogenesis in the rat olfactory bulb. *Experimental Brain Research, 30,* 329–340.

Brunjes, P. C., Schwark, H. D., & Greenough, W. T. (1982). Olfactory granule cell development in normal and hyperthyroid rats. *Developmental Brain Research, 5,* 149–159.

Cheal, M. L. (1975). Social olfaction: A review of the ontogeny of olfactory influences on vertebrate behavior. *Behavioral Biology, 15,* 1–25.

Cuschieri, A., & Bannister, L. H. (1975a). The development of the olfactory mucosa in the mouse: Light microscopy. *Journal of Anatomy, 119,* 277–286.

Cuschieri, A., & Bannister, L. H. (1975b). The development of the olfactory mucosa in the mouse: Electron microscopy. *Journal of Anatomy, 119,* 471–498.

Farbman, A. I., & Margolis, F. L. (1980). Olfactory marker protein during ontogeny. Immunohistochemical localization. *Developmental Biology, 74,* 205–215.

Friedman, B., & Price, J. L. (1984). Fiber systems in the olfactory bulb and cortex: A study in adult and developing rats, using the Timm method with light and electron microscope. *Journal of Comparative Neurology, 223,* 88–109.

Gesteland, R. C., Yancey, R. A., & Farbman, A. I. (1982). Development of olfactory receptor neuron selectivity in the rat fetus. *Neuroscience, 7,* 3127–3136.

Getchell, T. V., & Shepherd, G. M. (1975). Short-axon cells in the olfactory bulb: Dendo-dendritic synaptic interactions. *Journal of Physiology, 251,* 523–548.

Greer, C. A. (1984). A Golgi analysis of granule cell development in the neonatal rat olfactory bulb (Abstract). *Proceedings of the Society of Neuroscience, 10,* 531.

Greer, C. A., & Shepherd, G. M. (1982). Mitral cell degeneration and sensory function in the neurological mutant mouse Purkinje cell degeneration (PCD). *Brain Research, 235,* 156–161.

Greer, C. A., Stewart, W. B., Teicher, M. H., & Shepherd, G. M. (1982). Functional development of the olfactory bulb and a unique glomerular complex in the neonatal rat. *Journal of Neuroscience, 2*, 1744–1759.

Haberly, L. B. (1985). Neuronal circuitry in olfactory cortex: Anatomy and functional implications. *Chemical Senses, 10*, 219–238.

Halasz, N., & Shepherd, G. M. (1983). Neurochemistry of the vertebrate olfactory bulb. *Neuroscience, 10*, 579–619.

Henneman, E. (1968). Organization of the spinal cord. In V. B. Mountcastle (Ed.), *Medical physiology* (Vol. 2, pp. 1717–1732). St. Louis: Mosby.

Hinds, J. W. (1968a). Autoradiographic study of histogenesis in the mouse olfactory bulb: I. Time of origin of neurons and neuroglia. *Journal of Comparative Neurology, 134*, 287–304.

Hinds, J. W. (1968b). Autoradiographic study of histogenesis in the mouse olfactory bulb: II. Cell proliferation and migration. *Journal of Comparative Neurology, 132*, 305–322.

Hofer, M. A. (1981). *The roots of human behavior: An introduction to the psychobiology of human development.* San Francisco: W. H. Freeman.

Jastreboff, P. J., Pedersen, P. E., Greer, C. A., Stewart, W. B., Kauer, J. S., Benson, T. B., & Shepherd, G. M. (1984). Specific olfactory receptor populations projecting to identified glomeruli in the rat olfactory bulb. *Proceedings of the National Academy of Sciences 81*, 5250–5254.

Iwahara, S. Oishi, H., Sano, K., Yang., K., & Takahashi, T. (1973). Electrical activity of the olfactory bulb in the postnatal rat. *Japanese Journal of Physiology, 23*, 361–370.

Kaplan, J. N., Cubicciotti, D., & Redican, W. K. (1977). Olfactory discrimination of squirrel monkey mothers by their infants. *Developmental Psychobiology, 7*, 15–19.

Keveter, G. A., & Winans, S. S. (1981). Connections of the corticomedial amygdala in the golden hamster: I. Efferents of the "vomeronasal amygdala." *Journal of Comparative Neurology, 197*, 81–98.

Kratzing, J. (1976). The fine structure of the sensory epithelium of the vomeronasal organ in suckling rats. *Australian Journal of Biological Sciences, 24*, 787–796.

Lance-Jones, C., & Landmesser, L. (1980). Motoneuron projection patterns in embryonic chick limbs following partial deletions of the spinal cord. *Journal of Physiology, 302*, 559–580.

Leon, M. (1983). Chemical communication in mother–young interactions. In J. G. Vandenbergh (Ed.), *Pheromones and reproduction in mammals* (pp. 39–77). New York: Academic Press.

Macfarlane, A. (1975). Olfaction in the development of social preferences in the human neonate. In *Parent–infant interaction* (pp. 103–113). (Ciba Foundation Symposium 33). New York: Elsevier.

Macrides, F., & Davis, B. J. (1983). The olfactory bulb. In P. C. Emson (Ed.), *Chemical neuroanatomy* (pp. 391–426). New York: Raven.

Mair, R. G., & Gesteland, R. C. (1982). Response properties of mitral cells in the olfactory bulb of the neonatal rat. *Neuroscience, 7*, 3105–3116.

Math, F., & Davrainville, J. L. (1980). Electrophysiological study on the postnatal development of mitral cell activity in the rat olfactory bulb. *Brain Research, 190*, 243–247.

Monti Graziadei, G. A., Stanley, R. S., & Graziadei, P. P. C. (1980). The olfactory marker protein in the olfactory system of the mouse during development. *Neuroscience, 5*, 1239–1252.

Mori, K., Kishi, K., & Ojima, H. (1983). Distribution of dendrites of mitral, displaced mitral, tufted and granule cells in the rabbit olfactory bulb. *Journal of Comparative Neurology, 219,* 339–355.

Orona, E., Scott, J. W., & Rainer, E. C. (1983). Different granule cell populations innervate superficial and deep regions of the external plexiform layer in rat olfactory bulb. *Journal of Comparative Neurology, 217,* 227–237.

Pedersen, P. E., & Benson, T. B. (1986). Projection of septal organ receptor neurons to the main olfactory bulb in rats. *Journal of Comparative Neurology, 252,* 555–562.

Pedersen, P. E., & Blass, E. M. (1981). Olfactory control over suckling in albino rats. In R. N. Aslin, J. R. Alberts, & M. R. Peterson (Eds.) *Development of perception: Psychobiological perspectives* (Vol. 1, pp. 359–381). New York: Academic Press.

Pedersen, P. E., & Blass, E. M. (1982). Prenatal and postnatal determinants of the first suckling episode in the albino rat. *Developmental Psychobiology, 15,* 349–356.

Pedersen, P. E., Greer, C. A., & Shepherd, G. M. (1986). Early development of olfactory function. In E. M. Blass (ed.), *Handbook of behavioral neurobiology: Vol. 8. Developmental psychobiology and developmental psychobiology* (pp. 163–203). New York: Plenum.

Pedersen, P. E., Greer, C. A., Stewart, W. B., & Shepherd, G. M. (1982). A 2DG study of behavioral plasticity in odor dependent suckling. (Abstract) *Association for Chemoreception Sciences,* 22.

Pedersen, P. E., Jastreboff, P. J., Stewart, W. B., & Shepherd, G. M. (1986). Mapping of an olfactory receptor population that projects to a specific region in the rat olfactory bulb. *Journal of Comparative Neurology, 250,* 93–108.

Pedersen, P. E., Stewart, W. B., Greer, C. A., & Shepherd, G. M. (1983). Evidence for olfactory function *in utero. Science, 221,* 478–480.

Porter, R. H., Cernoch, J. M., & Balogh, R. D. (1985). Odor signatures and kin recognition. *Physiology and Behavior, 34,* 445–448.

Porter, R. H., Cernoch, J. M., & McLaughlin, F. J. (1983). Maternal recognition of neonates through olfactory cues. *Physiology and Behavior, 30,* 151–154.

Powers, J. B., & Winans, S. S. (1975). Vomeronasal organ: Critical role in mediating sexual behavior of the male hamster. *Science, 187,* 961–963.

Rall, W., Shepherd, G. M., Reese, T. S., & Brightman, M. W. (1966). Dendrodendritic synaptic pathway for inhibition in the olfactory bulb. *Experimental Neurology, 14,* 44–56.

Rosenblatt, J. S. (1983). Olfaction mediates developmental transition in the altricial newborn of selected species of mammals. *Developmental Psychobiology, 16,* 347–376.

Salas, M., Guzman-Flores, C., & Schapiro, S. (1969). An ontogenetic study of olfactory bulb electrical activity in the rat. *Physiology and Behavior, 4,* 699–703.

Scalia, F., & Winans, S. S. (1975). The differential projections of the olfactory bulb and accessory olfactory bulb in mammals. *Journal of Comparative Neurology, 161,* 31–56.

Schwob, J. E., & Price, J. L. (1978). The cortical projections of the olfactory bulb: Development in fetal and neonatal rats correlated with quantitative variations in adults rats. *Brain Research, 151,* 369–374.

Schwob, J. E., & Price, J. L. (1984a). The development of axonal connections in the central olfactory system of rat. *Journal of Comparative Neurology, 223,* 177–202.

Schwob, J. E., & Price, J. L. (1984b). The development of lamination of afferent fibers to the olfactory cortex in rats, with additional observations in the adult. *Journal of Comparative Neurology, 223,* 203–222.

Scott, J. W., McBride, R. L., & Schneider, S. P. (1980). The organization of projections from the olfactory bulb to the piriform cortex and olfactory tubercle in the rat. *Journal of Comparative Neurology, 194,* 519–534.

Shepherd, G. M. (1971). Physiological evidence for dendrodendritic synaptic interactions in the rabbit's olfactory glomerulus. *Brain Research, 32,* 212–217.

Shepherd, G. M. (1979). *The synaptic organization of the brain.* New York: Oxford University Press.

Stone, J., & Fukuda, Y., (1974). Properties of cat retinal ganglion cells: A comparison of W-cells with X- and Y-cells. *Journal of Neurophysiology, 37,* 722–748.

Teicher, M. H., & Blass, E. M. (1977). The role of olfaction and amniotic fluid in the first suckling response of newborn albino rats. *Science, 198,* 635–636.

Teicher, M. H., Stewart, W. B., Kauer, J. S., & Shepherd, G. M. (1980). Suckling pheromone stimulation of a modified glomerular region in the developing rat olfactory bulb revealed by the 2-deoxyglucose method. *Brain Research, 194,* 530–535.

Westrum, L. E. (1975). Electron microscopy of synaptic structures in olfactory cortex of early postnatal rats. *Journal of Neurocytology, 4,* 713–732.

White, L. E. (1973). Synaptic organization of the mammalian olfactory glomerulus: New findings including an intraspecific variation. *Brain Research, 60,* 299–313.

# 7

## Neural and Behavioral Plasticity Induced by Early Olfactory Learning

MICHAEL LEON, ROBERT COOPERSMITH,
SUZANNE LEE, REGINA M. SULLIVAN,
DONALD A. WILSON, and CYNTHIA C. WOO
*Department of Psychobiology*
*University of California*
*Irvine, California 92717*

## I. Introduction

### A.  Maternal Olfactory Attractant

Over a decade ago, we found that young Norway rats reliably (99%) come to approach the odor of their mother (Leon & Moltz, 1971, 1972). This behavior pattern has now been reported in more than a dozen species, ranging from crayfish (Little, 1975, 1976) to humans (MacFarlane, 1975; Russell, 1976). Norway rat pups are normally exposed to low concentrations of the maternal odor early in life (Leon, 1983). They orient toward the maternal odor (Altman, Sudarshan, Das, McCormick, & Barnes, 1971) and then approach it when they are mobile enough to leave the nest (Leon & Moltz, 1971). This olfactory preference facilitates mother–young reunions at a time when the mobile young still require their mother's milk (see Leon, 1983, for a review).

### B.  Experiential Basis for Attraction to Maternal and Other Odors

The principal source of the odor is the cecotrophe portion of the mother's anal excreta, (Leon, 1974). Cecotrophe is differentiated from the feces in the cecum, a large gastrointestinal structure located at the junction between the small and large intestines. Synthesis of the cecal odor depends on cecal bacterial function (Leon, 1974, 1975). Since enteric bacterial populations and their metabolic products differ with different diets (Draser et al., 1973; Lampen & Peterjohn, 1951; Porter & Rettger, 1940), it seemed possible that the cecal odor would also differ with different maternal diets. Indeed, it did. Leon (1975) found that pups raised with mothers on one diet were attracted only to mothers eating that diet. Pups must therefore acquire their attraction to the odor that they will approach postnatally, since no single "maternal" odor is invariably present in maternal anal excreta. Daily exposure to either a maternal or another odor induces a preferential approach response by the pups (Alberts, 1978; Brunjes & Alberts, 1979; Leon, 1974; Leon, Galef, & Behse, 1977).

## C.   Enhanced Olfactory Bulb Response

We considered the possibility that experience with a specific odor would induce the developing olfactory bulb to have a special, perhaps enhanced, response to that odor. If one accepts the reasonable assumptions that elevated glucose use reflects activity and that the uptake of the glucose analogue 2-deoxyglucose (2-DG) reflects elevated neuronal glucose use, then [14]C-labeled 2-DG autoradiography is a powerful technique for localizing areas of differentially active cells (see Gallistel, Piner, Allen, Adler, Yadin, & Negin, 1982; Mata et al., 1980; Sokoloff, 1981; Yarowski & Ingvar, 1981). It also should be noted that the metabolic pathways of different cell types have not been identified in the developing olfactory bulb, and it is not completely clear what proportion of neural activity is accounted for by this method in each type of cell.

An artificial odor was chosen as the olfactory stimulus, since its presentation could be controlled more precisely than the maternal odor. Peppermint was the odor of choice because, after repeated exposure, rat pups would approach it to the same extent as they would approach maternal odors (Leon et al., 1977). We used [14]C 2-DG autoradiography to map the response of the olfactory bulbs of 19-day-old rat pups during a 45-min test exposure to peppermint odor after the pups had been exposed to either peppermint or fresh air for 18 days. The olfactory experience occurred during daily 10-min sessions when the pups were held in either the peppermint or fresh airstream. Pups received perineal stimulation while exposed to the odor during the 10-min exposures (but not during the 45-min test on Day 19) because similar stimulation has been shown to facilitate odor-preference acquisition in neonatal rats (Pedersen & Blass, 1982; Pedersen, Williams, & Blass, 1982; Sullivan, Hofer, & Brake, 1986).

Autoradiographs of 20-$\mu$m coronal sections of the olfactory bulb were made using standard techniques. During development of the autoradiographs, the tissue was accompanied by $^{14}C$ standards that had previously been calibrated to $^{14}C$ uptake in similar brain sections. To analyze the autoradiographs, we employed a digital image-processing system which digitized and stored the image of the brain on the autoradiograph by assigning an 8-bit gray level to each element of the pixel array. A calibration function was then constructed by plotting the gray values of the exposure standards against their previously determined $^{14}C$-labeled tissue equivalents. This curve was then fitted to a linear function. A new image of the brain section was then constructed from this calibration function. Concentrations of $^{14}C$ could then be determined for any specified area of the section.

We found that both groups had a reliably high level of uptake in a specific area of the glomerular layer, lateral and 1.5–2.2 mm from the rostral pole. This uptake pattern presumably reflects a normal olfactory response to the peppermint odor present during the period of 2-DG uptake. The odor-experienced pups, however, had a significantly greater level of uptake (64%) in those areas (see Fig 1; Coopersmith & Leon, 1984). Neither the level of uptake in the periventricular core nor the uptake in other portions of the glomerular layer differed between groups, indicating that the response was not due to a generalized increase in neural activity.

Other investigators have found that when rats are exposed to different odors, the olfactory bulb reliably shows qualitatively different uptake patterns that are largely restricted to the glomerular layer (Astic & Saucier, 1982; Greer, Stewart, Kauer, & Shepherd, 1981; Greer, Stewart, Teicher, & Shepherd, 1982; Jourdan, Duveau, Astic, & Holley, 1980; Sharp, Kauer, & Shepherd, 1975; Stewart, Kauer, & Shepherd, 1979; Teicher, Stewart, Kaver, & Shepherd, 1980). We found that while there is no change in the qualitative pattern of 2-DG uptake after early experience with an odor, there is a quantitative difference in the relative response of the olfactory bulb to the same concentration of the same odor.

D.  Lack of Differential Respiration

The possibility existed, however, that the familiar odor induced the animals to increase their respiration rate, thereby increasing the stimulus intensity, during the test exposure. The increase in olfactory bulb activity could then be attributable to an increase in stimulus intensity (Greer *et al.*, 1981). No statistical differences were found between groups in the number of respirations or the distribution of respiratory frequencies either

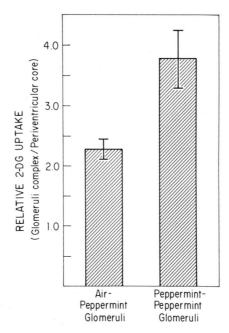

**Fig. 1.** Mean relative ¹⁴C 2-DG uptake in specific glomerular areas that are lateral and 1.5–2.2 mm from the rostral pole of the olfactory bulb in peppermint-peppermint (odor-familiar) and air-peppermint (odor-unfamiliar) pups on postnatal Day 19. Means and SEMs are shown in these graphs. From Coopersmith & Leon (1984), *Science, 225,* 849–851. Copyright 1984 by the AAAS.

during the entire 45-min test exposure period or in any of eight shorter intervals (Fig. 2; Coopersmith & Leon, 1984; unpublished observations). These data suggest that the enhanced response may be due to a reorganization of the olfactory system itself rather than to a behavioral difference between groups.

## E.   The Enhanced Response Is Odor-specific

It is possible that familiarity with one odor would increase the olfactory bulb response to any odor. That is, the enhanced neural response may be nonspecific. We therefore familiarized pups with either peppermint or cyclohexanone and tested their 2-DG uptake patterns in response to peppermint while their respiration frequency was being analyzed on Day 19.

The 2-DG uptake of peppermint-familiar pups replicated almost exactly the uptake levels reported by Coopersmith and Leon (1984). In addition, peppermint-familiar pups showed significantly higher 2-DG uptake than

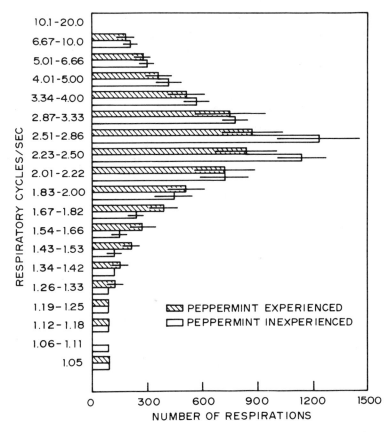

**Fig. 2.**   Number of respirations of different frequencies by peppermint-familiar and peppermint-unfamiliar pups during peppermint odor presentation on postnatal Day 19 during a 45-min test period.

cyclohexanone-familiar pups in the same area of the bulb described above (Coopersmith, Henderson, & Leon, 1986). No differences were found in respiration frequency patterns between the groups. The enhanced neural response therefore is specific to the odor with which the pup is familiar, although there may also be a nonspecific component of the response.

We then studied the effects of cyclohexanone experience on subsequent responsiveness to cyclohexanone. When tested on Day 19 with cyclohexanone, cyclohexanone-familiar pups had an enhanced neural response in a glomerular area different from that identified for peppermint. The glomerular area with particularly high 2-DG uptake is medial and caudal to the identified peppermint area (2.5–3.0 mm from the rostral pole of the bulb). The cyclohexanone-familiar pups had an enhanced response to cyclohexanone compared with that of cyclohexanone-unfamiliar (air-exposed) pups. The enhanced response was also not accompanied by changes in respiratory pattern.

## F.  The Enhanced Response is Long-Lasting

Rats exposed to peppermint odor and stroking from days 1–18 were tested for 2-DG uptake in their olfactory bulb in response to that odor on day 90. We found that such animals still had an enhanced glomerular uptake of 2-DG compared with air/stroking controls (Coopersmith and Leon, 1986). Exposure of adults to odor/stroking stimulation did not induce a subsequent enhanced response to that odor (Woo and Leon, 1987).

## G.  Familiarity Alone Is Insufficient to Produce the Enhanced Response

We then went on to find that simple odor exposure was insufficient to induce both odor attraction and the enhanced 2-DG uptake in the olfactory bulb. Recall that we routinely stroked the back or perineum of the pups with a small brush to mimic maternal licking during both odor and fresh air exposure because Pedersen et al. (1982) reported that similar stimulation facilitated odor-preference acquisition in perinates. To determine the importance of such stimulation in our situation, we exposed pups for 10 min/day to peppermint odor with stroking, odor without stroking, or stroking only or left them with their mothers until the test.

On Day 19, all groups of pups were tested for their olfactory preference; identical groups were exposed to peppermint odor following 2-DG injection. As can be seen in Fig. 3, only pups that were simultaneously stroked and exposed to peppermint had an increased preference and an enhanced neural response to the odor (Sullivan & Leon, 1986). These data suggest that simple odor familiarity is not sufficient to induce odor preferences or the enhanced glomerular response. Sullivan and Hall (1987) have recently shown that stroking acts as a reinforcer. In fact, their data indicate that stroking is as reinforcing to pups in learning situations as is milk. These data therefore suggest that the enhanced neural response develops after early olfactory learning rather than after other kinds of olfactory experience.

Several laboratories have previously found that the development of behavioral preferences for odors by young rats is greatly facilitated by stimulation of some sort during odor exposure. Such manipulations in-

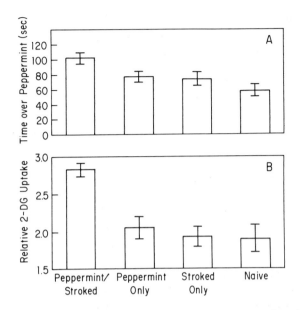

**Fig. 3.** Relative 2-DG uptake and behavioral preference for peppermint odor on Day 19 after being exposed to peppermint odor accompanied by perineal and back stroking, exposed to the odor alone, simply stroked, or left undisturbed during Days 1–18. From Sullivan & Leon (1986).

clude intraoral milk infusions (Brake, 1981; Johanson & Hall, 1979; Johanson, Hall, & Polefrone, 1984; Johanson & Teicher, 1980; Sullivan & Hall, 1987), stroking the ventral and dorsal areas of pups (Pedersen *et al.*, 1982; Sullivan, Hofer, & Brake, 1986), stroking the perineal area (Coopersmith & Leon, 1984), tail pinching (Sullivan, Brake, Hofer, & Williams, 1986), amphetamine injection (Pedersen *et al.*, 1982), morphine injection (Kehoe & Blass, 1986), prolonged isolation (Leon *et al.*, 1977), huddling with conspecifics (Alberts & May, 1984), or placing the young in a warm ambient temperature (Alberts & May, 1984; Pedersen *et al.*, 1982). These varied stimuli may mimic the stimuli, or the pup responses to the stimuli, provided by the mother during their interactions. Pups may normally develop olfactory preferences only when they are being cared for by the mother in the nest, thereby restricting the olfactory experience of the pups to maternal odors at the time in their lives when the pups must develop an olfactory preference only to their mother's odor.

We next determined whether the enhanced glomerular response would be found after any type of olfactory learning. Specifically, we wondered whether odors experienced in conjunction with aversive consequences would produce an enhanced response. We therefore trained pups to avoid peppermint odor on Day 18 by exposing them to either peppermint odor or fresh air for 30 min and then subjecting them to toxicosis (Coopersmith, Lee, & Leon, 1986). Five min after the beginning of the odor exposure, pups were injected IP with LiCl or with saline. All pups were given a 2-DG test with peppermint odor on Day 19. The efficacy of the aversion training was assessed with another pup from the same litter by its avoidance of the odor during a 3-min odor preference test.

The enhanced response is absent to familiar odors experienced with aversive consequences, even if that odor is behaviorally relevant to the pup. Those pups experiencing toxicosis in the presence of the odor avoided it, spending 26% of the test time in the presence of peppermint odor, while both control groups had a neutral response to peppermint (47%). Odor/toxicosis pups had significantly less 2-DG uptake in the identified glomerular areas than the odor/no toxicosis pups and were no different from the air/toxicosis pups. There is a slight, but significant, enhancement of 2-DG uptake in pups after only one brief experience with peppermint that was not followed by toxicosis. Again, differences in the pattern of respiration did not account for the difference in 2-DG uptake. The depressive action of LiCl on the brain also did not seem to account for the data collected 24 hr after toxicosis. While these pups did not have a number of olfactory experiences equivalent to the pups that developed an attraction to the odor over 18 days, they did learn a behavioral avoidance of the odor, and this learned response was not accompanied by the enhanced neural response.

## II.  Mechanisms for the Development of the Enhanced Glomerular Response

### A.  Structural Changes

While we are continuing to investigate the experiential circumstances under which the enhanced glomerular response develops, we also have become interested in determining its mechanism. Indeed, it has been our hope that the phenomenological results would either suggest or rule out possible mechanisms. Both the magnitude of the enhancement and the fact that it lasts into adulthood suggested that we might see a major structural change associated with the area in which the enhanced neural responses are observed. We first wanted to examine the glomerular area to determine whether the glomeruli associated with the enhanced 2-DG uptake had any obvious structural modification. We stained the brain sections with the Goshgarian modification of the Palmgren stain to delineate the fibers in the glomerular layer (Woo, Coopersmith, & Leon, 1987).

We also reacted the bulbs of odor-familiar and odor-unfamiliar pups for the mitochondrial enzymes, succinic dehydrogenase (SDH) and cytochrome oxidase (CO) following a 2-DG test with odor presentation (Woo, Coopersmith, & Leon, 1987). Every third section was used for 2-DG autoradiography, with the other two sections used to react for SDH and CO. The SDH and CO sections were then aligned with the autoradiographs, using the image analysis system.

Figure 4 shows our striking finding. The peppermint-familiar pups had enlarged glomeruli in the area generating the increased activity while the same area of odor-unfamiliar pups had no modified glomerular complex. In fact, areas of increased 2-DG uptake invariably have a modified glomerular complex, whereas we have not observed such structures in any odor-unfamiliar pup in the identified areas of the glomerular layer. The modified glomerular complexes have a characteristic orientation, protruding from the glomerular layer into the external plexiform layer.

It should be noted that we observed these clusters in other, particularly medial, parts of the bulb which are not associated with the focal areas of 2-DG uptake. These complexes may reflect the fact that the pups are exposed to other odors. Wherever there is an area of enhanced 2-DG uptake, however, there is a modified glomerular complex.

Morphometric analysis of these glomerular areas confirmed the observations of a structural modification in this lamina. The glomerular layer underlying the focuses of high 2-DG uptake in peppermint-familiar animals was about 30% wider than that in peppermint-unfamiliar animals. Baseline measurements from areas adjacent to these focuses were virtually identical in peppermint-familiar and peppermint-unfamiliar animals. While the number of glomeruli did not differ between groups, the cross-sectional area of peppermint-familiar pups was about 21% greater than for peppermint-unfamiliar pups. If one assumes that the glomeruli are ball shaped, such an increase would result in a 33% increase in glomerular size. This phenomenon, coupled with the concentration of two or three glomeruli in a small area, may account for the enhanced 2-DG uptake that we observed in the autoradiographs.

There are some data that lend at least some indirect support to this hypothesis. First, there is enormous cell death in the olfactory bulb early in life. During the first few weeks postpartum, approximately half of the mitral cells die (Rosselli-Austin & Altman, 1979). Without olfactory stimulation in early life, though, more mitral cells and even more tufted cells die (Brunjes & Borror, 1983; Laing & Panhuber, 1978; Meisami & Safari, 1981). Restriction of young animals to a single odor produces different

154  Michael Leon et al

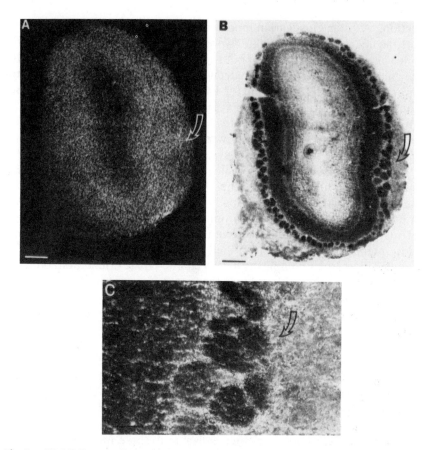

**Fig. 4.** (A) 2-DG autoradiograph of peppermint-familiar pups exposed to peppermint, with an arrow showing a glomerular area of heightened activity. (B) Adjacent section stained for succinic dehydrogenase with the arrow pointing to the same area. (C) Magnified view of this area showing the modified glomerular cluster shown in B. 20 μm sections. Scale bar: A and B = 400 μm; C = 100 μm.

patterns of mitral cell degeneration (Doving & Pinching, 1973; Laing & Panhuber, 1978; Pinching & Doving, 1974) and reduced sensitivity to other odors (Laing & Panhuber, 1978; but see Dalland & Doving, 1981). Other cell types within the olfactory bulb may also die if they are not stimulated at some minimal level. At the other extreme, high levels of olfactory stimulation by a particular odor may prevent many neurons from dying. The glomeruli formed by these neurons may crowd each other into the external plexiform layer. This process of selective cell death, possibly regulated by differential peripheral input, has been suggested to participate in the development of neural circuitry in other brain systems (Cowan, 1973; Guillery, 1972).

It is also possible that the modified glomerular complexes are the result, not of a failure to die, but of a differential arborization of the glomeruli that are there, since developing mitral cells arborize as they grow (Scheibel & Scheibel, 1975). Differential dendritic arborization with differential stimulation has been shown in other brain areas (see Greenough & Volkmar, 1973; Globus, Rosenzweig, Bennett, & Diamond, 1973).

Graziadei and his co-workers (Graziadei, Levine, & Monti Graziadei, 1978; Graziadei & Monti Graziadei, 1978; Graziadei & Samanen, 1980) have shown that incoming olfactory receptor axons will induce the formation of glomeruli in incompletely lesioned olfactory bulbs and even in cortical tissue. Increased local receptor stimulation by peppermint may allow more axons to penetrate and/or induce the formation of glomeruli in the olfactory bulb in the identified portions of the bulb. Indeed, some receptor axons normally penetrate into the external plexiform layer early in development (Hinds & Hinds, 1976; Monti Graziadei, Stanley, & Graziadei, 1980) and could induce the formation of enlarged glomeruli if they are stimulated.

## B.  Do Mitral Cells Mediate the Enhanced Glomerular Response?

To this point, our implicit assumption has been that the enhanced glomerular response is caused by differential mitral cell activity. Specifically, we have assumed that an increase in glomerular activity increases the firing rate of the mitral cells, which then relay this increased activity to the piriform cortex. This assumption, however, appears to be wrong.

We recorded single-unit activity from mitral cells associated with the identified glomerular areas of peppermint-familiar and peppermint-unfamiliar Day 19 pups (Wilson, Sullivan, & Leon, 1985; 1987). Mitral cells ($N = 111$) were isolated and identified by location and/or antidromic stimulation from the piriform. We found that mitral cells of peppermint-familiar pups had significantly fewer excitatory and significantly more suppressive responses to peppermint than the mitral cells of odor-unfamiliar pups. No differences in response pattern were found to orange odor in these mitral cells associated with peppermint-responsive glomeruli (Fig. 5). Again, odor experience without reinforcing tactile stimulation was not effective in changing olfactory system responses (Wilson et al., 1987).

These data suggest that early olfactory experience alters the neural signal emanating from the olfactory bulb. The signal appears to be a reversed pattern of excitatory and suppressive responses transmitted to

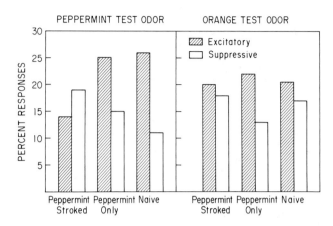

**Fig. 5.** Percentage of excitatory and suppressive responses of mitral cells associated with the peppermint-responsive glomerular area of peppermint-stroked, peppermint only, and peppermint-naive pups to peppermint or orange odor.

the olfactory cortex. Such an inhibition may serve as a unique stimulus for recognition of an odor that has acquired attractive qualities for the pups. Since this is, to our knowledge, the first time that anyone has recorded unit activity from mitral cells in areas activated by a specific odor, these data should have important implications for the understanding of olfactory coding.

Although neonatal odor exposure selectively alters subsequent mitral cell responsiveness to the odor, the changes are not what one would predict if the enhanced glomerular activity was localized in the mitral cell dendrites or in the olfactory neuron axons synapsing in mitral cell glomeruli. Clearly, mitral cell activity did not increase according to expectations.

There are, however, at least two circumstances under which odor familiarity might actually induce greater mitral cell responsiveness but which would make detection of this increase difficult with the sampling technique used here. First, tonic levels of mitral cell excitation in specific glomeruli may be greater in odor-familiar pups than in odor-unfamiliar pups. This could make excitatory responses more difficult to detect and inhibitory responses easier to detect. A comparison of baseline firing rates, however, makes this explanation unlikely, since there was no difference in baseline firing rates between the familiar and unfamiliar groups (Wilson et al., 1985).

A second possibility is that a few mitral cells may have been intensely excited by the familiar odor, and this intense excitation induced an equally powerful surrounding region of inhibition via inhibitory granule

cells. This inhibitory surround could suppress neighboring, weakly excited mitral cell responses and increase the number of inhibitory responses likely to be recorded. One might expect, then, that those few
excitatory responses that were recorded in odor-familiar pups would, on
average, be more intense than excitatory responses in unfamiliar pups.
We therefore compared the magnitude of excitatory responses to peppermint for the odor-familiar and odor-unfamiliar groups. The magnitude of
excitation was calculated as ([spikes/second during odor]/[baseline
spikes/second]) × 100. The magnitude of excitatory responses to peppermint revealed no difference between groups, suggesting that this possibility was unlikely to produce the observed mitral cell response (Wilson *et
al.*, 1985).

These results suggest that activity in neurons other than mitral cells
may be responsible for the enhanced glomerular 2-DG uptake to familiar
odors. Thus, a familiar odor may increase the activity of glomerular-layer
neurons (either periglomerular and/or external tufted cells), which may
then decrease mitral cell activity. The decrease in mitral cell activity to
attractive familiar odors may result in a unique, sharpened signal to the
piriform cortex.

## C. Glomerular-Layer Neurons

Our data demonstrate that mitral cell responses to an odor are altered
by the pup's previous experience with that odor. The direction of this
change in mitral cell responses (decreased excitation, increased inhibition), however, differs from what might be expected if the enhanced
glomerular uptake of 2-DG reflects increased activity in the mitral cell
dendrites. It seems likely, therefore, that another class of neuron increases its firing rate to attractive familiar odors, and these neurons directly or indirectly suppress mitral cell activity.

Macrides, Schoenfeld, Marchand, and Clancy (1985) have recently suggested that the external tufted cells become particularly active during
olfactory stimulation and that the activity of these cells may be reflected
in increased 2-DG uptake. They go on to suggest that the increased activity of tufted cells may mediate the sort of contrast enhancement or gain-
setting functions in olfactory processing that we have found. A subset of
tufted cells form topographically organized intra bulbar associational connections with the opposite side of the ipsilateral bulb (Macrides *et al.*,
1985). That is, laterally situated tufted cells project to the internal plexiform layer of the medial side of the same bulb. A close examination of the
spatial pattern of 2-DG uptake to odor reveals a similar lateral-medial
relationship (Jourdan *et al.*, 1980; Skeen, 1977; Wilson *et al.*, 1987).

Another population of tufted cells synapse on granule cells in the ipsilateral internal plexiform layer (Orona *et al.,* 1984). Thus, an increase in activity of this population of external tufted cells could lead to increased local mitral cell inhibition. Superficial tufted cells are far more responsive to olfactory nerve stimulation and have a greater tendency to have inhalation-related firing patterns than mitral cells and internal tufted cells (Onoda & Mori, 1980; Schneider & Scott, 1983).

All of these characteristics make the superficial tufted cells likely candidates to mediate the glomerular 2-DG patterns observed in both odor-unfamiliar and odor-familiar animals. In fact, the mutant mouse strain PCD (Purkinje cell degeneration) has no mitral cells but still has normal patterns of 2-DG uptake in response to an odor (Greer & Shepherd, 1982). The observed glomeruli were smaller than those normally seen in mice with their mitral cell complement. These data are consistent with the idea that the tufted cells had formed these 2-DG–responsive glomeruli.

It is also possible that the periglomerular cells increase their firing rate to odors and produce the increase in 2-DG uptake in the identified glomeruli. These cells receive input directly from the olfactory receptor neurons and via dendrodendritic synapses with mitral and tufted cells, and they appear to mediate interglomerular inhibition (Macrides & Davis, 1983). Increased activation of these cells by external tufted cell glomeruli may then decrease mitral cell firing.

Both external tufted cells and periglomerular cells are small neurons located in the glomerular region. Although these cell types can be distinguished by their size and presence or lack of dendritic spines, they cannot be definitively distinguished by extracellular electrophysiological criteria alone, since no periglomerular cells, and only a subset of external tufted cells, project out of the bulb (Getchell & Shepherd, 1975; Macrides *et al.,* 1985; Onoda & Mori, 1980; Scott, 1981).

If there is normally a die-off of tufted cells, and these neurons are even more sensitive to olfactory deprivation than mitral cells (Meisami & Safari, 1981), the increased activation of specific tufted cells by odor experience in the identified areas might prevent their death. The increased number of tufted cells responding to the familiar odor would then activate granule cells in the internal plexiform layer and inhibit neighboring mitral cells. If this model is correct, then one might expect to see increased numbers of tufted cells in association with the modified glomerular complexes. One might also expect increased activity of granule cells in line with these glomeruli in the internal plexiform layer of odor-familiar pups. We investigated the first possibility by using a silver fiber stain and counterstaining for Nissl substance to be able to localize cell bodies near the modified glomerular complexes. In some sections, we found that there were groups of what may be tufted cells in association with the modified glomeruli. We are currently quantifying these observations.

Close examination of the 2-DG autoradiographs suggested that there may have been an increased uptake in the internal plexiform or granule cell layer in odor-familiar pups. To determine whether there is increased activity in the granule cells in the ipsilateral internal plexiform layer, we used a technique that could give us a measure of relative activity with cellular resolution. We reasoned that if the granule cells or the tufted cells mobilize stored glycogen into glucose during increased firing, we should be able to detect the presence of the active form of the enzyme that promotes this reaction and thereby gain a measure of differential cellular activity. Such neurons exist, for example, in the spinal cord (Woolf, Chong, & Rashdi, 1985) and have been shown in somatosensory cortical whisker barrels in mice (Wallace, 1983). We aligned 2-DG autoradiographs with alternate sections stained for glycogen phosphorylase in odor-familiar and odor-unfamiliar pups. In only odor-familiar pups exposed to peppermint did we see increased activity in the internal plexiform layer aligned with the identified glomerular areas (Fig. 6). A restricted line of increased activity can be seen aligned with the modified glomerular complex only in peppermint-familiar pups tested with peppermint odor (Coopersmith & Leon, in press).

As it happens, astrocytes are known to contain and use glycogen (Phelps, 1972; Sotelo & Palay, 1968), and it was possible that the cells that we identified were not neurons. Indeed, Benson, Burd, Greer, Landis, and Shepherd (1985) have reported that glia have the greatest uptake of 2-DG of the cells identified in the olfactory bulb using a high-resolution technique. To distinguish between these possibilities, we used immunohistochemical procedures for marking the presence of glial fibrillary acidic protein (GFAP), a protein present only in astrocytes (Bignami & Dahl, 1977; Ludwin, Kosek, & Eng, 1976; Schachner, Hedley-Whyte, Hsu, Schoonmaker, & Bignami, 1977). We obtained excellent staining for GFAP and observed that the presumed astrocytes were in the same area as the highest levels of cells with glycogen phosphorylase activity (Coopersmith, Anderson, Cotman, & Leon, unpublished observations). These data support the idea that glia in the bulb have an important, energy-dependent role in the coding of olfactory cues.

A model of how olfactory experience may affect neural coding for familiar odors is summarized in Fig. 7. Differential olfactory experience increases the size and configuration of glomeruli in the olfactory bulb, perhaps because there is an increase in the number of tufted cells avoiding an early death in that area. The additional tufted cells would increase granule cell activation in the internal plexiform layer, which would inhibit

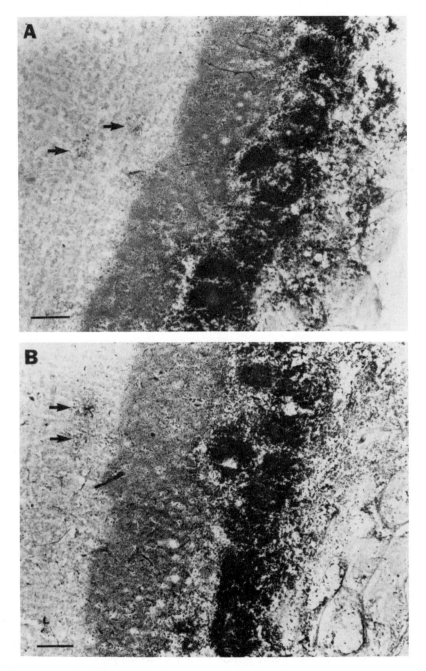

**Fig. 6.** Glycogen phosphorylase activity in the olfactory bulbs of peppermint-familiar pups in response to peppermint odor. Arrows point to enzyme activity associated with granule cells deep to the modified glomerular clusters that display enhanced 2-DG uptake. 20 μm coronal sections. Scale bar = 100 μm. From Coopersmith & Leon (in press).

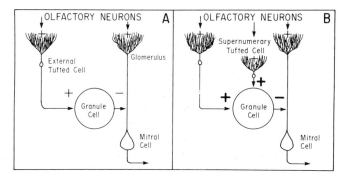

**Fig. 7.**  A model for the development of the enhanced neural response and its consequences for the neural coding of familiar odors. (A) Odor-unfamiliar pups may have many of their external tufted cells die, and the remaining cells may not be able to inhibit neighboring mitral cells via granule cell activation. (B) Early olfactory learning may allow an increased number of external tufted cells to survive in the stimulated area. Their increased activation of granule cells in response to the attractive odor would then inhibit neighboring mitral cells.

neighboring mitral cells. It is also possible that an increase in periglomerular cell inhibition could mediate the decrease in mitral cell activity. It is interesting to note that high-resolution 2-DG autoradiography demonstrated increased activity in response to olfactory stimulation in each of the cell types that we suggest may be involved in mediating early olfactory learning (Lancet, Greer, Kauer, & Shepherd, 1982).

Recall that there is also a subset of external tufted cells that form point-to-point, reciprocal connections between opposite regions of the medial and lateral bulb (Schoenfeld, Marchand, & Macrides, 1985), a pattern that correlates with 2-DG uptake. It seems possible that increased tufted cell input to granule cells from the contralateral side of the same bulb could also mediate the observed decrease in mitral cell activity.

## III.  Prospectus

We expect the future to bring a focus on normally occurring individual differences in the brain that underlie differences in behavior. Since the fields of behavioral ecology and of personality development have focused around the concepts of individual differences, an appreciation of such differences in neurobehavioral analyses may bring these areas closer to a reductionistic analysis. It should also be noted that the differences may be largely inherent or may be based on specific postnatal experiences. This research raises the possibility that there can be different courses for normal brain development.

The second focus for future research may well be the neurobiology of the learning that occurs in mammalian neonates. The neural basis for such learning may be relatively simple and may allow much progress to be made on the question. The developing mammal learns a few very important things about its environment that are critical for survival. Young mammals may be specially adapted for this sort of learning and may have the rather large changes that we have found in the brain as their consequence. Such large and permanent changes make the system amenable for analysis in the same way as the use of animals with few neurons make some types of neurobiological analyses possible. This developmental approach has allowed progress to be made in similar questions in birds and fish (Cooper & Hasler, 1973; Nottebohm, 1980).

The third prospect for the future is an increase in the appreciation of the olfactory system for providing an opportunity to understand plastic changes during development and in adulthood. Both olfactory neurons and olfactory bulb granule cells continue to be formed into adulthood (Graziadei & Monti Graziadei, 1978; Hinds, Hinds, & McNelly, 1984; Hinds & McNelly, 1981; Kaplan & Hinds, 1977). These plastic changes may represent an unusual capability of the olfactory system for change. The olfactory system also appears to subserve the type of complex learning used by humans (Nigrosh, Slotnick, & Nevin, 1975; Slotnick & Kaneko, 1981; Slotnick & Katz, 1974; Staubli, Ivy, & Lynch, 1984). Haberly (1985) and Lynch (1986) argue persuasively that the basis for this capacity may reside in the particular kind of neural network that constitutes the piriform cortex. The olfactory system may therefore even hold the key to understanding the neurobiology of human cognition.

## Acknowledgments

This work has been supported, in part, by grant NS21484 from the National Institute of Neurological and Communication Disorders and Stroke and BNS 8606786, as well as an equipment grant BNS 80-2310 from the National Science Foundation to M.L., who holds Research Scientist Development Award MH00371 from the National Institute for Mental Health. R.M.S. is supported by postdoctoral fellowship HD06818 from the National Institute for Child Health and Human Development. We thank Foteos Macrides for his insightful discussions.

## References

Alberts, J. R. (1978). Huddling by rat pups: Multisensory control of contact behavior. *Journal of Comparative and Physiological Psychology, 92,* 220–230.
Alberts, J. R., & May, B. (1984). Nonnutritive, thermotactile induction of filial huddling in rat pups. *Developmental Psychobiology, 17,* 161–181.

Altman, J., Sudarshan, K., Das, G. D., McCormick, N., & Barnes, D. (1971). The influence of nutrition on neural and behavioral development: III. Development of some motor, particularly locomotor, patterns during infancy. *Developmental Psychobiology, 4,* 97–114.

Astic, L., & Saucier, D. (1982). Metabolic mapping of functional activity in the olfactory projections of the rat: An ontogenetic study. *Developmental Brain Research, 2,* 141–156.

Benson, T. B., Burd, G. D., Greer, C. A., Landis, D. M., & Shepherd, G. M. (1985). High-resolution 2-deoxyglucose autoradiography in quick-frozen slabs of neonatal rat olfactory bulb. *Brain Research, 339,* 67–78.

Bignami, A., & Dahl, D. (1977). Specificity of the glial fibrillary acidic protein for astroglia. *Journal of Histochemistry and Cytochemistry, 256,* 466–469.

Brake, S. C. (1981). Suckling infant rats learn a preference for a novel olfactory stimulus paired with milk delivery. *Science, 211,* 506–508.

Brunjes, P. C., & Alberts, J. R. (1979). Olfactory stimulation induces filial preferences for huddling in rat pups. *Journal of Comparative and Physiological Psychology, 93,* 548–555.

Brunjes, P. C., & Borror, M. J. (1983). Unilateral odor deprivation: Differential effects due to time of treatment. *Brain Research Bulletin, 11,* 501–503.

Cooper, J. C., & Hasler, A. D. (1973). Electroencephalographic evidence for retention of olfactory cues in homing Coho salmon. *Science, 183,* 336–338.

Coopersmith, R., Henderson, S. R., & Leon, M. (1986). Odor specificity of the enhanced neural response following early odor exposure. *Developmental Brain Research, 27,* 191–197.

Coopersmith, R., Lee, S., & Leon, M. (1986). Olfactory bulb responses after odor aversion learning by young rats. *Developmental Brain Research, 24,* 271–277.

Coopersmith, R., & Leon, M. (1984). Enhanced neural response to familiar olfactory cues. *Science, 225,* 849–851.

Coopersmith, R., & Leon, M. (1986). Enhanced neural response by adult rats to odors experienced early in life. *Brain Research, 371,* 400–403.

Coopersmith, R., & Leon, M. (1987). Glycogen phosphorylase activity in the olfactory bulb of the young rat. *Journal of Comparative Neurology,* in press.

Cowan, W. M. (1973). Neuronal death as a regulative mechanism in the control of cell numbers in the nervous system. In M. E. Rockstein & M. L. Sussman (Eds.), *Development and aging in the nervous system* (pp. 19–41). New York: Academic Press.

Dalland, T., & Doving, K. B. (1981). Reaction to olfactory stimuli in odor-exposed rats. *Behavioral and Neural Biology, 32,* 79–88.

Doving, K. B., & Pinching, A. J. (1973). Selective degeneration of neurones in the olfactory bulb following prolonged odour exposure. *Brain Research, 52,* 115–129.

Draser, B. S., Crowther, J. S., Goddard, P., Hawksworth, G., Hill, M. J., Peach, S., & Williams, R. E. O. (1973). The relationship between diet and gut microflora in man. *Proceedings of the Nutrition Society, 32,* 49–52.

Gallistel, C. R., Piner, C. T., Allen, T. O., Adler, N. T., Yadin, E., & Negin, M. (1982). Computer assisted analysis of 2-DG autoradiographs. *Neuroscience and Biobehavioral Reviews, 6,* 409–420.

Getchell, T. V., & Shepherd, G. M. (1975). Short-axon cells in the olfactory bulb: Dendro-dendritic synaptic interactions. *Journal of Physiology, 251,* 523–548.

Globus, A., Rosenzweig, M. R., Bennett, E. L., & Diamond, M. C. (1973). Effects of differential experience on dendritic spine counts in rat cerebral cortex. *Journal of Comparative and Physiological Psychology, 82,* 175–181.

Graziadei, P. P. C., Levine, R. R., & Monti Graziadei, G. A. (1978). Regeneration of olfactory axons and synapse formation in the forebrain after bulbectomy. *Proceedings of the National Academy of Science, 75*, 5230–5234.

Graziadei, P. P. C., & Monti Graziadei, G. A. (1978). Continuous nerve cell renewal in the olfactory system. In M. Jacobsen (Ed.), *Handbook of sensory physiology* (Vol. 9, pp. 55–83). New York: Springer-Verlag.

Graziadei, P. P. C., & Samanen, D. W. (1980). Ectopic glomerular structures in the olfactory bulb of neonatal and adult mice. *Brain Research, 187*, 467–472.

Greenough, W. T., & Volkmar, F. R. (1973). Pattern of dendrite branching in occipital cortex of rats reared in complex environments. *Experimental Neurology, 40*, 491–504.

Greer, C. A., & Shepherd, G. M. (1982). Mitral cell degeneration and sensory function in the neurological mutant mouse Purkinje cell degeneration (PCD). *Brain Research, 235*, 156–161.

Greer, C. A., Stewart, W. B., Kauer, J. S., & Shepherd, G. M. (1981). Topographical and laminar localization of 2-deoxyglucose uptake in rat olfactory bulb induced by electrical stimulation of olfactory nerves. *Brain Research, 217*, 279–293.

Greer, C. A., Stewart, W. B., Teicher, M. H., & Shepherd, G. M. (1982). Functional development of the olfactory bulb and a unique glomerular complex in the neonatal rat. *Journal of Neuroscience, 2*, 1744–1759.

Guillery, R. W. (1972). Binocular competition in the control of geniculate cell growth. *Journal of Comparative Neurology, 144*, 117–127.

Haberly, L. B. (1985). Neuronal circuitry in olfactory cortex: Anatomy and functional implications. *Chemical Senses, 10*, 219–238.

Hinds, J. W., & Hinds, P. L. (1976). Synapse formation in the mouse olfactory bulb. *Journal of Comparative Neurology, 169*, 15–40.

Hinds, J. W., Hinds, P. L., & McNelly, N. A. (1984). An autoradiographic study of the mouse olfactory epithelium: Evidence for long-lived receptors. *Anatomical Record, 210*, 375–383.

Hinds, J. W., & McNelly, N. A. (1981). Aging in the rat olfactory system: Correlation of changes in the olfactory epithelium and olfactory bulb. *Journal of Comparative Neurology, 203*, 441–453.

Johanson, I. B., & Hall, W. G. (1979). Appetitive learning in 1-day-old rat pups. *Science, 205*, 419–421.

Johanson, I. B., Hall W. G., & Polefrone, J. M. (1984). Appetitive conditioning in neonatal rats: Conditioned ingestive responding to stimuli paired with oral infusions of milk. *Developmental Psychobiology, 17*, 357–381.

Johanson, I. B., & Teicher, M. H. (1980). Classical conditioning of an odor preference in 3-day-old rats. *Behavioral and Neural Biology, 29*, 132–136.

Jourdan, F., Duveau, A., Astic, L., & Holley, A. (1980). Space distribution of 14C-2-deoxyglucose uptake in the olfactory bulbs of rats stimulated with two different odours. *Brain Research, 188*, 139–154.

Kaplan, M. S., & Hinds, J. W. (1977). Neurogenesis in the adult rat: Electron microscopic analysis of light radioautographs. *Science, 197*, 1092–1094.

Kehoe, P., & Blass, E. M. (1986). Behaviorally functional opioid systems in infant rats: I. Evidence for olfactory and gustatory classical conditioning. *Behavioral Neuroscience, 100*, 359–367.

Laing, D. G., & Panhuber, H. (1978). Neural and behavioural changes in rats following continuous exposure to an odour. *Journal of Comparative Physiology, 124*, 259–265.

Lampen, J. A., & Peterjohn, H. R. (1951). Studies on the specificity of the fermentation of pentoses by *Lactobacillus* pentoses. *Journal of Bacteriology, 62*, 281–292.

Lancet, D., Greer, C. A., Kauer, J. S., & Shepherd, G. M. (1982). Mapping of odor-related neuronal activity in the olfactory bulb by high-resolution 2-deoxyglucose autoradiography. *Proceedings of the National Academy of Sciences, 79,* 670–674.

Leon, M. (1974). Maternal pheromone. *Physiology and Behavior, 13,* 441–453.

Leon, M. (1975). Dietary control of maternal pheromone in the lactating rat. *Physiology and Behavior, 14,* 311–319.

Leon, M. (1983). Chemical communication in mother-young interactions. In J. Vandenbergh (Ed.), *Pheromones and reproduction in mammals* (pp. 39–77). New York: Academic Press.

Leon, M., Galef, B. G., Jr., & Behse, J. H. (1977). Establishment of the pheromonal bonds and diet choice by odor pre-exposure. *Physiology and Behavior, 18,* 387–391.

Leon, M., & Moltz, H. (1971). Maternal pheromone: Discrimination by preweaning albino rats. *Physiology and Behavior, 7,* 265–267.

Leon, M., & Moltz, H. (1972). The development of the pheromonal bond in the albino rat. *Physiology and Behavior, 8,* 683–686.

Little, E. E. (1975). Chemical communication in maternal behavior of crayfish. *Nature, 225,* 400–401.

Little, E. E. (1976). Ontogeny of maternal behavior and brood pheromone in crayfish. *Journal of Comparative Physiology, 112,* 133–142.

Ludwin, S. K., Kosek, J. C., & Eng, L. F. (1976). The topographical distribution of S-100 and GFA proteins in the adult rat brain: An immunohistochemical study using horseradish peroxidase-labelled antibodies. *Journal of Comparative Neurology, 165,* 197–208.

Lynch, G. (1986). Synapses, circuits and the beginnings of memory. In *Cognitive neurobiology.* Cambridge: MIT Press.

MacFarlane, A. (1975). Olfaction in the development of social preferences in the human neonate. In *The human neonate in parent–infant interaction* (pp. 103–117). Amsterdam: Ciba Foundation.

Macrides, F., & Davis, B. J. (1983). The olfactory bulb. In P. C. Emson (Ed.), *Chemical neuroanatomy* (pp. 391–426). New York: Raven.

Macrides, F., Schoenfeld, T. A., Marchand, J. E., & Clancy, A. N. (1985). Evidence for morphologically, neurochemically and functionally heterogeneous classes of mitral and tufted cells in the olfactory bulb. *Chemical Senses, 10,* 175–202.

Mata, M., Fink, D., Gainer, H., Smith, C., Davidsen, L., Savaki, H., Schwartz, W., & Sokoloff, L. (1980). Activity-dependent energy metabolism in rat posterior pituitary primarily reflects sodium pump activity. *Journal of Neurochemistry, 34,* 213–215.

Meisami, E., & Safari, L. (1981). A quantitative study of the effects of early unilateral olfactory deprivation on the number and distribution of mitral and tufted cells and of glomeruli in the rat olfactory bulb. *Brain Research, 221,* 81–107.

Monti Graziadei, G. A., Stanley, R. S., & Graziadei, P. P. C. (1980). The olfactory marker protein in the olfactory system of the mouse during development. *Neuroscience, 5,* 1239–1252.

Nigrosh, B. J., Slotnick, B. M., & Nevin, J. A. (1975). Olfactory discrimination, reversal learning, and stimulus control in rats. *Journal of Comparative and Physiological Psychology, 89,* 285–294.

Nottebohm, F. (1980). Brain pathways for vocal learning in birds. In J. M. Sprague & A. N. Epstein (Eds.), *Progress in psychobiology and physiological psychology* (pp. 86–125). New York: Academic Press.

Orona, E., Rainer, E. C., & Scott, J. W. (1984). Dendritic and axonal organization of mitral and tufted cells in the rat olfactory bulb. *Journal Comparative Neurology, 226,* 346–356.

Onoda, N., & Mori, K. (1980). Depth distribution of temporal firing patterns in olfactory bulb related to air-intake cycles. *Journal of Neurophysiology, 44,* 29–39.

Pedersen, P. E., & Blass, E. M. (1982). Prenatal and postnatal determinants of the first suckling episode in albino rats. *Developmental Psychobiology, 15,* 349–355.

Pedersen, P. E., Williams, C. L., & Blass, E. M. (1982). Activation and odor conditioning of suckling behavior in 3-day-old albino rats. *Journal of Experimental Psychology: Animal Behavior Processes, 8,* 329–341.

Phelps, C. H. (1972). Barbiturate-induced glycogen accumulation in brain: An electron microscopic study. *Brain Research, 39,* 225–234.

Pinching, A. J., & Doving, K. B. (1974). Selective degeneration in the rat olfactory bulb following exposure to different odors. *Brain Research, 82,* 195–204.

Porter, J. R., & Rettger, L. F. (1940). Influence of diet on the distribution of bacteria in the stomach, small intestine and caecum of the white rat. *Journal of Infectious Diseases, 66,* 104–110.

Rosselli-Austin, L., & Altman, J. (1979). The postnatal development of the main olfactory bulb of the rat. *Journal of Developmental Physiology, 1,* 295–313.

Russell, M. (1976). Human olfactory communication. *Nature, 260,* 520–522.

Schachner, M., Hedley-Whyte, E. T., Hsu, D. W., Schoonmaker, G., & Bignami, A. (1977). Ultrastructural localization of glial fibrillary acidic protein in mouse cerebellum by immunoperoxidase labeling. *Journal of Cell Biology, 75,* 67–73.

Scheibel, M. E., & Scheibel, A. B. (1975). Dendrite bundles, central programs and the olfactory bulb. *Brain Research, 95,* 407–421.

Schneider, S. P., & Scott, J. W. (1983). Orthodromic response properties of rat olfactory bulb mitral and tufted cells correlate with their projection patterns. *Journal of Neurophysiology, 50,* 358–378.

Schoenfeld, T. A., Marchand, J. E., & Macrides, F. (1985). Topographic organization of tufted cell axonal projections in the hamster main olfactory bulb: An intrabulbar associational system. *Journal of Comparative Neurology, 235,* 503–518.

Scott, J. W. (1981). Electrophysiological identification of mitral and tufted cells and distributions of their axons in the olfactory system of the rat. *Journal of Neurophysiology, 46,* 918–931.

Sharp, F., Kauer, J. S., & Shepherd, G. M. (1975). Local sites of activity related glucose metabolism in the rat olfactory bulb during olfactory stimulation. *Brain Research, 98,* 596–600.

Skeen, L. C. (1977). Odor-induced patterns of deoxyglucose consumption in the olfactory bulb of the tree shrew, *Tupia glis. Brain Research, 124,* 147–153.

Slotnick, B. M., & Kaneko, N. (1981). Role of mediodorsal thalamic nucleus in olfactory discrimination learning in rats. *Science, 214,* 91–92.

Slotnick, B. M., & Katz, H. M. (1974). Olfactory learning-set formation in rats. *Science, 185,* 796–798.

Sokoloff, L. (1981). Localization of functional ability in the cerebral nervous system by measurement of glucose utilization with radioactive glucose. *Journal of Cerebral Blood Flow and Metabolism, 1,* 7–36.

Sotelo, C., & Palay, S. L. (1968). The fine structure of the lateral vestibular nucleus in the rat: I. Neurons and neuroglial cells. *Journal of Cell Biology, 36,* 151–179.

Staubli, U., Ivy, G., & Lynch, G. (1984). Hippocampal denervation causes rapid forgetting of olfactory information in rats. *Proceedings of the National Academy of Sciences, 81,* 5885–5887.

Stewart, W. B., Kauer, J. S., & Shepherd, G. M. (1979). Functional organization of rat olfactory bulb analyzed by the 2-deoxyglucose method. *Brain Research, 185,* 715–734.

Sullivan, R. M., Brake, S. C., Hofer, M. A., & Williams, C. L. (1986). Huddling and independent feeding of neonatal rats can be facilitated by a conditional change in behavioral state. *Developmental Psychobiology, 19,* 625–635.

Sullivan, R. M., & Hall, W. G. (1987). Reinforcers in infancy: Classical conditioning using stroking or intraoral infusions of milk as USC. *Developmental Psychobiology,* in press.

Sullivan, R. M., Hofer, M. A., & Brake, S. C. (1986). Olfactory-guided orientation in neonatal rats is enhanced by a conditioned change in behavioral state. *Developmental Psychobiology, 19,* 615–624.

Sullivan, R. M., & Leon, M. (1986). Early olfactory learning induces an enhanced olfactory bulb response in young rats. *Developmental Brain Research, 27,* 278–282.

Teicher, M. H., Stewart, W. B., Kaver, J. S., & Shepherd, G. M. (1980). Suckling pheromone stimulation of a modified glomerular region in the developing rat olfactory bulb revealed by the 2-deoxyglucose method. *Brain Research, 194,* 530–535.

Wallace, M. N. (1983). Organization of the mouse cerebral cortex: A histochemical study using glycogen phosphorylase. *Brain Research, 267,* 201–216.

Wilson, D. A., Sullivan, R. M., & Leon, M. (1985). Odor familiarity alters mitral cell response in the olfactory bulb of neonatal rats. *Developmental Brain Research, 22,* 314–317.

Wilson, D. A., Sullivan, R. M., & Leon, M. (1987). *Single unit analysis of postnatal olfactory learning: Modified olfactory bulb output response patterns.* Manuscript submitted for publication.

Woo, C. C., Coopersmith, R., & Leon, M. (1987). *Localized changes in olfactory bulb morphology associated with early olfactory learning.* Manuscript submitted for publication.

Woo, C. C., & Leon, M. (1987). *Sensitive period for neural and behavioral response development to learned odors.* Manuscript submitted for publication.

Woolf, C. J., Chong, M. S., & Rashdi, T. A. (1985). Mapping increased glycogen phosphorylase activity in dorsal root ganglia and in the spinal cord following peripheral stimuli. *Journal of Comparative Neurology, 234,* 60–76.

Yarowski, P. J., & Ingvar, D. H. (1981). Neuronal activity and energy metabolism. *Federation Proceedings, 40,* 2353–2362.

# 8

# Early Motivation, Reward, Learning, and Their Neural Bases: Developmental Revelations and Simplifications

W. G. HALL
*Department of Psychology*
*Duke University*
*Durham, North Carolina 27706*

Developmental analysis may reveal simple organizational principles of emerging neurobehavioral systems. At the same time, it can provide opportunities to trace these systems as ontogenetic processes add increasing complexity. A developmental strategy should be especially useful in the behavioral and neural analysis of those adaptive processes we think of as motivation, reward, and learning. Such behavioral processes are known to be present in infant mammals, often in rudimentary (and perhaps more easily understood) forms, and may provide a starting point for making sense of the more behaviorally and neurobiologically complex adult animal. Here, I illustrate the application of the developmental approach by describing the beginning neurobiologic analysis of a system of appetitive behavior, reward, and learning in infant rats.

## I. A Motivational System in Infants

Ingestive behavior represents an appealing appetitive system for developmental analysis because it is available for study, continuously, from birth to adulthood. For such studies, rats, despite their overrepresenta-

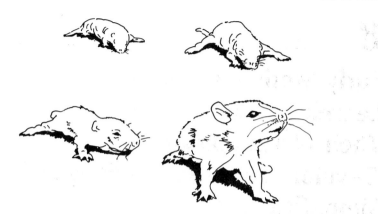

**Fig. 1.** Drawing of rat pups of 5, 10, 15, and 20 days of age, showing their rapid postnatal development from relatively primitive neonates.

tion in behavioral studies, are particularly appropriate subjects because they are born very immature but then develop rapidly (Fig. 1). However, for infant rats and perhaps other mammals, the first form of feeding is suckling, a form of feeding that is neither behaviorally nor neurally continuous with the ingestive system of adults (Blass & Cramer, 1982; Drewett, 1978; Epstein, in press; Hall & Williams, 1983). Analysis of suckling can provide only limited information about later ingestive systems. Fortunately for our interests in the early origins of later behavior, this problem can be avoided because a system of active ingestive behavior does exist independent of suckling in rat pups (Hall, 1979b; Wirth & Epstein, 1976). This second system appears to be the precursor to adult ingestion (Hall & Williams, 1983; Hall, 1985) and has therefore become the basis for an ontogenetic analysis of ingestion and ingestion-related reward and learning.

This other approach to the analysis of ingestion-based appetite, reward, and learning is based on the finding that rat pups as young as 1 day of age will actively ingest milk and other diets infused into their mouths (Fig. 2; Hall, 1979a, 1979b; Wirth & Epstein, 1976) or spread on the floor of their test container (Hall & Bryan, 1980) as long as they are fed in a warm ambiance (Johanson & Hall, 1980; Wirth & Epstein, 1976). Intake volumes are related to the length of time that pups have been deprived of the mother and food. Moreover, in deprived pups less than 9 days of age, a revealing response to milk infusions occurs. In these pups, infusions of milk elicit a profound behavioral activation (Fig. 3; Hall, 1979a, 1979b). Pups not only vigorously mouth and lick the milk, but they immediately crawl, probe, tumble, and climb about their test container and continue to

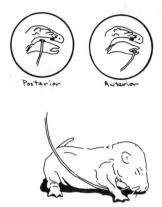

**Fig. 2.** Drawing of a 6-day-old rat pup receiving oral infusions of milk. Infusion cannulas can be placed in either anterior or posterior locations (inserts). Infusions of liquids at posterior locations trigger reflex swallowing; infusions at anterior locations spill out pups' mouths unless they actively lap, mouth, and swallow. From Hall (1985).

do this for the entire test period. Pups exhibit behaviors that appear related to suckling and feeding, as well as many others that are not; it is as if milk infusions release all the behavioral fragments in pups' repertoires. Pups older than 9 days of age no longer display this general behavioral activation; rather, their behavior is more directed and specifically ingestive.

## II. Early Activation, Reward, and Appetitive Learning

The activational component of the pup's response to food suggested to us that, in addition to ingestive behavior, pups were exhibiting evidence of primitive appetitive functioning and perhaps of milk-elicited reward—here externalized and made obvious in this form of excited activity. Unfortunately, the rat pup's lack of motoric competence and low level of spontaneous activity had made it difficult to evaluate appetitive reward and adaptive behavior during the first week of life. It was not known whether these immature animals were capable of rewarded learning.

Procedures developed in studies of early ingestion offered the potential to remedy this situation. Using small oral infusions of milk as reinforcers, we were able to demonstrate operant conditioning in pups as young as 1 day of age (Fig. 4; Johanson & Hall, 1979). Newborn pups would learn to probe into a paddle above their heads to receive a small milk infusion (with each such infusion setting off a flurry of activity just as we had seen

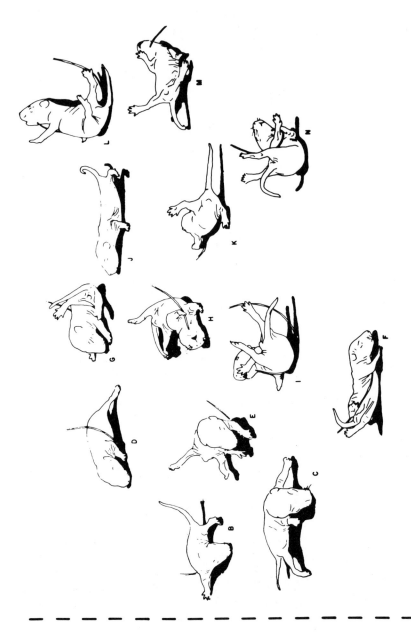

Before
diet infusion

With diet infusions

in experiments described above). In this operant setting, these very immature animals would even learn a two-choice olfactory discrimination. Besides showing that newborn pups were capable of fairly complex appetitive learning, these findings confirmed the suggestion that milk infusions were rewarding and indicated that the accompanying behavioral activation might also contribute to reward.

Oral milk infusions also seemed to act as reinforcers in a classical conditioning paradigm. If a novel odor (the CS) was paired several times with an infusion of milk (the US), pups would come to prefer the odor and orient toward it (Fig. 5; Johanson & Hall, 1982) even if the odor was normally aversive (as is the cedar odor used in many of these experiments). In addition, these repeated pairings led to a conditioning of specific responses that normally occurred with milk infusion, for example, increased activity, mouthing, and probing of the floor (Fig. 6; Johanson, Hall, & Polefrone, 1984). In each case, conditioning was specific to the paired odor and did not occur with various control procedures. More importantly, we found that conditioning did not occur in certain conditions in which behavioral activation was not elicited by the milk-infusion US (e.g., in dehydrated pups or in nondeprived pups, though these pups did show other responses such as mouthing during presentation of the US). That is, activation seemed to predict the occurrence or effectiveness of reinforcement.

The effectiveness of activation in producing reward has been demonstrated by manipulating pups in other ways that independently induce increases in general activity (e.g., familiar odors, Pederson & Blass, 1982; Terry & Johanson, in press; stroking with a soft brush, Sullivan, Hofer, & Brake, 1986). But perhaps the most revealing demonstration has been provided by Moran and co-workers. These investigators showed that electrical stimulation of the medial forebrain bundle (MFB) will reward paddle probing by young pups (i.e., as in Fig. 4; Moran, Lew, & Blass, 1981). Their interesting additional finding was that MFB stimulation in young pups produced a behavioral activation very similar to that seen with milk infusions (Moran et al., 1983); and, like the response to milk, overt activation diminished and behavior became more specific as pups

---

**Fig. 3.** Examples of the profound behavioral activation stimulated in young, deprived pups receiving oral infusions. Pups engage in behaviors that resemble feeding and suckling as well as in other forms of vigorous activity including locomotion, rolling, wall climbing, tumbling, grooming, and responses that resemble lordosis and pelvic thrusting. From Hall (1979). Similar activated responses are seen in young pups receiving medial forebrain bundle stimulation (Moran, Schwartz, & Blass, 1983) or receiving naturally relevant odors (Terry & Johanson, in press). From Hall (1979). Copyright 1979 by the American Psychological Association.

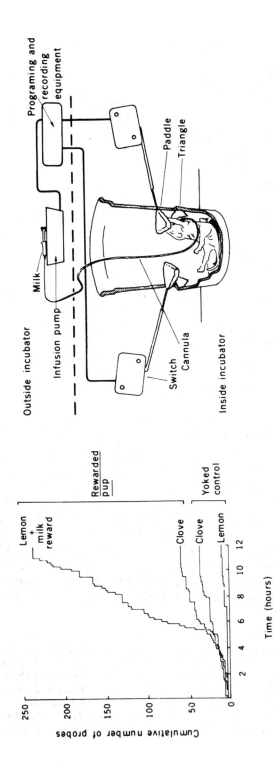

**Fig. 4.** Cumulative record of 1-day-old rewarded pup and yoked control (left) in an operant discrimination task with two odor-labeled paddles (right). Probing into one paddle produced a small oral infusion of milk; probing the other paddle had no effect. The operant chamber is a Styrofoam coffee cup, shown cut-away here. From Johanson & Hall (1979), *Science, 205,* 419–421. Copyright 1979 by the AAAS.

grew older. At 15 days of age, pups no longer showed the generalized activational response to MFB stimulation, though they would still work for MFB stimulation reward. That is, stimulation was still rewarding, but the reward process was no longer externalized. These forebrain reward effects fit with findings that pups require an intact forebrain for milk-elicited behavioral activation, though not for ingestive responses (cf. Kornblith & Hall, 1979; Grill & Norgren, 1978, for adult decerebrate rats). Indeed, the waning of activation in older pups may reflect forebrain maturation, particularly cortical maturation, in that it corresponds to the ages when spreading cortical depression first affects behavior (Hicks & D'Amato, 1975). The results of this group of studies argue that early

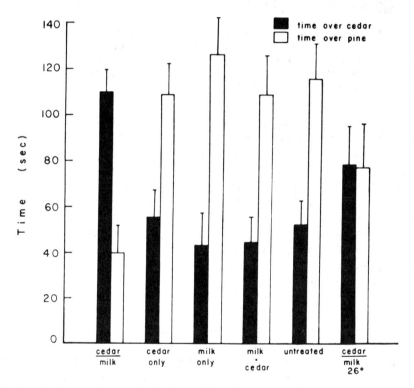

**Fig. 5.** Preference of pups classically conditioned to prefer cedar odor during 20 training pairings. Pups were placed on a screen over a floor with cedar-scented bedding on one side and unscented bedding on the other. Conditioned preference is indicated by a relative difference in the proportion of time spent over cedar. Conditioned pups are the two left-most bars; other values are for various control groups. Each pup received five 1-min trials. From Johanson & Hall (1982), *Developmental Psychobiology, 15,* 379–397. Copyright © 1982 and reprinted by permission of John Wiley & Sons, Inc.

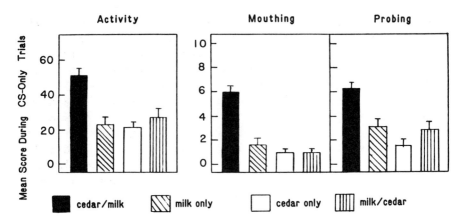

**Fig. 6.** Conditioned responding shown by 6-day-old pups to cedar odor during a CS-only test, 1 hr after training. Increases in activity, mouthing, and probing are seen in the forward conditioned group in comparison to the various controls. Redrawn from Johanson, Hall, & Polefrone (1984), *Developmental Psychobiology, 17,* 357–381. Copyright © 1984 and reprinted by permission of John Wiley & Sons, Inc.

feeding and certain other forms of stimulation are tapping into a generalized substrate for activation and reward, which in the young pup is more obvious and available for analysis. This system of ingestion-related early appetitive behavior, along with the restricted range and frequency of the immature rodent's behavior and its relatively limited previous experience, make for an ideal mammalian preparation in which to study the origins of appetitively based adaptive behavior. While providing a simplified starting point for initial analysis, there remains the opportunity to trace an increasingly complex system as neural maturation and the organism's interaction with its environment deposit successive layers of organizational control and intrigue.

## III. Neural Systems Involved in Early Appetitive Learning

To this system of early feeding-related reward and learning in infant rats, my co-workers and I have been applying the technique of $^{14}C$ 2-DG autoradiography (e.g., Sokoloff, Reivich, Kennedy, Des Rosiers, Patlak, & Pettigrew, 1977) to globally explore its neural substrate. Our first approach has been to carry out a general survey or mapping of brain systems showing activity changes during ingestion-related rewarding and conditioning experiences. 2-DG autoradiograms are used for sampling relative regional metabolic activity during relevant behavioral events. Briefly, radioactive 2-DG is injected into pups. This antimetabolite of glucose is taken up by cells, neurons for example, in the same manner and at the same rate as glucose but accumulates in the cell as 2-deoxyglucose-6-phosphate (Sokoloff *et al.,* 1977; though see Hawkins & Miller, 1978, and Sacks, Sacks, Badalamenti, & Fleischer, 1982, who question the fate of 2-DG—primarily a concern when actual rates of glucose utilization are being quantified). When brains are sectioned and placed on x-ray film, the resulting images reveal areas of greatest 2-DG incorporation (that is, those areas with the greatest metabolic activity during the incorporation period) as the areas of greatest darkness. Local metabolic activity has been shown to vary with neural activity (see Sokoloff, 1982, for review), and it is assumed that the two are monotonically related. These differences in activity are apparent by visual inspection of autoradiograms or in computer-enhanced versions (Fig. 7) and can be measured densitometrically (e.g., Gallistel, Piner, Allen, Adler, Yadin, & Negin, 1982; Plum, Gjedde, & Samson, 1976; density data reported here are of the type considered "semiquantitative," for they are expressed relative to other regions of the brain rather than transformed to actual metabolic rate; the caption to Fig. 9 provides a further explanation of the procedures). When density measurements are made in an extensive number of areas, the properties of 2-DG autoradiography can provide a descriptive map of the relative activity of regions throughout the brain. In work described here, 140 neural areas (Table I) were sampled from the front to the back of 6-day-old pups' brains. We were then able to compare these relative activities between groups of animals experiencing different conditions during the 2-DG uptake period.

## IV.  Neural Activity during the Unconditioned Response

In following sections, I present preliminary data from our neural mapping studies of the effects of oral infusions of milk and of appetitive classical conditioning of oral responses in 6-day-old pups. In some cases, the number of subjects in each group is small and the data merely suggestive; however, this material is intended as an example of an approach, not as a final or complete analysis.

### A.  Response Component

First, as an assessment of the working of the method, we attempted to map regions involved in the unconditional response (UR) of mouthing and licking in response to orally infused milk. We injected 2-DG into nonde-

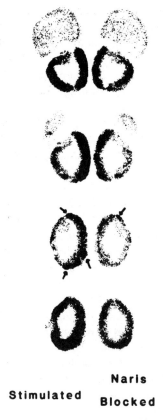

**Naris**

**Stimulated**  **Blocked**

**Fig. 7.** Olfactory system structures in pups receiving unilateral olfactory stimulation shown in 2-DG autoradiograms. Naris on the right was plugged. Increased activity is apparent in the olfactory bulb and anterior olfactory nucleus; specific focuses of activity are apparent as well. This figure replicates similar work by Sharp, Kauer, & Shepherd (1975) in adults and demonstrates the operation of the 2-DG method with olfactory function in the young rat pup (see text for reference to other 2-DG developmental studies on olfaction).

prived pups that then simply received the milk US in small repeated infusions during the 1-hr 2-DG incorporation period (in all of these experiments infusions of milk were made through cannulas located on the posterior portion of pup's tongues so that similar reflexive mouthing and swallowing would be triggered in all groups; repeated infusions were made to maximally stimulate the neural systems of interest during the 2-DG incorporation period). Measurements of 2-DG incorporated in the brains of these pups were compared to those of brains from a group of control

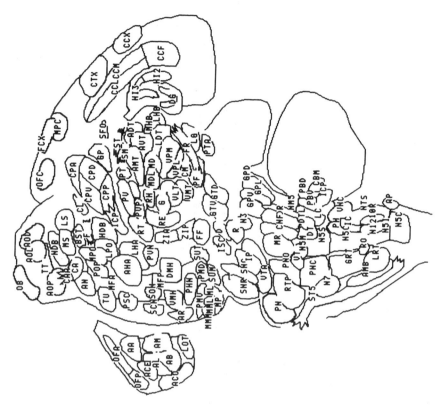

**Fig. 8.** Legend for schematic depiction of changes in regional activity in pup autoradiograms. Areas measured are plotted in a two-dimensional caricature of their location in the brain. Length of the region provides a relative index of the number of sections from which samples were obtained. Abbreviations used are in Table I.

pups, also nondeprived, that received no stimulation during the incorporation period. Comparisons between groups were based on contrasts of area means generated by transformation of the individual optical density measurements for each brain into Z scores; these scores were then averaged over groups and compared in terms of their individual variability (e.g., Gallistel *et al.*, 1982). They are presented on a summary schematic (Fig. 8) representing, in an anterior–posterior fashion, a densitometric mapping of differences in relative brain activity between the two groups.

In brains of pups that were receiving the US (in comparison to controls), increases in activity occurred in the hindbrain (Fig. 9), primarily in cranial nerve motor and sensory nuclei associated with ingestive re-

## Table I

Neural Regions Measured and Their
Abbreviations

| | |
|---|---|
| 10L | dors.motor nu.vagus, left |
| 10R | dors.motor nu.vagus, right |
| AA | ant.amygdaloid area |
| AB | basal amygdaloid nu. |
| ACE | cent.amygdaloid nu. |
| ACO | cortical amygdaloid nu. |
| ADT | anterodors.thal.nu. |
| AHA | ant.hypothal.area |
| AL | lat.amygdaloid nu. |
| AM | med.amygdaloid nu. |
| AMB | ambiguus nu. |
| AMT | anteromed.thal.nu. |
| AN | accumbens nu. |
| AOD | ant.olf.nu., dors. |
| AOL | ant.olf.nu., lat. |
| AOP | ant.olf.nu., post. |
| AP | area postrema |
| AR | arcuate nu. |
| AVT | anterovent.thal.nu. |
| BST | bed nu.stria terminalis |
| CA | ant.commissure |
| CAA | ant.commissure, ant. |
| CBM | med.cerebellar nu. |
| CCF | corpus callosum, forceps major |
| CCL | corpus callosum, lat. |
| CCM | corpus callosum, med. |
| CCX | cingulate cortex |
| CL | claustrum |
| CM | cent.med.thal.nu. |
| CNF | cuneiform nu. |
| CPA | caudate putamen, ant. |
| CPD | caudate putamen, dors. |
| CPP | caudate putamen, post. |
| CPV | caudate putamen, vent. |
| CTX | frontoparietal cortex |
| D | nu.of Darkschewitsch |
| DG | dentate gyrus |
| DMH | dorsomed.hypothal.nu. |
| DR | dors.raphe nu. |
| DT | dors.tegmental nu. |
| DTL | laterodors.tegmental nu. |
| F | fornix |
| FCX | frontoparietal cortex, ant. |
| FF | nu.fields of Forel |
| FR | fasciculus retroflexus |
| G | gelatinosus thal.nu. |
| GP | globus pallidus |

**Table I** *Continued*

| | |
|---|---|
| GPD | cent.gray, pons, dors. |
| GPL | cent.gray, pons, lat. |
| GPV | cent.gray, pons, vent. |
| GRT | gigantocellular reticular nu. |
| GTD | cent.gray, thal., dors. |
| GTV | cent.gray, thal., vent. |
| HDB | nu.horz.limb diagonal band |
| HI2 | hippocampus, CA2 |
| HI3 | hippocampus, CA3 |
| IC | intercalated nu. |
| ICP | internal capsule |
| IP | interpeduncular nu. |
| ISC | intersitital nu.of Cajal |
| LC | locus ceruleus |
| LDT | laterodors.thal.nu. |
| LG | lat.geniculate nu. |
| LHA | lat.hypothal.area |
| LHB | lat.habenular nu. |
| LOT | nu.lat.olf.tract |
| LPO | lat.preoptic nu. |
| LRT | lat.reticular nu. |
| LS | lat.septal nu. |
| MD | mediodors.thal.nu. |
| MDL | mediodors.thal.nu., lat. |
| MFA | med.forebrain bundle, ant. |
| MFP | med.forebrain bundle, post. |
| MHB | med.habenular nu. |
| ML | lat.mammillary nu. |
| MML | med.mammillary nu., lat. |
| MMM | med.mammillary nu., med. |
| MP | post.mammillary nu. |
| MPC | med.prefrontal cortex |
| MPO | med.preoptic nu. |
| MR | median raphe |
| MS | med.septal nu. |
| N12 | hypoglossal nu. |
| N3 | oculomotor nu. |
| N5C | spinal trigem.nu., caudal |
| N5I | spinal trigem.nu., interpositus |
| N5M | trigem.motor nu. |
| N5O | spinal trigem.nu., oral |
| N5S | principal trigem.sensory nu. |
| N7 | facial nu. |
| NDB | nu.diagonal band |
| NM5 | mesenceph.trigeminal nu. |
| NTS | nu.solitary tr. |
| OB | olf.bulb, med.mitral cell layer |
| OFA | olfactory cortex, ant. |
| OFC | orbitofrontal cortex |
| OFP | olfactory cortex, post. |

*(continued)*

**Table I** *Continued*

| | |
|---|---|
| PBD | dors.parabrachial nu. |
| PBV | vent.parabrachial nu. |
| PF | parafascicular thal.nu. |
| PH | prepositus hypoglossal nu. |
| PHN | post.hypothal.nu |
| PMD | premammillary nu., dors. |
| PMV | premammillary nu., vent. |
| PN | pontine nuclei |
| PNC | pontine reticular nu., caudal |
| PNO | pontine reticular nu., oral |
| POP | preoptic periventricular nu. |
| PSC | preoptic suprachiasmatic nu. |
| PT | paratenial thal.nu. |
| PTA | prectectal area |
| PV | paraventricular thal.nu. |
| PVN | paraventricular nu., magnocel. |
| PVP | paraventricular thal.nu., post |
| R | red nu. |
| RE | reuniens thal.nu. |
| RH | rhomboid thal.nu. |
| RO | nu.of Roller |
| RT | reticular thal.nu. |
| RTP | reticulotegmental nu., pons |
| SCN | suprachiasmatic nu. |
| SFO | subfornical organ |
| SM | stria medullaris |
| SNC | substantia nigra, compact |
| SNR | substantia nigra, reticular |
| SON | supraoptic nu. |
| ST | stria terminalis |
| STS | spinal tr.trigem.nerve |
| SUM | supramammillary nu. |
| SUT | subthal.nu. |
| TT | tenia tecta |
| TU | olf.tubercle |
| VLT | ventrolat.thal.nu. |
| VMH | ventromed.hypothal.nu. |
| VMT | ventromed.thal.nu. |
| VNC | vestibular nuclear complex |
| VPL | ventropost.thal.nu., lat. |
| VMP | ventropost.thal.nu., med. |
| VT | vent.tegmental nu. |
| VTA | vent.tegmental area |
| WML | cerebellar white matter, left |
| WMR | cerebellar white matter, right |
| ZIA | zona incerta, ant. |
| ZIP | zona incerta, post. |

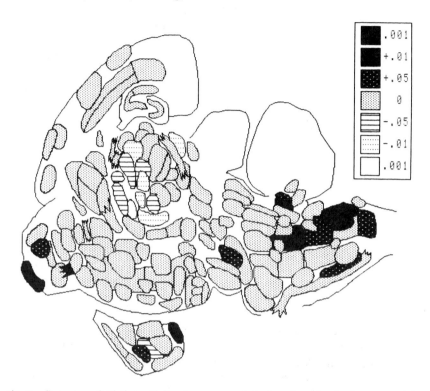

**Fig. 9.** Summary of relative activity changes seen in brains of nondeprived pups receiving oral infusions compared to control pups. Measurements for each brain were first expressed as standard scores and were then averaged between groups. After finding a significant overall difference between brains (by ANOVA), individual comparisons were made for each area. They are plotted here in terms of increasing levels of statistical confidence (i.e., in terms of the area's variability between subjects). Areas showing increased relative metabolic activity compared to control values are plotted with increasing darkness. Areas of decreased relative activity are increasingly light. Areas showing no significant differences are stipled gray ($n$'s = 8).

sponses (e.g., the hypoglossal, ambiguus, and trigeminal nuclei, and nucleus of the solitary tract). This activity presumably reflects the mouthing and swallowing that occurred during milk infusions. Increased activity was also apparent in parabrachial nuclei and the central amygdaloid nucleus (probably reflecting taste and other oral sensory effects; e.g., Norgren, 1983) as well as in some olfactory regions (the nucleus of the lateral olfactory tract and part of the anterior commissure; milk infusions provided pups with odor stimulation). General decreases in activity were seen in the thalamus of these fed animals; these changes are perhaps a result of the fact that control animals were typically asleep during the incorporation period, whereas pups receiving the US were repeatedly stimulated and awake and alert (metabolic changes related to sleep have been observed in the thalamus of adult rats, Ramm & Frost, 1983). The main point here is that the mouthing response to infused milk, which becomes a part of the conditioned response (CR) (after appropriate experience), is reflected in brainstem activity of oral, sensory, and motor structures and is revealed by this application of the 2-DG method. Thus, while 2-DG autoradiography as applied here may have limited sensitivity and resolution, it is capable of detecting certain events (though probably not all) related to ingestive responding and thus may reveal components and effects of the conditioning process.

## B.  Substrates of Activation/Reward

Oral milk infusions only appear to be behaviorally activating and rewarding when provided to pups deprived of the mother and food (Bornstein, Terry, Browde, Assimon, & Hall, in press). Thus, in an appetitive conditioning situation in which deprived pups are receiving the milk US, not only are oral motor responses engaged, but so are those that subserve activation and, we presume, those that produce milk's reinforcing effect. Neural systems involved in activation might be identified by comparing autoradiographic measurements from brains of *deprived* pups that are receiving repeated milk infusions to those of brains of control pups (nondeprived, not fed). When this is done (Fig. 10), it can be seen that besides the ingestion-related increases in brainstem activity and thalamic activity already noted, profound changes in activity occur throughout the brain, particularly in the basal forebrain (e.g., the hypothalamus, amygdala, and MFB). These effects are consistent with the data for a basal forebrain role in the behavioral activation and reward to infant rodents, as discussed. The activated regions also overlap regions associated with brain stimulation reward, particularly those recently demonstrated using similar 2-DG methods (Yadin, Guarini, & Gallistel, 1983; Porrino, Esposito, Seeger, Crane, Pert, & Sokoloff, 1984; Roberts, 1980). Unfortunately, for our understanding of the critical features of reward, the situation is complicated here by the fact that some of these changes result from deprivation itself, but others result from the fact that deprived pups are feeding. A separation of these processes can be accomplished with comparisons to other appropriate groups. For example, the effects of deprivation alone can be compared to the effects of ingestion in deprived pups. This comparison would provide an indication of the activity changes that go on in the brains of deprived pups that are ingesting (i.e., changes in regional activity in addition to those produced by deprivation). Areas revealed would represent output components for the UR/CR as well as candidates

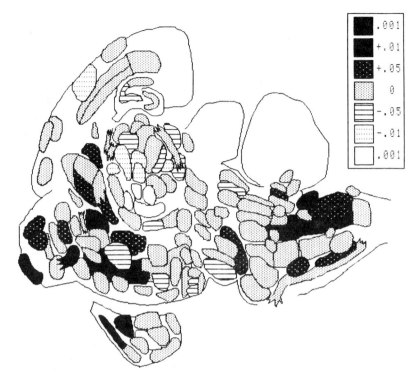

**Fig. 10.** Activity changes seen in brains of deprived pups receiving oral infusions compared to nondeprived, nonfed controls. (Note that this comparison contrasts pups in very different behavioral and metabolic states and as such may reveal some artifactual effects; $n$'s = 5.)

for systems involved with reinforcement. In addition, we have recently found that after deprivation with nonlactating mothers, pups show vigorous ingestion but no behavioral excitement (Bornstein *et al.*, in press). By comparing groups deprived with nonlactating foster mothers to incubator-deprived pups, the neural effects of deprivation that are responsible for activation may be identified. This ability to manipulate activation thus allows us to compare the brains of equivalently nutritionally deprived pups (either those that are ingesting or those that are not) whose systems for activation and, presumably, reward are not equivalently engaged.

## V. The CS and Results of CS/US Pairings

In the appetitive classical conditioning paradigm that we have been studying (e.g., Fig. 5 and 6), a novel odor that is initially somewhat aversive to pups and elicits no obvious ingestive responses comes to be preferred and to elicit mouthing, probing, and activity after only a few pairings with milk. I have shown how a 2-DG autoradiographic analysis can be used to map systems involved in producing ingestive responses and in behavioral activation. Metabolic mapping may also be useful in tracking the neural effects of an odor stimulus in the brains of pups that have had different recent experiences. Such a use of 2-DG has been pioneered by Coopersmith and Leon (1984) to evaluate the effects of extensive early odor experiences in olfactory structures. These methods have also been effectively applied to auditory classical conditioning in rats (Gonzalez-Lima & Scheich, 1984), but there has been limited analysis of the process of appetitive conditioning. Our strategy has been to evaluate the effect of the odor stimulus, both before and after pups have had experience with it. At the most straightforward level, the idea is to map the different or additional structures that are activated in pups that have received conditioning experiences.

## A. CS Alone

As indicated by Fig. 7, odor stimulation with novel odors activates olfactory structures in the bulb and anterior olfactory nuclei (a finding already well documented for adults, e.g., Sharp *et al.*, 1975, and Stewart, Kauer, & Shepherd, 1979, and for pups, e.g., Astic & Saucier, 1982; Greer, Stewart, Teicher, & Shepherd, 1982). In preliminary analyses, we also have seen that stimulation with a novel odor produces a general decrease in thalamic and supraoptic activity as well as an increased activity in the frontal cortex, subfornical organ, substantia nigra, and pontine reticular regions. The comparison controls were brains of similarly deprived pups receiving no stimulation. Thus, in response to a novel odor, pups show changes in neural activity in primary and some secondary olfactory structures as well as other regions that may be involved in orienting toward or away from novel odors. These descriptive findings provide a baseline against which to assess the effects of conditioning on responsiveness to the odor.

## B. Effects of Previous Conditioning

Analysis of the effects of odor stimulation in brains of pups that have experienced olfactory conditioning provide the most intriguing information in this series of analyses. Figure 11 contrasts brains of groups of three pups that an hour earlier had received either forward olfactory conditioning or backward pairings. Both groups, then, during the 2-DG incorporation period, received the same CS (in the absence of other stimulation)

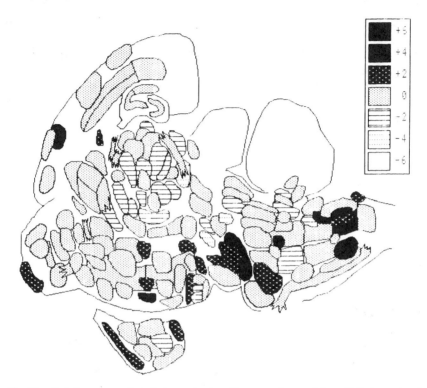

**Fig. 11.** Relative comparison between brains of groups of pups (*n*'s = 3) that previously received either forward training trials or backward training trials that were experiencing the CS alone during the 2-DG uptake period. Because of the small sample, differences are expressed in terms of the number of SEMs separating means rather than as significance values.

and thus only differed in the nature of previous odor and milk pairings (as well as in their response to the CS only). Note, first, that the effects of conditioning reach the brainstem motor response system (e.g., the hypoglossal, vagal, and trigeminal motor nuclei). What was apparent in pups' behavior thus also appears represented as changes in neural activity: Motor systems for ingestive responses are engaged by the CS. Second, while odor produces some common metabolic changes in olfactory structures that are thus not apparent in the figure, other olfactory structures are preferentially activated in conditioned pups (e.g., the medial posterior olfactory bulb, olfactory cortex, and nucleus of the lateral olfactory tract). Moreover, there are activity differences in measured regions of the thalamus, midbrain, basal forebrain, and frontal cortex.

These comparisons provide a global, if somewhat irresolute, impression of the effects of conditioning and the expression of learning. In the brains of untrained pups, the effects of olfactory stimulation with the CS are somewhat limited. In particular, they do not appear to gain access to the forebrain, midbrain, or hindbrain regions that show altered activity in response to the same stimulus after conditioning. These regions may be involved in mediating the effects of learning or in producing the CR (or feedback from it). Further analysis will be required to identify their relative roles.

Unfortunately, our application of the 2-DG method only speaks strongly about discovered effects. The survey method may be insensitive to other relevant or informative changes in localized regions of sampled areas, or we may have failed to sample critical regions. These are thus only initial steps toward understanding the effects of learning in this simple appetitive conditioning system. The approach is promising, however, to the extent that further analysis and identification of activated pathways can be accomplished, particularly those differentiating initial responses to odor stimulation by the untrained brain, on the one hand, and those recruiting the motor-neuron-pool output system in conditioned brains, on the other.

## VI.  What Happens during Conditioning?

A parallel 2-DG analysis involves studying the neural activity of brains of pups that are in the process of learning (as opposed to studying the results of learning as above). This involves comparing brains of animals undergoing forward conditioning training to those that are undergoing backward or random conditioning experiences (i.e., 2-DG injected just before a 1-hr period of training). In all cases, pups receive equivalent CS/odor and US/milk infusion stimulation during the incorporation period, and all pups show equivalent behavior and ingestion. The only differences between the groups is in the timing of the experiences; in the case of forward versus backward conditioning, there is simply a 10-s difference in the onset to the CS. Our previous behavioral analysis of this form of early conditioning (e.g., Johanson *et al.*, 1984) indicated that learning was apparent after only 5–10 pairings of the CS/US. Thus learning should be occurring around the time of maximal 2-DG incorporation, and the differences between the brains of these groups should reflect primarily differences in stimulus timing that produce the observed conditioning. (This is not to suggest that there are not other effects—e.g., other forms of learning—occurring in control pups but that the behavioral distinction between classical conditioning of ingestive responses represents a relevant distinction between them.)

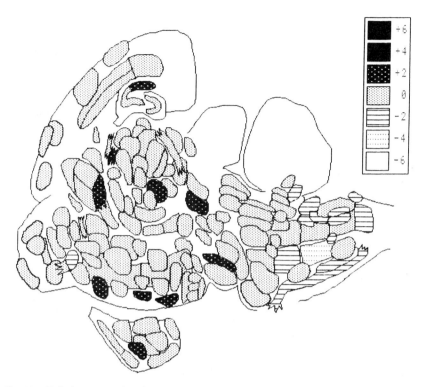

**Fig. 12.** Relative comparison between brains of groups of pups (*n*'s = 4) in which 2-DG was being incorporated during forward versus backward training. Differences are again expressed in terms of SEMs of difference.

Figure 12 depicts the differences in surveyed regional brain activity between groups of four pups receiving forward conditioning versus backward conditioning training. What is revealed here are detectable neural activity increases, primarily in the basal forebrain, thalamus, and hippocampus, due only to ongoing difference in the CS/US relationship. Structures showing changes similar to those detected *after* conditioning were the suprachiasmatic nucleus, substantia nigra, and pontine reticular nucleus. Several other areas also showed differences in both comparisons, though in opposite directions: the ventrolateral thalamic, hypoglossal, and vagal nuclei and the area postrema. Because of their involvement during both training and later recognition, both of these categories of regions become particularly interesting candidates for substrates of the conditioning process. In addition, note that in this comparison of brains undergoing training, several olfaction-related structures were differentially activated (e.g., the olfactory tubercle, hippocampus, and central amygdaloid nucleus), though none of these were common to olfactory structures that were differentially activated by the CS after conditioning. Systems showing such separable effects may play roles in detecting differences among the training conditions and the processes responsible for encoding their effects but may not participate during later expression of the learned responses.

As noted earlier, a major problem with the 2-DG technique is its insensivity. Failure to see an effect in a given area cannot be confidently taken as a demonstration that no effect occurred. Moreover, because 2-DG effects may represent activities of cell bodies or of terminal regions (e.g., Lippe, Steward, & Rubel, 1980), there may be more overlap in activated systems between training and testing conditions than is initially apparent. Note, as well, that the sample sizes were small in these last two experiments and that these data are presented primarily for illustrative purposes.

## VII.  The Process of Simple Appetitive Conditioning in Rat Pups

I have attempted to illustrate the manner in which characteristics of infant rodents make them particularly valuable in the analysis of the ontogeny of appetitive behavior and perhaps in understanding appetitively based conditioning processes. These advantages accrue, first, from the fact that young pups are normally inactive and do few things to confound neurobehavioral analyses and, second, because rapid and reliable appetitive classical conditioning can be obtained in them. More significantly, operation of their reward or reinforcement system is behaviorally obvious, apparently undifferentiated, and available for analysis. These characteristics permit the use of broad mapping techniques, like 2-DG autoradiography as a starting point for characterizing the neural effects of ingestive, activational, and conditioning stimuli and pairings of these stimuli. As shown here, effects of such ongoing activity can be seen pervasively across the brain. With further refinement of metabolic mapping techniques, both spatially and temporally, and careful application of specific behavioral manipulations to this behavioral system of infants, it should be possible to isolate and identify means by which experiences alter appetitive responses.

### Acknowledgments

I am grateful to D. Kucharski, C. Phifer, and L. Terry, for comments on an earlier draft of this paper, and to D. Kucharski and J. Browde for collecting and analyzing much of the 2-DG data.

## References

Astic, L., & Saucier, D. (1982). Ontogenesis of the functional activity of rat olfactory bulb: Autoradiographic study with the 2-deoxyglucose method. *Developmental Brain Research, 2,* 243–256.

Blass, E. M., & Cramer, C. P. (1982). Analogy and homology in the development of ingestive behavior. In A. R. Morrison & P. L. Strick (Eds.), *Changing concepts of the nervous system* (pp. 503–523). New York: Academic Press.

Bornstein, B., Terry, L., Browde, J. A., Jr., Assimon, S. A., & Hall, W. G. (in press). Sensory and nutritional contributions to rat pups' early activational response to ingestion.

Coopersmith, R., & Leon, M. (1984). Enhanced neural response to familiar olfactory cues. *Science, 225,* 849–851.

Drewett, R. F. (1978). The development of motivational systems. *Progressive Brain Research, 48,* 407–417.

Epstein, A. N. (in press). The ontogeny of ingestive behaviors: Control of milk intake by suckling rats and the emergence of feeding and drinking at weaning. In R. Ritter, S. Ritter, & C. D. Barnes (Eds.), *Neural and humoral controls of food intake.* Academic Press, New York.

Gallistel, C. R., Piner, C., Allen, T. O., Adler, N. T., Yadin, E., & Negin, M. (1982). Computer assisted analysis of 2-deoxyglucose autoradiographs. *Neuroscience and Biobehavioral Reviews, 6,* 409–420.

Gonzalez-Lima, F., & Scheich, H. (1984). Neural substrates for tone-conditioned bradycardia demonstrated with 2-deoxyglucose. I. Activation of auditory nuclei. *Behavioral Brain Research, 14,* 213–233.

Greer, C. A., Stewart, W. B., Teicher, M. H., & Shepherd, G. M. (1982). Functional development of the olfactory bulb and a unique glomerular complex in the neonatal rat. *Journal of Neuroscience, 2,* 1744–1759.

Grill, H. J., & Norgren, R. (1978). The taste reactivity test: II. Mimetic responses to gustatory stimuli in chronic thalamic and chronic decerebrate rats. *Brain Research, 143,* 281–297.

Hall, W. G. (1979a). Feeding and behavioral activation in infant rats. *Science, 205,* 206–209.

Hall, W. G. (1979b). The ontogeny of feeding in rats: I. Ingestive and behavioral responses to oral infusions. *Journal of Comparative and Physiological Psychology, 93,* 977–1000.

Hall, W. G. (1985). What we know and don't know about the development of independent ingestion in rats. *Appetite, 6,* 333–356.

Hall, W. G., & Bryan, T. E. (1980). The ontogeny of feeding in rats: II. Independent ingestive behavior. *Journal of Comparative and Physiological Psychology, 94,* 746–756.

Hall, W. G., & Williams, C. L. (1983). Suckling isn't feeding, or is it? A search for developmental continuities. In J. S. Rosenblatt, R. A. Hinde, C. Beer, & M. C. Busnel (Eds.), *Advances in the study of behavior* (Vol. 13, pp. 218–254). New York: Academic Press.

Hawkins, R. A., & Miller, A. L. (1978). Loss of radioactive 2-deoxy-D-glucose-6-phosphate from brains of conscious rats. *Neuroscience, 3,* 251–258.

Hicks, S. P., & D'Amato, C. J. (1975). Moto-sensory cortex-corticospinal system and developing locomotion and placing in rats. *American Journal of Anatomy, 143,* 1–42.

Johanson, I. B., & Hall, W. G. (1979). Appetitive learning in 1-day-old rat pups. *Science, 205,* 419–421.

Johanson, I. B., & Hall, W. G. (1980). The ontogeny of feeding in rats: III. Thermal determinants of early ingestive behavior. *Journal of Comparative and Physiological Psychology, 94*, 977–992.

Johanson, I. B., & Hall, W. G. (1982). Appetitive conditioning in neonatal rats: Conditioned orientation to a novel odor. *Developmental Psychobiology, 15*, 379–397.

Johanson, I. B., Hall, W. G., & Polefrone, J. M. (1984). Appetitive conditioning in neonatal rats: Conditioned ingestive responding to stimuli paired with oral infusions of milk. *Developmental Psychobiology, 17*, 357–381.

Kornblith, C., & Hall, W. G. (1979). Neurological separation of ingestion and behavioral activation in neonatal rats. *Journal of Comparative and Physiological Psychology, 93*, 1109–1117.

Lippe, W. R., Steward, O., & Rubel, E. W. (1980). The effect of unilateral basilar papilla removal upon nuclei laminaris and magnocellularis of the chick examined with ($^3$H)2-deoxy-D-glucose autoradiography. *Brain Research, 196*, 43–58.

Moran, T. H., Lew, M. F., & Blass, E. M. (1981). Intracranial self-stimulation in 3-day-old rats. *Science, 214*, 1366–1368.

Moran, T. H., Schwartz, G. J., & Blass, E. M. (1983). Organized behavioral responses to lateral hypothalamic electrical stimulation in infant rats. *Journal of Neuroscience, 3*, 10–19.

Norgren, R. (1983). Afferent interactions of cranial nerves involved in ingestion. *Journal of the Autonomic Nervous System, 9*, 67–77.

Pedersen, P. E., & Blass, E. M. (1982). Prenatal and postnatal determinants of the 1st suckling episode in albino rats. *Developmental Psychobiology, 15*, 349–355.

Plum, F., Gjedde, A., & Samson, F. E. (Eds.). (1976). Neuroanatomical functional mapping by the radioactive 2-deoxy-D-glucose method. *Neuroscience Research Program Bulletin, 14*, 457–518.

Porrino, L. J., Esposito, R. U., Seeger, T. F., Crane, A. M., Pert, A., & Sokoloff, L. (1984). Metabolic mapping of the brain during rewarding self-stimulation. *Science, 224*, 306–309.

Ramm, P., & Frost, B. J. (1983). Regional metabolic activity in the rat brain during sleep–wake activity. *Sleep, 6*, 196–216.

Roberts, W. W. (1980). ($^{14}$C)Deoxyglucose mapping of first order projections activated by stimulation of lateral hypothalamic sites eliciting gnawing, eating, and drinking in rats. *Journal of Comparative Neurology, 194*, 617–638.

Sacks, W., Sacks, S., Badalamenti, A., & Fleischer, A. (1982). A proposed method for the determination of cerebral regional intermediary glucose metabolism in humans using specifically labeled $^{11}$C-glucose and PETT. *Journal of Neuroscience Research, 7*, 57–69.

Sharp, F., Kauer, J. S., & Shepherd, G. M. (1975). Local sites of activity related glucose metabolism in the rat olfactory bulb during olfactory stimulation. *Brain Research, 98*, 596–600.

Sokoloff, L. (1982). The radioactive DG method: Theory, procedure, and applications for the measurement of local glucose utilization in the CNS. In B. W. Agranoff & M. H. Aprison (Eds.), *Advances in neurochemistry* (Vol. 4, pp. 1–82).

Sokoloff, L., Reivich, M., Kennedy, C., Des Rosiers, M. H., Patlak, C. S., Pettigrew, K. D., Sakurada, O., Shinohara, M. (1977). The (14C)deoxyglucose method for the measurement of local cerebral glucose utilization. *Journal of Neurochemistry, 28*, 897–916.

Stewart, W. B., Kauer, J. S., & Shepard, G. M. (1979). Functional organization of rat olfactory bulb analyzed by 2-deoxyglucose method. *Journal of Comparative Neurology, 185*, 715–734.

Sullivan, R. M., Hofer, M. A., & Brake, S. C. (1986). Olfactory-guided orientation in neonatal rats is enhanced by a conditioned change in behavioral state. *Developmental Psychobiology, 19*, 615–623.

Terry, L. M., & Johanson, I. B. (in press). *The development of the olfactory mediation of the ingestive behavior of infant rats.*

Wirth, J. B., & Epstein, A. N. (1976). The ontogeny of thirst in the infant rat. *American Journal of Physiology, 230*, 188–198.

Yadin, E., Guarini, V., & Gallistel, C. R. (1983). Unilaterally activated systems in rats self-stimulating at sites in the medial forebrain bundle, medial prefrontal cortex, or locus coeruleus. *Brain Research, 266*, 39–50.

# 9

# Experience Effects on the Developing and the Mature Brain: Dendritic Branching and Synaptogenesis

WILLIAM T. GREENOUGH
*Departments of Psychology and Anatomical Sciences
and Neural and Behavioral Biology Program
University of Illinois at Urbana–Champaign
Champaign, Illinois 61820*

## I. Introduction

Most people would agree with the first premise of this chapter, which is that the neural substrates for many effects of experience on early brain development differ from the substrates of learning in the adult. A second premise, with which fewer might agree, is that the neural substrates really look quite a lot like each other and may differ more in how they are regulated than in the underlying processes at the cellular level. Specifically, at least some forms of developmental information storage and adult learning appear to be similar in that they involve the selective preservation of synaptic connections from a larger, previously generated population of connections. However, the two types of information storage appear to differ in the role that experience plays in the *generation* of the larger population of connections—often little or no role of experience seems to be involved in generating connections in early development, whereas experience, through its neural consequences, may play a primary role in the case of adult learning.

Perinatal Development:
A Psychobiological Perspective

**195**

196                                                      William T. Greenough

## II. Synapse Overproduction and Selective Preservation in Developing Sensory and Motor Systems

There is considerable evidence that synapses are produced in early development in significantly larger numbers than ultimately survive to maturity in the innervation of peripheral autonomic and skeletal musculature (e.g., Purves & Lichtman, 1980). Which synapses survive appears to depend upon relative activity in at least some cases, since blockage of activity can slow the elimination of supernumerary connections (W. Thompson, Kuffler, & Jansen, 1979), and increased activity can speed elimination and selectively increase the number of surviving synapses of the stimulated fibers (Ridge & Betz, 1984; W. Thompson, 1983).

An analogous process appears to be widespread in the developing CNS. Perhaps the best evidence that neural activity plays a role in selective preservation of central synapses comes from studies of developing feline and primate visual systems (LeVay, Wiesel, & Hubel, 1980; Wiesel & Hubel, 1963). In these species, projections from corresponding parts of the visual field in the two eyes terminate in adjacent bands, termed *columns,* in the primary visual cortex, and their integration provides the basis for stereoscopic depth perception. As first shown in monkeys, the

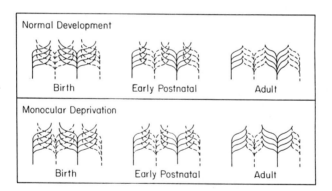

**Fig. 1.**  Highly schematized depiction of ocular dominance column development in normally reared or monocularly deprived monkeys. There is extensive overlap of the axonal branches from the two eyes at birth (left panels). In normal development (top), the competitive interactions result in equal pruning back of axons from each eye in the adult (right panels). After monocular deprivation, however, axons from the nondeprived eye (solid lines) retain more branches, but the axons from the deprived eye (dashed lines) retain fewer branches. From "Age-related Aspects of Experience Effects upon Brain Structure" by W. T. Greenough and H. D. Schwark, 1984, in R. N. Emde and R. J. Harmon (Eds.), *Continuities and Discontinuities in Development,* Hillsdale, NJ: Plenum. Copyright 1984 by Plenum Publishing. Reprinted by permission.

projections overlap one another initially and gradually withdraw to form the well-defined columns of the adult (LeVay *et al.*, 1980; see Fig. 1). Several lines of evidence indicate that axons from the two eyes compete for control of visual cortex neurons and that activity provides an advantage in the competition. The first evidence came from experiments in which patterned vision in one eye was prevented during a sensitive period of development, usually by monocular suture. The physiological and behavioral result was that the deprived eye lost control over the visual cortex: Many fewer visual cortex neurons were activated by stimulation of the deprived eye, and the animal lost visual ability in that eye, the severity of the effects depending upon the timing and duration of the deprivation. A number of mechanisms are involved in the loss of visual control, including inhibition dependent upon activity of the nondeprived eye (Burchfiel & Duffy, 1981; Hubel & Wiesel, 1970; Kratz, Spear, & Smith, 1976; Sherman, Guillery, Kaas, & Sanderson, 1974), but the primary mechanism appears to be a relative loss of visual cortex territory innervated by the deprived eye. The columns of axon termination, normally of equivalent width for the two eyes, become shrunken for the deprived eye and correspondingly expanded for the nondeprived eye (LeVay *et al.*, 1980). The involvement of *patterned* neural activity has been indicated by experiments in which retinal input is blocked pharmacologically and the optic nerves are stimulated. If both nerves are stimulated synchronously, segregation of cortical inputs is retarded; with asynchronous stimulation, columns form; if only one eye's input is blocked, the result is similar to that of eye closure (Stryker, 1981; Stryker & Strickland, 1984).

This process probably involves both the loss of preexisting connections and the formation of new ones, given that there is some reversal if the nondeprived eye is sutured and the deprived eye is opened later in development (reversibility decreases with age), but it is clear that a primary mechanism is the overproduction of synapses involved in the initially overlapping columns and the subsequent failure of the deprived eye to maintain its normal complement of connections. Other studies have shown that the number of synapses per neuron reaches a peak at a time roughly corresponding to the sensitive period and that some of these synapses are subsequently lost (e.g., Boothe, Greenough, Lund, & Wrege, 1979; Cragg, 1975; Rakic, Bourgeois, Eckenhoff, Zecevic, & Goldman-Rakic, 1986; Winfield, 1981). The axons of the deprived eye have fewer synapses than those of the experienced eye, as would be expected (Tieman, 1984). Similar patterns of "exuberant" synaptogenesis followed by elimination are sufficiently widespread to support the assertion that intrinsically generated sytemwide overproduction followed by

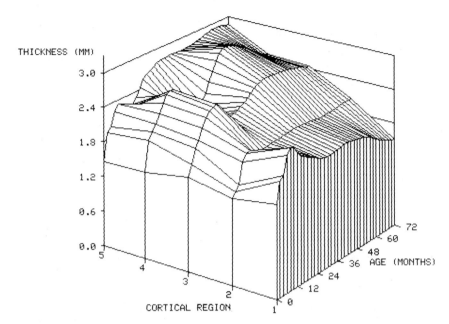

**Fig. 2.** Cortical thickness in humans as a function of age and area (data from Conel, 1939–1967). Postnatal changes in cortical thickness indirectly reflect the addition or deletion of brain components such as synapses, neurons and supporting cells, and blood vessels. The postcentral gyrus (region 1), involved in sensing touch and position for the trunk region, gains most of its thickness around 15 months and then drops off. The striate cortex (region 2), involved in basic visual processing, appears to be growing slowly past 6 years of age. Both the angular gyrus (region 3), involved in spatial perception, and the inferior temporal lobe (region 4), involved in recognition of objects, show a peak thickness at 2 years and then appear to decline before reaching a second peak at 4 years. Prefrontal cortex (region 5), involved in planning and sequencing activities, is adding substantial thickness at 6 years of age. Figure redrawn from "Effects of Experience on Brain Development," by W. T. Greenough, J. E. Black, and C. S. Wallace, *Child Development* (in press).

activity-dependent selective preservation or elimination of synapses is a general feature of early CNS development in mammals (e.g., Brunjes, Schwark, & Greenough, 1982; Ivy & Killackey, 1982; Miriani & Changeaux, 1981).

Rakic *et al.* (1986) have argued, based upon studies of the developing monkey brain, that the overproduction and selection process is synchronous across diverse neocortical regions. They suggest that a "single genetic or humoral signal" may orchestrate the process throughout the brain. Other studies, however, contradict this view. For example, some older, not very well known data on human cerebral cortex development (Conel, 1939–1967), summarized in Fig. 2, indicate rather striking differences in the pattern of growth among different brain regions. The postcentral gyrus, for example, appears to peak in cortical thickness relatively early and then to decline after the 2nd year, whereas the prefrontal cortex appears to grow continuously thicker throughout the first 6 years of life. In what appears to be a parallel to this asynchrony in a macroscopic growth index, Huttenlocher, de Courten, Garey, and Van der Loos (1982) reported that synapse density in the human visual cortex peaked several years before the peak in the human frontal cortex described by Huttenlocher (1979). Stable adult values in the frontal cortex were not achieved until between 7 and 15 years of age, whereas synapse density stablized in the visual cortex by about age 2. There may also be a metabolic parallel to these reports. Chugani and Phelps (1986) reported that glucose utilization in human infants was initially highest in the sensorimotor cortex and only later rose in the frontal cortex. Both the Huttenlocher results suggesting asynchronous synapse stabilization processes and the Rakic *et al.* work suggesting synchrony are based upon synapse density measurements. As illustrated later, a more appropriate measure of rates of synapse formation and elimination when the number of neurons remains constant is the number of synapses per neuron.

This issue is not merely a technical controversy; an important question regarding brain development is involved. Turkewitz and Kenny (1982; see also Black & Greenough, 1986) suggested that brain maturation occurred in a sequential manner, such that information incorporated in earlier maturing structures could be utilized in the organization of new ones. If synapse overproduction and loss were determined to be synchronous across most of the cerebral cortex, this proposal would seem improbable.

The issue of *why* developing systems are so labile to the whim of experience is an important one. Would it not be better to have one's sensory systems impervious to potential environmental insult? With the exception of many mammalian and possibly some avian species, this appears to be the case, but it may be that the detailed pattern and stereoscopic capabilities of visual systems of higher mammals require more precision in their organization than intrinsic mechanisms can provide. In the absence of neuroscientists, their normal environments provide a range of stimuli that can be used to fine-tune and integrate sensory and motor systems. Since these qualities of the rearing environment have been relatively stable throughout the evolutionary history of the species, they have evolved mechanisms, such as synapse overproduction and selection, to take advantage of environmental information. We have previously termed this form of developmental storage of environmentally originating information *experience-expectant* (Black & Greenough, 1986) to reflect the concept that the developing nervous system expects that certain qualities of stimulation will be provided by the environment at the time they are needed. If abnormal patterns of stimulation are provided, an abnormal pattern of neural organization results because the temporally locked synapse overproduction and preservation–loss process is specified by whatever experiences occur.

What causes the initial overproduction of synapses is uncertain, but the impulse activity of the neurons involved seems insufficient to account for it. Both peripheral and central synapses appear capable of forming in the absence of activity, although the number of synapses may be reduced and their properties altered (e.g., Cohen, 1972; Van Huizen, Romijn, & Habets, 1985). There is evidence that the peak number of synapses per neuron reached during development in the cat visual cortex is reduced by visual deprivation (Winfield, 1981), suggesting that activity stimulates some synapse formation, although this may reflect loss of synapses at the same time that new ones are forming.

## III. Is Developmental Plasticity Modulated by Hormones or Neurotransmitters?

Given that neural activity is not a sufficient explanation, it is of much interest to know whether other intrinsic signals modulate the overproduction-selection process. The obvious candidates—hormones, neuromodulators, and neurotransmitters—are legion, and space limitations prevent a full discussion. (A more detailed discussion of known roles of a number of candidates appears in Lauder & Krebs, 1986.)

A hormone that appears to have some potential is thyroxine, given that it appears to perform some timing functions in amphibian maturation (Allen, 1938) and because it appears responsible for (or capable of) triggering the developmental shift from cell proliferation to migration and process extension in the cerebellum (Nicholson & Altman, 1972). Administration of excess neonatal thyroxine triggers precocious development of a number of basic behavioral patterns (Eayrs, 1964; Schapiro & Norman, 1967; Schapiro, Salas, & Vukovitch, 1970; Stone & Greenough, 1975) and sensory abilities, including olfaction (Brunjes & Alberts, 1980, 1981). We (Brunjes et al., 1982) examined effects of excess neonatal thyroxine administration on the postnatal process of overproduction and loss of dendritic material in olfactory bulb granule cells. As Fig. 3 indicates, there was no evidence that the rate of the overproduction–loss process was affected by excess thyroxine, suggesting, at least for this system, that it does not regulate developmental experience-expectant mechanisms.

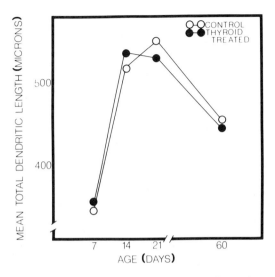

**Fig. 3.**   Dendritic fields of granule cells of the olfactory bulb reach a peak size during development and then decline to smaller adult size. Neonatal treatment with thyroxine did not noticeably affect either the overproduction of dendrites or the subsequent loss. From Brunjes, Schwark, & Greenough (1982). © 1982 by Elsevier.

A candidate neurotransmitter/neuromodulator that has come into some prominence recently as a possible regulator of developmental plasticity is norepinephrine (NE), following reports by Kasamatsu and Pettigrew (1976, 1979) that administration of 6-hydroxydopamine (6-OHDA), which destroys noradrenergic innervation, prevents the shift in eye dominance of visual cortical neurons that normally occurs in kittens when one eye is briefly deprived of vision. Several more recent studies have suggested that this phenomenon may be a result of toxic effects of local visual cortex 6-OHDA administration, since it does not occur with systemic or more general treatments or with different drugs that also deplete NE (Bear & Daniels, 1983; Daw, Robertson, Rader, Videen, & Coscia, 1984; Daw, Videen, Parkinson, & Rader, 1985). Bear and Singer (1986) have determined that the effects of 6-OHDA in the original studies may have been due to the drug's damaging both NE and Ach projections to the visual cortex, because they found, using a different procedure, that combined damage to both systems was necessary for the visual development effects. However, reports that manipulations thought to be selective to NE systems affect adult learning (Gold, 1984), late developmental plasticity (Mirmiran & Uylings, 1983; O'Shea, Saari, Pappas, Ings, & Stange, 1983), and the morphology of developing neurons (Felten, Hallman, & Jonsson, 1982) suggest that it may have a developmental role independent of ACh. Studies of the effects of short-term noradrenergic manipulations on the adult brain suggest that NE may truly act as a "modulator" of neural responsiveness, suppressing "spontaneous" or background activity while enhancing evoked responses to activation of inhibitory or excitatory afferents (Foote, Bloom, & Aston-Jones, 1983; Waterhouse & Woodward, 1980). Such a role might be more compatible with effects on the preservation or stabilization process itself than with effects on the generation of connections. If preservation involved the oft-invoked Hebb (1949) synapse concept, in which correlated pre- and postsynaptic activity was necessary to bring about change, then a modulator of this sort could increase the organizing influences of active afferents while suppressing consequences of less systematic local background activity.

Some recent data from our laboratory supports this prediction. Loeb, Chang, and Greenough (1986) examined the effects of neonatal 6-OHDA administration upon the organization of the somatosensory cortical barrels that subserve initial cortical information processing from the large facial whiskers, or mystacial vibrissae, in mice and certain other mammals (Welker & Woolsey, 1974; Woolsey & Van der Loos, 1970). Each barrel is associated primarily with a single vibrissa, and deletion of the vibrissa and its follicle in the periphery during early development disrupts the process of organization of the barrel (Harris & Woolsey, 1981; Killackey, Belford, Ryugo, & Ryugo, 1976; Van der Loos & Woolsey, 1973). The barrels are organized into rows corresponding to the rows of vibrissae on the face (Simons & Woolsey, 1979; Welker, 1971), and deleting a row of vibrissae results in the transformation of a presumptive row of barrels into an elongated, relatively undifferentiated structure termed a *barreloid*. Barrels have their appearance because the nerve cells comprising them tend to be grouped in the walls of a cylindrically shaped structure in Layer IV of the cortex and to extend much of their dendrite into the central hollow, where the thalamic afferent fibers are concentrated (Killackey & Leshin, 1975; White, 1978; Woolsey, Dierker, & Wann, 1975).

We reasoned that if the normal developmental role of NE was to sharpen the distinction between somatosensory (thalamic) afferent and background activity, then its absence would lead to a more loosely organized barrel, because the degree to which these afferents influenced its organization would be reduced. To test this, we examined barrels of adult mice that had been treated neonatally with 6-OHDA, which reduced somatosensory cortical NE levels by 96–98%. The results generally agreed with this hypothesis. First, there was no difference in the size of nerve cell dendritic fields in the treated and control groups, suggesting that NE does not promote synaptogenesis, at least of a type that is permanent.

Second, barrels in 6-OHDA–treated mice had a basically normal cellular organization, as Lidov and Molliver (1982) previously reported. The consequence of 6-OHDA treatment was that barrels had a less rigidly organized dendritic pattern than in controls. Dendrites of the spiny non-

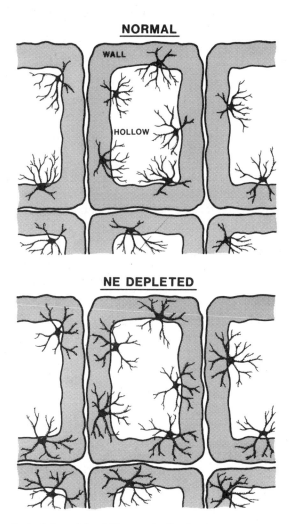

**Fig. 4.** Schematic depiction of dendritic organization in mouse somatosensory cortex barrels of controls or after 6-OHDA treatment that destroys NE-containing nerve terminals (after Loeb, Chang, & Greenough, 1986). Normally, dendrites exhibit a strong tendency to grow into the hollows of the barrels, whether the cell bodies from which they arise are in the hollow or the cell-rich wall. After 6-OHDA treatment, this tendency is reduced. The effect is overemphasized for clarity in this depiction.

pyramidal cells that receive most specific thalamic afferent input in barrels simply "showed less respect" for the boundary between the wall and hollow in the drug-treated case (Fig. 4). Details of the results rule out any general attractiveness of the NE fibers for barrel dendrites as an alternate explanation of these results. Thus the results suggest that the role of NE in development is one of promoting afferent-dependent synapse stabilization, rather than of governing the synapse generation process.

## IV. Changes in the Pattern of Synaptic Connections in Later Development and Adulthood

Considerable evidence suggests that more specific sorts of information storage similarly involve changes in the pattern of synaptic connections. Much of the early evidence sprang from the complex environment paradigm pioneered by Hebb (1949) and the subsequent pioneering studies of the brain effects of complex, or "enriched," laboratory environments by Rosenzweig, Bennett, and Diamond (e.g., 1972) and their colleagues. These investigators showed that several regions of the neocortex, particularly the occipital or visual cortex, grew thicker and heavier in rats placed in a complex environment than in rats placed individually or in small groups in standard laboratory cages. Subsequent studies indicated that neuronal somata were larger in the complex-environment rats' visual cortices, that there appeared to be more glial cells, and that metabolic indexes reflected a higher general level of carbohydrate catabolism and protein synthetic activity per neuron. Behavioral studies indicated that rats reared in complex environments tended to learn complex, appetitively rewarded tasks as well as a variety of other types of problems more rapidly than rats from individual or group laboratory cages. This implied that they had stored information that improved their performance as a result of their housing conditions (see Black & Greenough, 1986, and Greenough, 1976, for reviews). While much of the earlier work focused upon postweaning rats, similar structural and biochemical patterns were also described in adult rats placed in complex environments (Diamond, Rosenzweig, Bennett, Lindner, & Lyon, 1972).

Subsequent research indicated that one component of the effect of housing in a complex environment was an increase in the number of synaptic connections made by neocortical neurons. Initial demonstrations of more extensive visual cortical dendritic fields in rats reared in complex environments (Greenough & Volkmar, 1973; Holloway, 1966) have been supported by more recent EM demonstrations that rats reared in complex environments have more synapses per neuronal cell body in the visual cortex than their laboratory cage counterparts (Turner & Greenough, 1985). The results of this study are presented in Fig. 5. A particularly important point to note is that the *density* of synapses, that is, the number per unit volume of brain tissue, does not differ statistically across the three differentially reared groups. What differs is the number of synapses per neuron—the ratio of synapse density to the density of neuronal nuclei. It appears that, when additional synapses are put into place, other tissue components, such as dendritic, axonal, glial, and vascular tissue necessary for the existence and maintenance of the synapses tend to push both synapses and neuronal cell bodies further apart, such that the density of synapses remains relatively constant and the density of neuronal somata is decreased. This result exemplifies what was noted earlier: Conclusions from studies in which only the density of synapses is assessed may be misleading.

Similar, though smaller, differences in dendritic field dimensions resulting from differential environmental complexity have been described in other neocortical regions, and some neocortical regions appeared unaffected by differential rearing (Greenough, Volkmar & Juraska, 1973). Rearing environment-dependent dendritic field differences have also been described in some subcortical regions, such as the cerebellum (Pysh & Weiss, 1979) and hippocampus (Juraska, Fitch, Henderson, & Rivers, 1985), and similar differences in the cerebellum have also been described

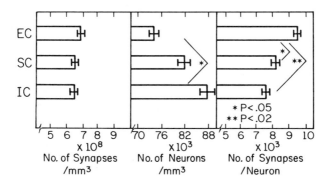

**Fig. 5.** Synaptic and neuronal density and synapses per neuron in the upper visual cortex of rats reared for 30 days after weaning in environmental complexity (EC), social cages (SC), or individual cages (IC). The lower density of neurons in EC and SC rats occurs because there are increases in other tissue components, such as synapses, axons, and dendrites. The greater number of synapses per neuron in the EC group confirms findings of Golgi stain studies that indicated a greater amount of dendrite per neuron. After Turner & Greenough (1985). Copyright 1984, Elsevier Science Publishers.

in monkeys (Floeter & Greenough, 1979). Differences quite similar to the
rat visual cortex synapse-per-neuron data have been reported in the visual
cortex of cats reared in complex environments compared to cats reared in
simple cages (Beaulieu & Colonnier, 1985). As with cortical weight and
thickness, visual cortex dendritic field differences between rats housed in
complex environments and those from standard cages have been found in
adult and middle-aged rats (Green, Greenough, & Schlumpf, 1983;
Juraska, Greenough, Elliott, Mack, & Berkowitz, 1980; Uylings, Kuypers, & Veltman, 1978). More extensive reviews of this work appear
elsewhere (Black & Greenough, 1986; Greenough & Chang, 1985).

The fact that many of these effects were not limited to prepubertal
developmental periods but occurred at seemingly any age led to more
direct studies of the possible role of such changes in specific tests of
memory. Our laboratory has performed three such studies. In the first,
rats were trained on a changing series of Hebb-Williams (1946) maze
patterns, one new pattern per day plus rehearsals of previous patterns,
over a 25-day period (Greenough, Juraska, & Volkmar, 1979). Controls
were given the sweetened-water maze reward in the experimenter's hands
when the trained group received maze trials. Results showed that Layer
IV and V occipital cortex pyramidal neurons had more extensive apical
dendritic fields in the trained animals. This indicated that the experience
of training could alter dendritic fields, and presumably associated patterns
of synaptic organization, although it did not indicate the aspect or aspects
of the training experience responsible for the dendritic effects.

A second study used a split-brain (corpus callosum transection) procedure combined with opaque eye occluders to direct visual input from the
same maze training procedure to one hemisphere, taking advantage of the
largely crossed nature of the rodent visual system (Chang & Greenough,
1982). In rats trained with the same eye each day, apical dendrites of
Layer V occipital cortex pyramidal neurons were more extensive in the
hemisphere receiving input from the trained eye than in the hemisphere
receiving occluded-eye input. This result ruled out many nonspecific features of the training procedure, such as stress, motor activity, and general
arousal, as sources of the training-dependent dendritic field differences.

A third experiment used a different learning paradigm to examine the
generality of the effects of training on dendritic field structure. The task,
devised by Peterson (1934), requires the rat to reach into a tube for bits of
highly desired food. Most rats prefer to reach with a particular forepaw,
although there is no general species bias toward right or left. Peterson
(1951) showed that, when the rat could not conveniently use the preferred
forepaw, the rat would learn to use the nonpreferred paw and, with sufficient training, would come to prefer to use that forepaw when given a free

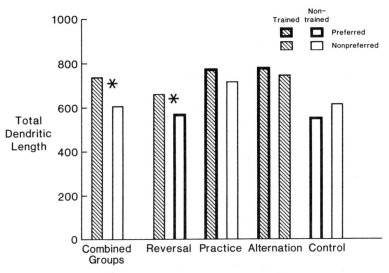

**Fig. 6.** Effect of training to reach for food on total length of the apical dendrite of neurons in the motor-sensory forelimb cortex (Greenough, Larson, & Withers, 1985). For "combined groups," the trained group includes both hemispheres of the alternation-trained group, and hemispheres opposite trained forelimbs in nonpreferred-forepaw and preferred-forepaw trained groups; the nontrained group includes both hemispheres of the untrained control group, and hemispheres opposite nontrained forelimbs in nonpreferred-forepaw and preferred-forepaw trained groups. *$p < .001$.

choice. The involvement of a relatively restricted region of the motor-sensory region of the neocortex in reaching and similar motor tasks has been confirmed by both lesion (Castro, 1972; Peterson & Devine, 1963) and electrophysiological (Dolbakyan, Hernandez-Mesa, & Bures, 1977; Donoghue & Wise, 1982) procedures. We (Greenough, Larson, & Withers, 1985) trained rats to reach in this manner with either the preferred, the nonpreferred, both, or neither forepaws and examined a region of the sensory-motor cortex which was activated, in terms of the uptake of the metabolic marker 2-DG, during performance of the reaching task in well-trained rats. The results of measurements of oblique branches from apical dendrites of Layer V pyramidal neurons in this region are presented in Fig. 6. Two effects are evident. First, training increased dendritic branching in the hemispheres opposite the trained forelimbs both within the unilaterally trained animals and in the bilaterally trained animals compared to nontrained controls. Second, there appeared to be some nonspecific effects of being trained, since dendritic fields in hemispheres opposite the nontrained forelimb in the unilaterally trained (preferred or nonpreferred) rats were larger than those in the nontrained animals. This effect was not due merely to being placed in the training apparatus, as this was also done with the nontrained animals. The first result is compatible with the maze-training experiments. In both cases, dendritic fields are larger in the hemisphere involved in the performance of the learned task. Moreover, the effects appear to be specific to the neocortical region within the hemisphere that actually mediates the behavior. When we examined apical dendritic fields of neurons in a sensory-motor region outside that activated during reach training, there were no consistent hemispheric differences in dendritic field dimensions between trained and nontrained hemispheres in the group trained with the nonpreferred forepaw (Simonson, Larson, & Greenough, 1984).

Taken together, the results of these three studies indicate that training increased dendritic field dimensions in neocortical regions involved in the performance of the tasks. Experiments utilizing quantitative Golgi/EM measures (Greenough & Volkmar, 1973; Turner & Greenough, 1985) have indicated, at least in the complex-environment paradigm, that increased dendritic field size accurately reflects increased numbers of synapses per neuron. Thus these results indicate that new synapses appear as a consequence of training. The results do not, of course, indicate what role these synapses play, but it seems reasonable to suggest that the altered patterns of neuronal organization may underlie aspects of memory for the learned tasks.

## V.  Connectivity Changes and Cerebellar Plasticity

Of more than passing interest, given the detailed and systematic body of work that has highlighted the role of the cerebellum in the generation of conditioned eye-blink responsiveness, is whether altered patterns of synaptic connectivity may also be involved in this phenomenon. This question has potentially broader application because the role of cerebellar mechanisms in motor learning has been a subject of intense investigation, and of parallel progress, in recent years. Although a complete answer is not available at this point, it is clear that altered patterns of cerebellar synaptic organization should be considered a possible substrate for some aspects of conditioning and motor learning.

The work of Thompson and his co-workers (see chap. 10, this volume) has implicated deep nuclei of the cerebellum, specifically the region of the dentate and interpositus nuclei, as a critical locus for an essential component of the CR. Electrophysiological studies have indicated that CR-correlated activity occurs in both the cerebellar cortex and deep nuclei (McCormick & Thompson, 1984b; R. F. Thompson et al., 1984). Lesions of the deep nuclei abolished CR without serious disruption of UR to airpuff stimuli (McCormick & Thompson, 1984a). Restricted lesions of the overlying cerebellar cortex that did not impinge upon the deep nuclei did not abolish CR selectively. Using a somewhat different procedure, Yeo, Hardiman, and Glickstein (1984, 1985a, 1985b, 1985c) argued that the cerebellar cortex is involved in elicitation of CR. Thus both regions may be involved, and the degree (or apparent degree) of involvement may vary with particular aspects of procedure.

The cerebellar cortex has proven attractive to theorists modeling motor learning (Albus, 1971; Eccles, 1977; Marr, 1969), and recent work has suggested that changes in the strength of connections between parallel fibers and Purkinje cell spiny branchlets occur during motor learning and simulations of it (Gilbert & Thatch, 1977; Ito, 1982). Theorists have tended to propose changes in the efficacy of previously existing connections, rather than formation or loss of connections, as the cellular mechanism underlying motor learning. However, it has been shown that the size of Purkinje cell dendritic fields, and specifically the size of spiny branchlets, varies as a function of the opportunity for sensory-motor activity afforded by the rearing environments of both rodents and primates (Floeter & Greenough, 1979; Pysh & Weiss, 1979). Recently, we have found that this plasticity is not unique to the developing cerebellum but in fact occurs in elderly rats (Greenough, McDonald, Parnisari, & Camel, 1986). We placed 2-year-old rats in environmentally complex (EC) or standard-cage (SC) housing for 4 1/2 months and compared them with baseline 2-year-old SC rats. Cerebellar Purkinje neurons in the EC rats had 20% more spiny branchlets than same-age SC rats and 17% more than the younger baseline rats (see Table I). Thus while we lack direct evidence, it seems plausible that changes in the pattern of parallel fiber connections on Purkinje cell spiny branchlets could mediate aspects of motor learning and associative eye-blink conditioning.

## VI. Possible Mechanisms of Synaptic Pattern Change in Later Development and Adulthood

The foregoing data, while they remain only correlative, make a strong case for the involvement of changes in the pattern of synaptic connections both in developmental plasticity and in adult memory processes. A crucial issue, if such changes are involved in memory, is the manner in which they occur. The early development work suggests one possibility, while some recent findings suggest an alternative:

1. *The intrinsic overproduction-activity–based selection process extends into adulthood.* As suggested by Changeaux and Danchin (1976) and

**Table I**

Measures of Purkinje neurons in elderly baseline rats at
26 months of age (BL) or after an additional 4 1/2 months
of housing in standard cages (SC) or environmental
complexity (EC).

| | Experimental group | | |
|---|---|---|---|
| Measure | EC | SC | BL |
| Mean number of spiny branchlets per neuron* | 68.38 | 57.00 | 58.33 |
| Mean dendrite length per spiny branchlet** | 100.04 | 107.97 | 134.96 |

*Note.* The number of spiny branchlets, the dendrites that receive most synapses on these neurons, is increased even in elderly rats as a consequence of
housing in a complex environment. The size of spiny branchlets declines from the
baseline level over 4 1/2 months in both environments, however (data from
Greenough, McDonald, Parnisari, & Camel, 1986). When SAS GLM analysis of
variance indicated significant group effects, group differences were assessed with
the Newman-Keuls test, alpha = .05.
* $p < .025$; EC > SC = BL.
** $p < .001$; BL > EC = SC.

others, synapses might continue to form more or less at random in the
brain or certain of its regions during later development and adulthood.
These synapses, like those described above for early development, would
not be permanent when formed but would require some sort of confirmation for long-term preservation. Those preserved would be the ones that
were in the right place at the right time relative to ongoing neural activity
or some combination of activity and neuromodulatory signals (e.g., the
*now print* of Kety, 1976). Thus the generation of a brain wiring diagram
containing increasing amounts of information would be a bit like clay
sculpture, in which unformed dabs of soft clay are added to the sculpture
and then the excess is scraped away.

2. *Synapses form actively in response to neural activity containing
information to be stored* (Kappers, 1917; Greenough, 1984). In contrast to
the first alternative, synaptogenesis is proposed to be experience dependent in this alternative, initiated by neural activity arising from an event to
be encoded or by some neuromodulatory signal triggered by that neural
activity. Synapses might still be formed more or less randomly, with a
selective preservation process determining the ultimate organizational
pattern, but they would form only when triggered to do so and only where
the triggering occurred. In the first alternative, by contrast, synaptogenesis would be continuous and widespread, independent of the quality of
experience or information to be stored.

The first alternative is attractive because it does not require a difference in the manner in which the cellular processes of synaptogenesis are regulated in development and adulthood. It would, however, be a metabolically more costly process, assuming that most synapses generated would turn over without ever being meaningfully used. Moreover, assuming that the synapses in the prestabilized state were capable of generating postsynaptic potentials, they might add to background noise in the nervous system.

The second alternative was unattractive in earlier forms because, aside from the proposal of Kappers (1917) that bioelectrical activity might influence neuronal process growth (for which there is some support: Jaffe & Poo, 1979), suggestions of ways in which nerve cells could get hooked up with the proper set of other ones to be part of a memory have been rare. The version above avoids this problem because it requires no specificity of initial connection patterns. The only specific suggestion is that elements activated by an event about which information is to be stored are the ones that will engage in synaptogenesis. Recipients need not be active, and a modified Hebb (1949) synapse view might suggest that subsequent selective preservation might involve which recipients had been active. A similar consequence of coactivation seems to be involved in the developmental overproduction–loss process described earlier.

Some recent findings have made the idea that *synapses form in response to a demand for memory* more attractive. One of these involves long-term potentiation (LTP), an increased postsynaptic responsiveness to afferent activity following brief trains of high-frequency stimuli that occurs in the hippocampal formation and a number of other CNS and (with some differences in details) peripheral regions (Teyler & Discenna, 1984). A number of mechanisms have been proposed to underlie LTP, and there may well be more than one, given that LTP appears to have multiple temporal phases (Racine, Milgram, & Hafner, 1983). One plausible mechanism is the formation of additional synapses between afferents and recipients in response to the high-frequency stimulation, which has been reported in hippocampal subfield CA1 following LTP-inducing stimulation (Lee, Oliver, Schottler, & Lynch, 1981; Lee, Schottler, Oliver, & Lynch, 1980). Chang and Greenough (1984) repeated this observation and noted that both shaft and sessile spine synapses form in relatively large numbers within 10–15 min of the eliciting stimulation and persist for at least 8 hr thereafter in the hippocampal slice in vitro. This study included two control procedures: (1) slices that received an equal number of stimuli within the same overall period of time used for LTP treatment but at a lower frequency that did not produce LTP and (2) slices that received much more high-frequency stimulation than the LTP group, but continuously, such that LTP did not occur. In neither of these control groups was there an increase in synapse formation, indicating that neural activity alone was insufficient to cause the effect and suggesting that the synaptic increase was specifically related to LTP. However, whether or not it is actually involved in the potentiation process, the fact that synapses can increase in numbers within a few minutes suggests that this was not mediated by a continuous turnover process but that active synapse formation occurred in response to the LTP-inducing electrical stimulation. Thus synaptogenesis can occur on a time scale compatible with the time course of long-term memory formation.

A second finding that has renewed our interest in active synapse formation as a possible memory mechanism is based upon reports that the location of polyribosomal aggregates may serve to identify newly forming or recently formed synapses. Steward (1983) noted that polyribosomal aggregates (PRAs) increased in frequency in spine heads and stems during reactive synaptogenesis in the dentate gyrus. At other times PRAs were more likely to be located in the dendrite proper, at the base of the spine. In support of his suggestion that PRA location in spines might be associated with synaptogenesis, Hwang and Greenough (1984) reported that the frequency of PRAs in spine heads and stems was 400% higher in the rat visual cortex during periods of peak postnatal synaptogenesis than in adulthood.

If PRAs located in spines are indicators of synaptogenesis, this offers a way to test whether the increased numbers of synapses that result from experience in a complex environment occur through active formation in response to experience or through selective preservation of a subpopulation of continuously forming synapses. The continuous-formation model predicts that information storage should affect the number of synapses preserved, but not the number formed, whereas the active formation model predicts that the number of synapses forming should increase in response to elevated information storage demands. Greenough, Hwang, and Gorman (1985) examined the relative frequency of spines containing PRAs in the visual cortex of rats housed from weaning for 30 days in EC, SC, or individual cage (IC) environments. The number was dramatically greater in the EC rats, in support of the active formation model.

Of course it is possible, perhaps likely, that PRAs may aggregate in spines to perform functions associated with increased activity or strength modifications. We must develop additional ways to identify newly forming synapses and also need to determine whether similar increases in such possible synaptogenic markers occur in adult animals during learning. The data to this point, however, suggest that synapses do form in response to experience, at least in the postweaning environmental complexity paradigm.

## VII. A Cautious Summary

This chapter has argued two primary points: (1) changes in the pattern of synaptic connections seem likely to be involved in a variety of types of CNS information storage, ranging from the effects of experience upon early sensory system development to adult learning and memory and (2) the primary distinction between these two extremes is that very early plastic developmental phenomena appear to involve intrinsically triggered synapse overproduction and extrinsically controlled synapse selection, whereas for adult learning, both synapse formation and synapse selection may be controlled by experience.

The distinction between intrinsically triggered and extrinsically triggered synaptogenesis seems likely to be real, but the extent to which ongoing synaptogenesis is governed *exclusively* by one or the other source at any point may rarely be as absolute as the distinction suggests. In early visual development, for example, both the potential for recovery following deprivation (LeVay *et al.,* 1980) and the fact that the peak number of synapses is reduced in deprived animals (Winfield, 1981) suggest that visual experience drives synapse formation to at least some degree. Visual experience can also drive synaptogenesis in previously deprived older animals (Cragg, 1967), although this may involve an adultlike extrinsically driven process. In older animals, a significant amount of synaptogenesis not obviously driven by experience is suggested by the presence of PRAs in many spines even in the IC animals (Greenough, Hwang, & Gorman, 1985), although it might be expected that some synapse formation might be driven by ongoing neural activity even when the external world is rather uninteresting. Nonetheless, the relative emphasis of intrinsically driven processes in early sensory and motor development, and the evidence for pronounced external driving of synaptogenesis in later development and in the adult hippocampal slice, suggest that the distinction is a meaningful one.

There is no intention to suggest here that synapse formation or selective preservation is likely to be the only mechanism of neural information storage in either early development or adulthood. As noted elsewhere (see Greenough, 1984), mammals are critically dependent for survival on the ability to retain information from their experiences, and it seems quite likely that multiple mechanisms would have evolved to optimize this ability. There is evidence for a variety of both presynaptic and postsynaptic phenomena that could affect efficacy of preexisting synapses (e.g., Cragg, 1967; Fifkova & Van Harreveld, 1977; Greenough, West, & DeVoogd, 1978; Kandel & Schwartz, 1982; Lynch & Baudry, 1984; Sirevaag & Greenough, 1985; Skrede & Malthe-Sorensen, 1981; Tieman, 1984; Vrensen & Cardozo, 1981; Wesa, Chang, Greenough, & West, 1982), and nonsynaptic mechanisms of information storage have been proposed as well (e.g., Alkon, 1982). Various mechanisms could be used independently or in concert, in various brain regions, to effect the storage of information. Such mechanisms might also be differentially involved in memories with different durations. It is interesting in this regard that an increased responsiveness to afferent stimulation in the hippocampal dentate gyrus (perhaps similar to LTP), which was apparent immediately after postweaning rearing in a complex environment, had entirely disappeared after 30 days' additional housing in individual cages (Green & Greenough, 1986). In contrast, dendritic branching differences induced in the visual cortex in this paradigm were relatively stable over the same period (Camel, Withers, & Greenough, 1986).

Thus the categories of experience-driven and intrinsically driven synaptogenesis proposed here, though likely to be involved in brain information storage, are unlikely to comprise a comprehensive description of the mechanisms underlying brain information storage. Nonetheless, the evidence that these processes are involved in at least some aspects of brain information storage, and in particular the evidence that synapse formation is associated with at least some forms of adult learning and memory, is becoming increasingly strong.

## Acknowledgments

Preparation of this paper and research not otherwise reported was supported by National Institute of Mental Health grants MH35321 and MH40631, National Institutes of Health Grant RR07030, Public Health Service grants 5 T-32EY07005 and 5 T-32GM7143, Office of Naval Research Grant N00014-85-K-0587, the Retirement Research Foundation, the System Development Foundation, and the University of Illinois Research Board.

## References

Albus, J. S. (1971). A theory of cerebellar function. *Mathematical Biosciences, 10,* 25–61.
Alkon, D. L. (1982). A biophysical basis for molluscan associative learning. In C. D. Woody (Ed.), *Conditioning: Representation of involved neural functions* (pp. 147–170). New York: Plenum.
Allen, B. M. (1938). The endocrine control of amphibian metamorphosis. *Biological Reviews, 13,* 1–19.

Bear, M. F., & Daniels, J. D. (1983). The plastic response to monocular deprivation persists in kitten visual cortex after chronic depletion of norepinephrine. *Journal of Neuroscience, 3,* 407–416.

Bear, M. F., & Singer, W. (1986). Modulation of visual cortical plasticity by acetylcholine and noradrenaline. *Nature, 320,* 172–176.

Beaulieu, C., & Colonnier, M. (1985). The effect of environmental complexity on the numerical density of neurons and on the size of their nuclei in the visual cortex of cat. *Society for Neuroscience Abstracts, 11,* 225.

Black, J. E., & Greenough, W. T. (1986). Induction of pattern in neural structure by experience: Implications for cognitive development. In M. E. Lamb, A. L. Brown, & B. Rogoff (Eds.), *Advances in developmental psychology* (Vol. 4, pp. 1–50). Hillsdale, NJ: Earlbaum.

Boothe, R. G., Greenough, W. T., Lund, J. S., & Wrege, K. (1979). A quantitative investigation of spine and dendritic development of neurons in visual cortex (area 17) of *Macaca nemestrina* monkeys. *Journal of Comparative Neurology, 186,* 473–490.

Brunjes, P. C., & Alberts, J. R. (1980). Precocious nasal chemosensitivity in hyperthyroid rat pups. *Hormones and Behavior, 14,* 76–85.

Brunjes, P. C., & Alberts, J. R. (1981). Early auditory and visual function in normal and hyperthyroid rats. *Behavioral and Neural Biology, 31,* 393–417.

Brunjes, P. C., Schwark, H. D., & Greenough, W. T. (1982). Olfactory granule cell development in normal and hyperthyroid rats. *Developmental Brain Research, 5,* 149–159.

Burchfiel, J. L., & Duffy, F. H. (1981). Role of intracortical inhibition in deprivation amblyopia: Reversal by microintophoretic bicuculline. *Brain Research, 206,* 479–484.

Camel, J. E., Withers, G. S., & Greenough, W. T. (1986). Persistence of visual cortex dendritic alterations induced by postweaning exposure to a ''superenriched'' environment in rats. *Behavioral Neuroscience, 100,* 810–813.

Castro, A. J. (1972). The effects of cortical ablations on digital usage in the rat. *Brain Research, 37,* 173–185.

Chang, F.-L. F., & Greenough, W. T. (1982). Lateralized effects of monocular training on dendritic branching in adult split-brain rats. *Brain Research, 232,* 283–292.

Chang, F.-L. F., & Greenough, W. T. (1984). Transient and enduring morphological correlates of synaptic activity and efficacy change in the rat hippocampal slice. *Brain Research, 309,* 35–46.

Changeaux, J.-P., & Danchin, A. (1976). Selective stabilization of developing synapses as a mechanism for the specification of neuronal networks. *Nature, 264,* 705–712.

Chugani, H. T., & Phelps, M. E. (1986). Maturational changes in cerebral function in infants determined by (18) FDG positron emission tomography. *Science, 231,* 840–843.

Cohen, M. W. (1972). The development of neuromuscular connexions in the presence of D-tubocurarine. *Brain Research, 41,* 457–463.

Conel, J. L. (1939–1967). *The postnatal development of the human cerebral cortex* (Vol. 1–8). Cambridge: Harvard University Press.

Cragg, B. G. (1967). Changes in visual cortex on first exposure of rats to light: Effect on synaptic dimensions. *Nature, 215,* 251–253.

Cragg, B. G. (1975). The development of synapses in the visual system of the cat. *Journal of Comparative Neurology, 160,* 147–166.

Daw, N. W., Robertson, T. W., Rader, R. K., Videen, T. O., & Coscia, C. J. (1984). Substantial reduction of cortical norepinephrine by lesions of adrenergic pathway does not prevent effects of monocular deprivation. *Journal of Neuroscience, 4,* 1354–1360.

Daw, N. W., Videen, T. O., Parkinson, D., & Rader, R. K. (1985). DSP-4 depletes noradrenaline in kitten visual cortex without altering the effects of monocular deprivation. *Journal of Neuroscience, 5,* 1925–1933.

Diamond, M. C., Rosenzweig, M. R., Bennett, E. L., Lindner, B., & Lyon, L. (1972). Effects of environmental enrichment and impoverishment on rat cerebral cortex. *Journal of Neurobiology, 3,* 47–64.

Dolbakyan, E., Hernandez-Mesa, N., & Bures, J. (1977). Skilled forelimb movements and unit activity in motor cortex and caudate nucleus in rats. *Neuroscience, 2,* 73–80.

Donoghue, J. P., & Wise, S. P. (1982). The motor cortex of the rat: Cytoarchitecture and microstimulation mapping. *Journal of Comparative Neurology, 212,* 76–88.

Eayrs, J. T. (1964). Effect of neonatal hyperthyroidism on maturation and learning in the rat. *Animal Behaviour, 12,* 195–199.

Eccles, J. C. (1977). An instruction-selection theory of learning in the cerebellar cortex. *Brain Research, 127,* 327–352.

Felten, D. L., Hallman, H., & Jonsson, G. (1982). Evidence for a neurotrophic role of noradrenaline neurons in the postnatal development of rat cerebral cortex. *Journal of Neurocytology, 11,* 119–135.

Fifkova, E., & Van Harreveld, A. (1977). Long-lasting morphological changes in dendritic spines of dentate granular cells following stimulation of the entorhinal area. *Journal of Neurocytology, 6,* 211–230.

Floeter, M. K., & Greenough, W. T. (1979). Cerebellar plasticity: Modification of Purkinje cell structure by differential rearing in monkeys. *Science, 206,* 227–229.

Foote, S. L., Bloom, F. E., & Aston-Jones, G. (1983). Nucleus locus ceruleus: New evidence of anatomical and physiological specificity. *Physiological Review, 63,* 844–914.

Gilbert, P. F. C., & Thatch, W. T. (1977). Purkinje cell activity during motor learning. *Brain Research, 128,* 309–328.

Gold, P. E. (1984). Memory modulation: Neurobiological contexts. In G. Lynch, J. L. McGaugh, & N. M. Weinberger (Eds.), *Neurobiology of learning and memory* (pp. 374–382). New York: Guilford.

Green, E. J., & Greenough, W. T. (1986). Altered synaptic transmission in dentate gyrus of rats reared in complex environments: Evidence from hippocampal slices maintained *in vivo*. *Journal of Neurophysiology, 55,* 739–750.

Green, E. J., Greenough, W. T., & Schlumpf, B. E. (1983). Effects of complex or isolated environments on cortical dendrites of middle-aged rats. *Brain Research, 264,* 233–240.

Greenough, W. T. (1976). Enduring brain effects of differential experience and training. In M. R. Rosenzweig & E. L. Bennett (Eds.), *Neural mechanisms of learning and memory* (pp. 255–278). Cambridge: MIT Press.

Greenough, W. T. (1984). Structural correlates of information storage in the mammalian brain: A review and hypothesis. *Trends in NeuroSciences, 7,* 229–233.

Greenough, W. T., & Chang, F.-L. F. (1985). Synaptic structural correlates of information storage in mammalian nervous systems. In C. W. Cotman (Ed.), *Synaptic plasticity and remodeling* (pp. 335–372). New York: Guilford.

Greenough, W. T., Hwang, H.-M., & Gorman, C. (1985). Evidence for active synapse formation, or altered postsynaptic metabolism, in visual cortex of rats reared in complex environments. *Proceedings of the National Academy of Sciences, 82,* 4549–4552.

Greenough, W. T., Juraska, J. M., & Volkmar, F. R. (1979). Maze training effects on dendritic branching in occipital cortex of adult rats. *Behavioral and Neural Biology, 26,* 287–297.

Greenough, W. T., Larson, J. R., & Withers, G. S. (1985). Effects of unilateral and bilateral training in a reaching task on dendritic branching of neurons in the rat motor-sensory forelimb cortex. *Behavioral and Neural Biology, 44,* 301–314.

Greenough, W. T., McDonald, J. W., Parnisari, R. M., & Camel, J. E. (1986). Environmental conditions modulate degeneration and new dendrite growth in cerebellum of senescent rats. *Brain Research, 380,* 136–143.

Greenough, W. T., & Volkmar, F. R. (1973). Pattern of dendritic branching in occipital cortex of rats reared in complex environments. *Experimental Neurology, 40,* 491–504.

Greenough, W. T., Volkmar, F. R., & Juraska, J. M. (1973). Effects of rearing complexity on dendritic branching in frontolateral and temporal cortex of the rat. *Experimental Neurology, 41,* 371–378.

Greenough, W. T., West, R. W., & DeVoogd, T. J. (1978). Subsynaptic plate perforations: Changes with age and experience in the rat. *Science, 202,* 1096–1098.

Harris, R. M., & Woolsey, T. A. (1981). Dendritic plasticity in mouse barrel cortex following postnatal vibrissa follicle damage. *Journal of Comparative Neurology, 196,* 357–376.

Hebb, D. O. (1949). The organization of behavior. New York: Wiley.

Hebb, D. O., & Williams, K. A. (1946). A method of rating animal intelligence. *Journal of Genetic Psychology, 34,* 59–65.

Holloway, R. L. (1966). Dendritic branching: Some preliminary results of training and complexity in rat visual cortex. *Brain Research, 2,* 393–396.

Hubel, D. H., & Wiesel, T. N. (1970). The period of susceptibility to the physiological effects of unilateral eye closure in kittens. *Journal of Physiology, 206,* 419–436.

Huttenlocher, P. R. (1979). Synaptic density in human frontal cortex: Developmental changes and effects of aging. *Brain Research, 163,* 195–205.

Huttenlocher, P. R., de Courten, C., Garey, L. J., & Van der Loos, H. (1982). Synaptogenesis in human visual cortex: Evidence for synapse elimination during normal development. *Neuroscience Letters, 33,* 247–252.

Hwang, H.-M., & Greenough, W. T. (1984). Spine formation and synaptogenesis in rat visual cortex: A serial section developmental study. *Society for Neuroscience Abstracts, 10,* 579.

Ito, M. (1982). Cerebellar control of vestibulo-ocular reflex—Around the flocculus hypothesis. *Annual Review of Neuroscience, 5,* 275–296.

Ivy, G. O., & Killackey, H. P. (1982). Ontogenetic changes in the projections of neocortical neurons. *Journal of Neuroscience, 2,* 735–743.

Jaffe, L. F, & Poo, M. M. (1979). Neurites grow faster towards the cathode than the anode in a steady field. *Journal of Experimental Zoology, 209,* 115–128.

Juraska, J. M., Fitch, J., Henderson, C., & Rivers, N. (1985). Sex differences in the dendritic branching of dentate granule cells following differential experience. *Brain Research, 333,* 73–80.

Juraska, J. M., Greenough, W. T., Elliott, C., Mack, K. J., & Berkowitz, R. (1980). Plasticity in adult rat visual cortex: An examination of several cell populations after differential rearing. *Behavioral and Neural Biology, 29,* 157–167.

Kandel, E. R., & Schwartz, J. H. (1982). Molecular biology of learning: Modulation of transmitter release. *Science, 218,* 433–443.

Kappers, C. U. A. (1917). Further contributions on neurobiotaxis: IX. An attempt to compare the phenomena of neurobiotaxis with other phenomena of taxis and tropism: The dynamic polarization of the neurone. *Journal of Comparative Neurology, 27,* 261–298.

Kasamatsu, T., & Pettigrew, J. D. (1976). Depletion of brain catecholamines: Failure of ocular dominance shift after monocular occlusion in kittens. *Science, 194,* 206–209.

218                                                    William T. Greenough

Kasamatsu, T., & Pettigrew, J. D. (1979). Preservation of binocularity after monocular deprivation in the striate cortex of kittens treated with 6-hydroxydopamine. *Journal of Comparative Neurology, 185,* 139–162.

Kety, S. S. (1976). Biological concomitants of affective states and their possible role in memory processes. In M. R. Rosenzweig & E. L. Bennett (Eds.), *Neural mechanisms of learning and memory* (pp. 321–326). Cambridge: MIT Press.

Killackey, H. P., Belford, G., Ryugo, R., & Ryugo, D. K. (1976). Anomalous organization of thalamocortical projections consequent to vibrissae removal in the newborn rat and mouse. *Brain Research, 104,* 309–315.

Killackey, H. P., & Leshin, S. (1975). The organization of specific thalamocortical projections to the posteromedial barrel subfield of the rat somatic sensory cortex. *Brain Research, 86,* 469–472.

Kratz, K. E., Spear, P. D., & Smith, D. C. (1976). Postcritical period reversal of effects of monocular deprivation on striate cortex cells in the cat. *Journal of Neurophysiology, 39,* 501–511.

Lauder, J. M., & Krebs, H. (1986). Do neurotransmitters, neurohumors, and hormones specify critical periods? In W. T. Greenough & J. M. Juraska (Eds.), *Developmental neuropsychobiology* (pp. 119–174). Orlando: Academic Press.

Lee, K., Oliver, M., Schottler, F., & Lynch, G. (1981). Electron microscopic studies of brain slices: The effects of high-frequency stimulation on dendritic ultrastructure. In G. A. Kerkut & H. V. Wheal (Eds.), *Electrophysiology of isolated mammalian CNS preparations* (pp. 189–211). New York: Academic Press.

Lee, K. S., Schottler, F., Oliver, M., & Lynch, G. (1980). Brief bursts of high-frequency stimulation produce two types of structural change in rat hippocampus. *Journal of Neurophysiology, 44,* 247–258.

LeVay, S., Wiesel, T. N., & Hubel, D. H. (1980). The development of ocular dominance columns in normal and visually deprived monkeys. *Journal of Comparative Neurology, 191,* 1–51.

Lidov, H. G. W., & Molliver, M. E. (1982). The structure of cerebral cortex in the rat following prenatal administration of 6-hydroxydopamine. *Developmental Brain Research, 3,* 81–108.

Loeb, E. P., Chang, F.-L. F., & Greenough, W. T. (in press). Effects of neonatal 6-hydroxydopamine treatment upon morphological organization of the posteromedial barrel subfield in mouse somatosensory cortex. *Brain Research.*

Lynch, G., & Baudry, M. (1984). The biochemistry of memory: A new and specific hypothesis. *Science, 224,* 1057–1063.

Mariani, J., & Changeaux, J.-P. (1981). Ontogenesis of olivocerebellar relationships: I. Studies by intracellular recording of the multiple innervation of Purkinje cells by climbing fibers in the developing rat. *Journal of Neuroscience, 1,* 696–702.

Marr, D. (1969). A theory of cerebellar cortex. *Journal of Physiology* (London), *202,* 437–470.

McCormick, D. A., & Thompson, R. F. (1984a). Cerebellum: Essential involvement in the classically conditioned eyelid response. *Science, 223,* 296–299.

McCormick, D. A., & Thompson, R. F. (1984b). Neuronal responses of the rabbit cerebellum during acquisition and performance of a classically conditioned nictitating membrane-eyelid response. *Journal of Neuroscience, 4,* 2811–2822.

Mirmiran, M., & Uylings, H. B. M. (1983). The environmental enrichment effect upon cortical growth is neutralized by concomitant pharmacological suppression of active sleep in female rats. *Brain Research, 261,* 331–334.

Nicholson, J. L., & Altman, J. (1972). Synaptogenesis in the rat cerebellum: Effects of early hypo- and hyperthyroidism. *Science, 176,* 530–532.

O'Shea, L., Saari, M., Pappas, B. A., Ings, R., & Stange, K. (1983). Neonatal 6-hydroxydopamine attenuates the neural and behavioral effects of enriched rearing in the rat. *European Journal of Pharmacology, 92,* 43–47.

Peterson, G. M. (1934). Mechanisms of handedness in the rat. *Comparative Psychology Monographs, 9,* 1–67.

Peterson, G. M. (1951). Transfers of handedness in the rat from forced practice. *Journal of Comparative and Physiological Psychology, 44,* 184–190.

Peterson, G. M., & Devine, J. V. (1963). Transfer of handedness in the rat resulting from small cortical lesions after limited forced practice. *Journal of Comparative and Physiological Psychology, 56,* 752–756.

Purves, D., & Lichtman, J. W. (1980). Elimination of synapses in the developing nervous system. *Science, 210,* 153–157.

Pysh, J. J., & Weiss, M. (1979). Exercise during development induces an increase in Purkinje cell dendritic tree size. *Science, 206,* 230–232.

Racine, R. J., Milgram, N. W., & Hafner, S. (1983). Long-term potentiation phenomena in the rat limbic forebrain. *Brain Research, 260,* 217–231.

Rakic, P., Bourgeois, J.-P., Eckenhoff, M. F., Zecevic, N., & Goldman-Rakic, P. (1986). Concurrent overproduction of synapses in diverse regions of the primate cerebral cortex. *Science, 232,* 232–235.

Ridge, R. M. A. P., & Betz, W. J. (1984). The effect of selective, chronic stimulation on motor unit size in developing rat muscle. *Journal of Neuroscience, 4,* 2614–2620.

Rosenzweig, M. R., Bennett, E. L., & Diamond, M. C. (1972). Chemical and anatomical plasticity of brain: Replications and extensions. In J. Gaito (Ed.), *Macromolecules and behavior* (2nd ed., pp. 205–278). New York: Appleton-Century-Crofts.

Schapiro, S., & Norman, R. J. (1967). Thyroxine: Effects of neonatal administration on maturation, development, and behavior. *Science, 155,* 1279–1281.

Schapiro, S., Salas, M., & Vukovitch, K. (1970). Hormonal effects on ontogeny of swimming ability in the rat: Assessment of central nervous development. *Science, 168,* 147–150.

Sherman, S. M., Guillery, R. W., Kaas, J. H., & Sanderson, K. J. (1974). Behavioral, electrophysiological, and morphological studies of binocular competition in the development of the geniculo-cortical pathways of cats. *Journal of Comparative Neurology, 158,* 1–18.

Simons, D. J., & Woolsey, T. A. (1979). Functional organization in mouse barrel cortex. *Brain Research, 165,* 207–245.

Simonson, L., Larson, J. R., & Greenough, W. T. (1984). Dendritic branching in hindlimb area of rat motor cortex. Unpublished study.

Sirevaag, A. M., & Greenough, W. T. (1985). Differential rearing effects on rat visual cortex synapses: II. Synaptic morphometry. *Developmental Brain Research, 19,* 215–226.

Skrede, K. K., & Malthe-Sorenssen, D. (1981). Increased resting and evoked release of transmitter following repetitive electrical tetanization in hippocampus: A biochemical correlate to long-lasting synaptic potentiation. *Brain Research, 208,* 436–441.

Steward, O. (1983). Polyribosomes at the base of dendritic spines of CNS neurons: Their possible role in synapse construction and modification. *Cold Spring Harbor Symposium on Quantitative Biology, 48,* 745–759.

Stone, J. M., & Greenough, W. T. (1975). Excess neonatal thyroxine: Effects on learning in infant and adolescent rats. *Developmental Psychobiology, 8,* 479–488.

Stryker, M. P. (1981). Late segregation of geniculate afferents to the cat's visual cortex after recovery from binocular impulse blockade. *Society for Neuroscience Abstracts, 7,* 842.

Stryker, M. P., & Strickland, S. L. (1984). Physiological segregation of ocular dominance columns depends on the pattern of afferent electrical activity. *Investigative Ophthalmology and Visual Science, 25,* (Suppl.) 278.

Teyler, T. J., & Discenna, P. (1984). Long-term potentiation as a candidate mnemonic device. *Brain Research Reviews, 7,* 15–28.

Thompson, R. F., Clark, G. A., Donegan, N. H., Lavond, D. G., Lincoln, J. S., Madden, J., IV, Mamounas, L. A., Mauk, M. D., McCormick, D. A., & Thompson, J. K. (1984). Neuronal substrates of learning and memory: A "multiple-trace" view. In G. Lynch, J. L. McGaugh, & N. M. Weinberger (Eds.), *Neurobiology of learning and memory* (pp. 137–164). New York: Guilford.

Thompson, W. (1983). Synapse elimination in neonatal rat muscle is sensitive to pattern of muscle use. *Nature, 303,* 614–616.

Thompson, W., Kuffler, D. P., & Jansen, J. K. S. (1979). The effect of prolonged, reversible block of nerve impulses on the elimination of polyneuronal innervation of newborn rat skeletal muscle fibers. *Neuroscience, 4,* 271–281.

Tieman, S. B. (1984). Effects of monocular deprivation on geniculocortical synapses in the cat. *Journal of Comparative Neurology, 222,* 166–176.

Turkewitz, G., & Kenny, P. A. (1982). Limitations on input as a basis for neural organization and perceptual development: A preliminary theoretical statement. *Developmental Psychobiology, 15,* 357–368.

Turner, A. M., & Greenough, W. T. (1985). Differential rearing effects on rat visual cortex synapses: I. Synaptic and neuronal density and synapses per neuron. *Brain Research, 329,* 195–203.

Uylings, H. B. M., Kuypers, K., & Veltman, W. A. M. (1978). Environmental influences on neocortex in later life. *Progress in Brain Research, 48,* 261–274.

Van der Loos, H., & Woolsey, T. A. (1973). Somatosensory cortex: Structural alterations following early injury to sense organs. *Science, 179,* 395–398.

Van Huizen, F., Romijn, H. J., & Habets, A. M. M. C. (1985). Synaptogenesis in rat cerebral cortex cultures is affected during chronic blockade of spontaneous bioelectric activity by tetrodotoxin. *Developmental Brain Research, 19,* 67–80.

Vrensen, G., & Cardozo, J. N. (1981). Changes in size and shape of synaptic connections after visual training: An ultrastructural approach of synaptic plasticity. *Brain Research, 218,* 79–98.

Waterhouse, B. D., & Woodward, D. J. (1980). Interaction of norepinephrine with cerebrocortical activity evoked by stimulation of somatosensory afferent pathways in the rat. *Experimental Brain Research, 67,* 11–34.

Welker, C. (1971). Microelectrode delineation of fine grain somatotopic organization of SmI cerebral neocortex in albino rat. *Brain Research, 26,* 259–275.

Welker, C., & Woolsey, T. A. (1974). Structure of layer IV in the somatosensory neocortex of the rat: Description and comparison with the mouse. *Journal of Comparative Neurology, 158,* 437–453.

Wesa, J. M., Chang, F.-L. F., Greenough, W. T., & West, R. W. (1982). Synaptic contact curvature: Effects of differential rearing on rat occipital cortex. *Developmental Brain Research, 4,* 253–257.

White, E. L. (1978). Identified neurons in mouse SmI cortex which are postsynaptic to thalamocortical axon terminals: A combined Golgi-electron microscopic and degeneration study. *Journal of Comparative Neurology, 181,* 627–662.

Wiesel, T. N., & Hubel, D. H. (1963). Single-cell responses in striate cortex of kittens deprived of vision in one eye. *Journal of Neurophysiology, 26,* 1003–1017.

Winfield, D. A. (1981). The postnatal development of synapses in the visual cortex of the cat and the effects of eyelid closure. *Brain Research, 206,* 166–171.

Woolsey, T. A., Dierker, M. L., & Wann, D. F. (1975). Mouse SmI cortex: Qualitative and quantitative classification of Golgi-impregnated barrel neurons. *Proceedings of the National Academy of Sciences, 72,* 2165–2169.

Woolsey, T. A., & Van der Loos, H. (1970). The structural organization of layer IV in the somatosensory region (SI) of the mouse cerebral cortex: The description of a cortical field composed of discrete cytoarchitectonic units. *Brain Research, 17,* 205–242.

Yeo, C. H., Hardiman, M., & Glickstein, M. (1984). Discrete lesions of the cerebellar cortex abolish the classically conditioned nictitating membrane response of the rabbit. *Behavioral Brain Research, 13,* 261–266.

Yeo, C. H., Hardiman, M., & Glickstein, M. (1985a). Classical conditioning of the nictitating membrane response of the rabbit: I. Lesions of the cerebellar nuclei. *Experimental Brain Research, 60,* 87–98.

Yeo, C. H., Hardiman, M., & Glickstein, M. (1985b). Classical conditioning of the nictitating membrane response of the rabbit: II. Lesions of the cerebellar cortex. *Experimental Brain Research, 60,* 99–113.

Yeo, C. H., Hardiman, M., & Glickstein, M. (1985c). Classical conditioning of the nictitating membrane response of the rabbit: III. Connections of cerebellar lobule HVI. *Experimental Brain Research, 60,* 114–126.

# 10

## Neural Circuitry of Basic Associative Learning and Implications for Ontogeny

RICHARD F. THOMPSON
*Department of Psychology*
*Stanford University*
*Stanford, California 94305*

How the brain codes, stores, and retrieves memories is among the most important and baffling questions in science. At the cellular level, there are two fundamental types of information coding. One of these is the familiar genetic code, shared by organisms from virus to man. In higher organisms, literally millions of bits of information are coded in the DNA of the cell nucleus. Over the course of evolution, a quite different kind of information coding has developed—the cellular encoding of acquired information in the brain. This coding is no less remarkable than the genetic code. It has been estimated that a well-educated adult human has millions of bits of acquired information stored in the brain.

The generic term for acquired information coding in the brain is the *memory trace*. The fundamental difference between the genetic code and the memory trace code is, of course, that each individual human's memory store is acquired through experience and learning. It is the biologic substrate for the growth of knowledge and civilization. The individual uniqueness of each human being is due largely to the memory store—the biologic residue of memory from a lifetime of experience.

In the past generation, understanding of the biologic basis of learning and memory has undergone a revolution. The earlier notion that memory is diffusely distributed in the brain has been largely discounted. It is now clear that various forms and aspects of learning and memory involve particular systems and circuits in the brain. This realization means that it is now both theoretically and technically possible to define these circuits, localize the sites of memory storage, and analyze the cellular and molecular mechanisms of memory.

The nature of the biologic substrate of learning and memory is a fundamental issue in the psychobiologic aspects of behavioral development. How the developing mammalian brain is organized to learn and the underlying neurobiologic processes involved are key themes. In order to understand how the developing brain is modified by experience, it is perhaps necessary to understand more generally how the brain is modified by experience—the neurobiologic substrates of learning and memory.

Given the fact that learning is certainly among the most important processes in the postnatal development of mammals (and even in prenatal development, Smotherman & Robinson, in press), it is astonishing that so little work has been done on relations between development of learning abilities and capacities and the development of mammalian brain structures. One of the few systematic attempts along these lines is the work of Amsel and associates on the ontogeny of paradoxical reward. One example of this phenomenon is the partial reinforcement extinction effect: With partial reinforcement during learning, extinction is more prolonged than after 100% reinforcement training in adult mammals, including humans, and in rats over 14 days of age. It is "paradoxical" because less reinforcement during training leads to better retention. But prior to 11 days of age, rat pups do not show the paradoxical effect. There is reason to believe that the hippocampus may play some role in this phenomenon, and there are marked and rapid developmental changes in the septohippocampal system at this period in the postnatal development of the rat brain (Amsel & Stanton, 1980).

A fundamental issue is identification of brain structures and systems essential for various aspects of learning and memory. If a given form of memory can be shown to be stored in a particular brain structure, then it will be possible to undertake a detailed comparative analysis of the postnatal development of this form of learning and of the brain structure. Much evidence points to the critical role of experience itself in shaping the fine-tuned synaptic organization of brain structures (chap. 9, this volume). So, if one knows where, and ultimately even how, a given form of learning and memory is stored in the brain, it will be possible to analyze in detail the interactions of genetic programming and experience in the developmental processes of memory storage in the brain. The key is localization of memory traces. In this chapter we overview recent work, primarily from our laboratory, building an increasingly strong case that the memory traces for a basic form of associative learning are stored in the cerebellum.

## I. The Model Biologic System Approach

Quinn offered this tongue-in-cheek sketch of the ideal preparation for analysis of neurobiologic substrates of learning and memory:

> The organism should have no more than three genes, a generation time of twelve hours, be able to play the cello or at least recite classical Greek, and learn these tasks with a nervous system containing only ten large, differently colored, and therefore easily recognizable neurons. (Cited as personal communication in Kandel, 1976, p. 45)

Quinn's preparation illustrates a number of features that an ideal model biologic system should possess. The model system approach to brain substrates of learning and memory was of course first developed by Pavlov and by Lashley. Lashley (1950) states the essence of the approach most simply in the following passage: "In experiments extending over the past 30 years, I have been trying to trace conditioned reflex paths through the brain or to find the locus of specific memory traces" (p. 455).

At the present time, the model system approach is perhaps the most promising research strategy for investigating the neural bases of behavior and changes in behavior, particularly for dealing with the problem of localization of memory traces (Alkon, 1980; Chang & Gelperin, 1980; Cohen, 1980; Ito, 1982; Kandel, 1976; Kandel & Spencer, 1968; Sahley, Rudy, & Gelperin, 1981; Thompson, 1983; 1986; Thompson *et al.*, 1976; Thompson, Berger, & Madden, 1983; Thompson, McCormick, & Lavond, 1986; Thompson & Spencer, 1966; Tsukahara, 1981; Woody, 1982). The strategy of this approach is to select an organism capable of exhibiting a range of behavioral phenomena that one wishes to explain and whose nervous system possesses properties that make neuroanatomic, neuropharmacological, and neurophysiological experimentation tractable. The goal is to work out in detail (to a cellular level) how a nervous system controls some type of behavior. This description then is taken to be a model of how the same and related behavioral phenomena are produced in other species. The tradeoff typically encountered is that the more complex the behavior one wishes to explain, the less tractable are the nervous systems of organisms capable of exhibiting such behavior. A chief advantage of model systems is that the facts gained from anatomic, physiological, biochemical, and behavioral investigations for a particular preparation are cumulative and tend to have synergistic effects on theory development and research.

Each approach and model preparation has particular advantages. The unique value of invertebrate preparations as model systems results from the fact that certain behavioral functions are controlled by ganglia containing relatively small numbers of large, identifiable cells—cells which can be consistently identified across individuals of the species (Alkon, 1980; Davis & Gillette, 1978; Hoyle, 1980; Kandel, 1976; Krasne, 1969). As a result of knowing the architecture of the system, one can begin to determine systematically which neurons of the system are responsible for the behavior under investigation. Upon defining such neural circuits, one can then evaluate how the functioning of the neurons in the circuit are affected by training procedures. Once the neurons exhibiting plasticity are known, it is possible to identify changes in their structure and function that are responsible for the observed changes in behavior. But the key question with simplified invertebrate models is of course the extent to which they can be generalized to the mammalian brain. The answer will not really be known until mechanisms have been analyzed in the mammalian brain.

With intact mammalian model systems, characterization of the neurobiologic substrates of learning and memory is a formidable task. One uses mammals for the simple reason that if one is to understand vertebrate nervous systems, one must at some point study them. In addition, if the behavior of interest is complex, it might be observed only in mammals. It is clear that they have developed increasing capacities for learning and have made use of these capacities in the development of adaptive behavior. It would seem that the evolution of the mammalian brain has resulted in systems especially well adapted for information processing, learning, and memory.

## II. Eyelid Conditioning: A Mammalian Model System

Some years ago we adopted a particularly clear-cut and robust form of associative learning in the intact mammal as a model biologic system: classical conditioning of the rabbit nictitating membrane (NM) and eyelid response to an acoustic or visual CS using a corneal airpuff US. Classical conditioning of the rabbit NM/eyelid response has a number of advantages for analysis of brain substrates of learning and memory, which have been detailed elsewhere (Thompson et al., 1976). Perhaps the greatest single advantage of this, and classical conditioning paradigms in general, is that the effects of experimental manipulations on learning versus performance can be more easily evaluated than in instrumental procedures.

Another advantage of the conditioned eyelid response is the fact that eyelid conditioning has become perhaps the most widely used paradigm for the study of basic properties of classical or Pavlovian conditioning of striated muscle responses in both humans and infrahuman subjects. It displays the same basic laws of learning in humans and other animals (Hilgard & Marquis, 1940). Consequently, it seems highly likely that neuronal mechanisms found to underlie conditioning of the eyelid response in rabbits will hold for all mammals, including humans. We view the conditioned eyelid response as an instance of the general class of discrete, adaptive behavioral responses learned to deal with an aversive event, and we adopt the working assumption that neuronal mechanisms underlying associative learning of the eyelid response will in fact be general for all such learning.

In the rabbit NM conditioning paradigm, considerably more than just NM extension becomes conditioned. Gormezano and associates first showed that eyelid closure, eyeball retraction, and NM extension all develop during conditioning in essentially the same manner (Deaux & Gormezano, 1963; Gormezano, Schneiderman, Deaux, & Fuentes, 1962; Schneiderman, Fuentes, & Gormezano, 1962). The efferent limb thus involves several cranial nerve nuclei. The total response is a coordinated defense of the eye involving primarily eyeball retraction (NM extension) and eyelid closure with some contraction of periorbital facial musculature (see McCormick, Lavond, & Thompson, 1982). Simultaneous recordings from the NM and eyelid during conditioning show essentially perfect correlations in both amplitude and latency of the conditioned responses as they develop over the course of training.

Recordings of neural activity from one of the critical motor nuclei (6th or abducens) simultaneously with measurement of NM extension or eyelid closure show that the pattern of increased neural unit response precedes and closely parallels the amplitude-time course of the behavioral NM response. The cross-correlation between the two responses is very high—typically over 0.90 (Cegavske, Thompson, Patterson, & Gormezano, 1976).

The amplitude-time course of the eyelid response thus mirrors the pattern of increased neuronal unit activity in the relevant motor nuclei with considerable precision on a trial-by-trial basis (except, of course, for onset latency differences). This is a great convenience. The extension of the NM eyelid across the eye reflects the change in neural unit activity in the final common path—a learned neuronal response that has the same properties in several motor nuclei. We adopted the working hypothesis that the neuronal system responsible for generation of the learned eyelid response will exhibit this same pattern of increased neuronal activity. Something must drive the several motor nuclei in a synchronous fashion. The amplitude-time course of the learned eyelid response provides a marker for the pattern of increased neuronal activity in the memory trace circuit.

In the standard conditioning paradigm, animals with the cerebral neocortex or hippocampus removed are able to learn (Oakley & Russell, 1972; Solomon & Moore, 1975), as are animals with all brain tissue above the level of the thalamus or midbrain removed (Esner, 1976; Norman, Buchwald, & Villablanca, 1977). Some caution must be exercised in drawing conclusions regarding the locus of the memory trace in the intact animal from results on reduced preparations. The fact that a decerebrate animal can learn the eyelid response does not necessarily mean that the memory trace is normally established in the intact animal below the level of the thalamus, only that the remaining tissue is capable of supporting learning. Oakley and Russell (1977) addressed this issue for the cerebral cortex by first training the animals, then decorticating them, allowing 5–10 weeks for recovery, and then continuing training. They found a transient depression in conditioned responding but a rapid recovery (marked savings), arguing that a substantial part of the memory trace established in the intact animal is below the level of the cerebral cortex.

Current work in our laboratory provides a dramatic demonstration that the essential memory trace for the standard short-delay eyelid CR is in fact established below the level of the thalamus in intact animals. (Our standard conditions are tone CS of 1 KHz, 85 dB, duration 350 ms; corneal airpuff US of 100-ms duration, coterminating with CS.) Rabbits were trained and overtrained. At the end of the overtraining session, they were anesthetized (with halothane) and decerebrated: All brain tissue above the caudal level of the thalamus was aspirated. They were allowed 3–4 hr of recovery following decerebration, and training was continued. The animals retained normal CR following decerebration (Mauk & Thompson, in press)!

It seems very likely that memory trace systems develop in higher regions of the brain in classical conditioning. Indeed, evidence to data argues strongly that a memory trace system develops in the hippocampus very early in training in classical conditioning of the rabbit eyelid response (Berger & Thompson, 1978a, 1978b, 1978c; Berger, Rinaldi, Weisz, & Thompson, 1983). However, this hippocampal memory trace system is not essential for learning or memory of the CR, although it does appear to become more critical when greater demands are placed on the memory system. The development of such "higher order" memory systems in basic learning paradigms may provide simplified models for the study of neuronal substrates of the more complex or cognitive functions of higher regions of the brain like the cerebral cortex and hippocampus (see also Amsel & Stanton, 1980; Thompson, Berger, & Madden, 1983).

In a series of studies described elsewhere (Thompson, McCormick, Lavond, Clark, Kettner, & Mauk, 1983), we have developed evidence against localization of the memory traces for these basic CR to several brain systems. One must distinguish between the essential memory trace circuit, here from the ear (tone CS) to the eyelid, and the memory traces themselves. In brief, our evidence argues against the memory traces being localized to the primary auditory relay nuclei (CS channel), to the motor nuclei, or to the more direct US reflex pathways. But some portions of these nuclei and pathways are of course a part of the essential memory trace circuit.

## III.  Cerebellum: The Locus of the Memory Trace?

From the above findings, the circuitry that might serve to code the primary memory trace for the eyelid CR in the standard delay paradigm could include much of the midbrain and brainstem and the cerebellum, excluding the primary CS channel (here the auditory relay nuclei), the reflex pathways, and the motor neurons. Since there was no a priori way of determining which of these regions and structures are involved in the memory trace, we undertook, beginning some years ago, to map the entire midbrain, brainstem, and cerebellum by systematically recording neuronal unit activity (unit cluster recording) in already trained animals (Cegavske, Patterson, & Thompson, 1979; McCormick, Lavond, & Thompson, 1983; Thompson, Berger, & Madden, 1983). For this purpose we developed a chronic micromanipulator system that permits mapping of unit activity in a substantial number of neural loci per animal. Increases in unit activity that form a temporal model within a trial of the learned behavioral response were prominent in certain regions of the cerebellum, as well as in certain other regions, and of course in the cranial motor nuclei engaged in generation of the behavioral response. The results of the mapping studies pointed to substantial engagement of the cerebellar system in the generation of the CR. An example is shown in Fig. 1 with unit recordings from the cerebellar interpositus nucleus ipsilateral to the trained eye. This animal was given unpaired training before acquisition began. Average histograms reveal that the unit activity showed only minimal responses to the tone and airpuff during the unpaired day of training. However, during acquisition, as the animal learned, the unit activity developed a model of the CR. Again, there is no clear model of the UR. The cerebellar unit model of the learned response precedes the behavioral response significantly in time. A neuronal model of the learned behavioral response appears to develop de novo in the cerebellar deep nuclear region. The course of development of the conditioned behavioral eyelid response and the concomitant growth in the neuronal unit "model" of the

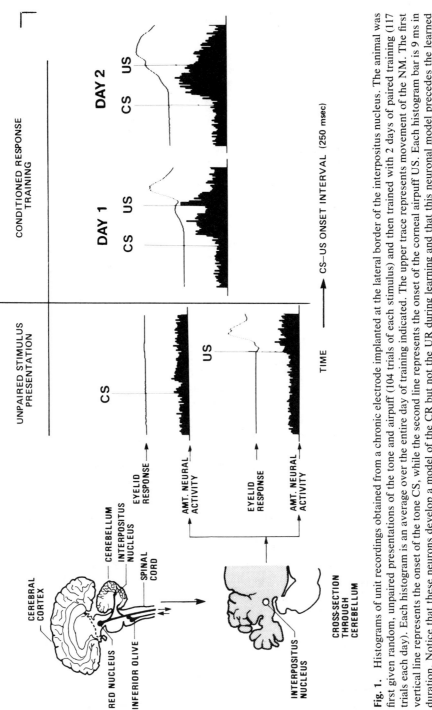

**Fig. 1.** Histograms of unit recordings obtained from a chronic electrode implanted at the lateral border of the interpositus nucleus. The animal was first given random, unpaired presentations of the tone and airpuff (104 trials of each stimulus) and then trained with 2 days of paired training (117 trials each day). Each histogram is an average over the entire day of training indicated. The upper trace represents movement of the NM. The first vertical line represents the onset of the tone CS, while the second line represents the onset of the corneal airpuff US. Each histogram bar is 9 ms in duration. Notice that these neurons develop a model of the CR but not the UR during learning and that this neuronal model precedes the learned behavioral response substantially in time. From McCormick and Thompson (1984b); reproduced by permission.

CR in the interpositus nuclear region show very high correlations (e.g., $r = .90$).

In current work, we have found that lesions ipsilateral to the trained eye in the neocerebellum (Fig. 2) permanently abolish the CR but have no

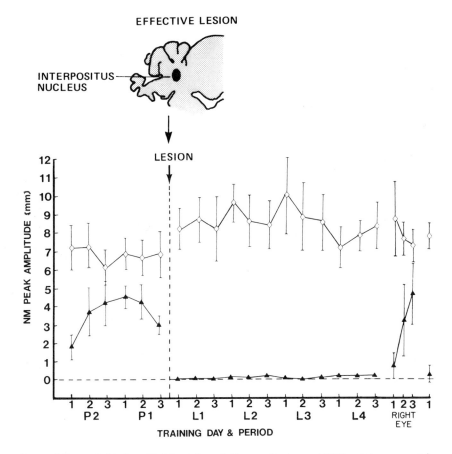

**Fig. 2.** Effects of ablation of left lateral cerebellum on the learned NM/eyelid response (six animals). Solid triangles: amplitude of CR; open diamonds; amplitude of UR. All training was to left eye (ipsilateral to lesion) except where labeled *right eye*. The cerebellar lesion completely and permanently abolished the CR of the ipsilateral eye but had no effect on the UR. P1 and P2 indicate initial learning on the 2 days prior to the lesion. L1–L4 are 4 days of postoperative training to the left eye. The right eye was then trained and learned rapidly, thus controlling for nonspecific lesion effects. The left eye was again trained and showed no learning. Numbers on abscissa indicate 40 trial periods, except for "right eye," which are 24 trial periods. From McCormick, Clark, Lavond, and Thompson (1982); reproduced by permission.

232 Richard F. Thompson

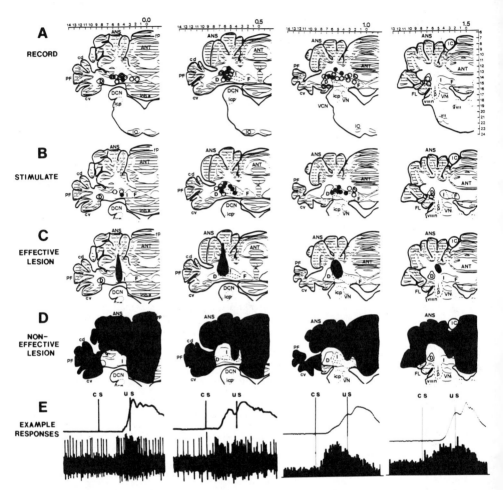

**Fig. 3.** Spatial distribution of recording, stimulating, effective, and noneffective lesion sites within the ipsilateral cerebellum. (A) Recording sites that did (filled circles) and did not (open circles) develop neuronal "models" (E) of the learned eyeblink response. Only the recording sites that developed robust responses or no response at all are plotted. The larger numbers above each section represent millimeters anterior to lambda, and the numbers to the side represent millimeters below bone at lambda. (B) Sites that, when stimulated, did (filled circles) and did not (open) elicit eyeblink responses. (C) An example of a lesion of the dentate and interpositus (D-I) nuclei which permanently abolished the learned response (3). (D) Composite from three animals of cortical lesions that were not effective in abolishing the learned eyeblink response. (E) Neuronal responses of four different recording sites within the cerebellum. The first recording is an example of multiple unit activity from the ansiform cortex. The second recording and the two histograms on the right were obtained from the D-I nuclei. The histograms are averages of an entire session of training. The first vertical line represents the onset of the tone, and the second represents the onset of the airpuff. Each

effect on the UR and do not prevent subsequent learning by the contralateral eye (Clark, McCormick, Lavond, Baxter, Gray, & Thompson, 1982; Clark, McCormick, Lavond, & Thompson, 1984; Lavond, McCormick, Clark, Holmes, & Thompson, 1981; McCormick, Lavond, Clark, Kettner, Rising, & Thompson; McCormick, Clark et al., 1982; McCormick, Guyer, & Thompson, 1982; McCormick & Thompson 1984a, 1984b; Thompson, 1983). If the lesion is made before training, no learning occurs (Lincoln, McCormick, & Thompson, 1982). The critical region is the lateral interpositus nucleus. Perhaps most dramatic is a recent study involving kainic acid (it destroys nerve cell bodies but not nerve fibers or terminals): Destruction of neurons in a region as small as a cubic millimeter in the lateral portion of the interpositus causes complete and permanent loss of the learned eyelid response (Lavond, Hembree, & Thompson, 1985).

Lesions of the cerebellar cortex do not abolish the basic conditioned eyelid response (McCormick & Thompson, 1984b). To date, we have removed all lobes of the ipsilateral cerebellar cortex except the flocculus in different groups of animals. However, our results to date to not exclude the possibility of a multiple trace in the cerebellar cortex represented in several lobes that project to the critical deep nuclear region.

Electrical stimulation through recording microelectrodes in the critical lateral interpositus nuclear region elicits a discrete eyelid response prior to training. Indeed, a range of discrete behavioral responses—eyelid closure, leg flexion, head turning—can be elicited by microstimulation of the interpositus, the type of response depending upon the exact location of the stimulating electrode.

Composite diagrams are shown in Fig. 3 indicating regions of the ipsilateral cerebellar deep nuclei from which the neuronal unit "model" of the learned behavioral response can be recorded (solid dots in A), regions from which electrical stimulation evokes on eyelid response (solid dots in B), the locus of lesions that permanently abolish the conditioned eyelid response (C), and large cerebellar cortical lesions that do not abolish the

---

histogram bar is 9 ms wide, and the length of the entire trace is 750 ms. The top trace in each set is the movement of the NM with "up" being extension across the eyeball. Abbreviations: ANS, ansiform lobule (crus I and crus II); ANT, anterior lobule; FL, flocculus; D, dentate nucleus; DCN, dorsal cochlear nucleus; F, fastigial nucleus; I, interpositus nucleus; IC, interior colliculus; I0, inferior olive; lob a, lobulus A (nodulus); PF, paraflocculus; VN, vestibular nuclei; cd, dorsal crus; cv, ventral crus; gVII, genu of the tract of the seventh nerve; icp, inferior cerebellar peduncle; VII, seventh (facial) nucleus; and VCN, ventral cochlear nucleus. From McCormick and Thompson (1984a); reproduced by permission.

conditioned eyelid response (D). Note that the sites of the neuronal
model, the sites of effective electrical stimulation, and the effective lesion
site are essentially identical, involving the lateral portion of the interpositus
nucleus. Importantly, a lesion placed more medially in the interpositus
nucleus selectively abolishes the learned hindlimb flexion response
(Donegan, Lowry, & Thompson, 1983).

These results indicate that the essential memory trace circuits for these
learned responses are extremely localized in the brain. How general is
this finding? Most of our work has been on the learned eyelid response,
but as noted above, we have shown that a different part of the interpositus
is essential for hindlimb flexion conditioning. We and our associated laboratories are now exploring the generality of our results across learning
paradigms and species. Particularly important are current results in collaboration with Michael Patterson at Ohio University. He developed a
procedure for eyelid conditioning in the cat and has now found that the
interpositus nucleus ipsilateral to the trained eye is essential for the
learned response in this species as well as in the rabbit. It would seem that
our results may be generalizable to all mammals. In other work, Patterson
developed a paradigm for instrumental avoidance learning of the eyelid
closure response in the rabbit, where eyelid closure to the tone CS before
onset of the corneal airpuff results in the airpuff not being delivered. He
found that lesions of the ipsilateral interpositus nucleus abolish this instrumental avoidance response as well as the classically conditioned response. Hence, we feel we can generalize our essential cerebellar circuit
to discrete, adaptive responses learned to deal with aversive stimuli in
both classical and instrumental avoidance learning paradigms in mammals.

In other work we have identified much of the efferent pathway from
interpositus nucleus to motor nuclei. Our results indicate that it courses
out the superior cerebellar peduncle (McCormick, Guyer, & Thompson,
1982), crosses to the contralateral side in the peduncle (Lavond *et al.*,
1981), relays in the magnocellular division of the red nucleus (Haley,
Lavond, & Thompson, 1983; Madden, Haley, Barchas, & Thompson,
1983), crosses back to the ipsilateral side, and projects to the lower brainstem as a part of the descending rubral pathway (Fig. 4). The essential CR
circuit we have so far defined could be called the *efferent limb* in that
destruction of any part of the circuit abolishes the CR to any CS (e.g.,
light or tone), but the association between CS and US/UR could very well
be formed in the cerebellum. Collectively, these results argue strongly for
the memory trace being in the cerebellum and/or in structures afferent to
it for which the cerebellum is a mandatory efferent.

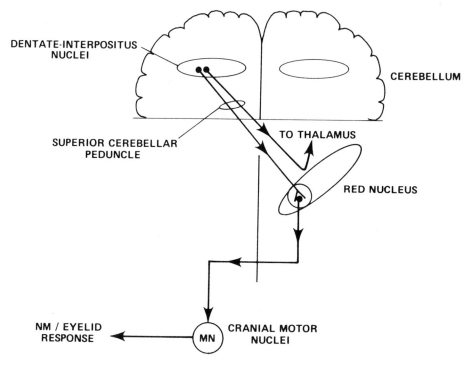

**Fig. 4.**  The efferent (output) pathway we hypothesize from the cerebellar memory trace system to motor nuclei.

## A.  A Hypothetical Model

In late 1983 we developed a hypothetical schema or model of how the cerebellar memory trace circuit might work (Fig. 5), based on the well-known anatomy of the system, on our results described above, and on theories of how the cerebellum might function as a learning machine. The cerebellar cortex has great appeal to theoreticians and modelers because of its elegant uniformity and simplicity and because of the striking fact of two quite different inputs to each Purkinje cell: a mossy fiber–granule cell–parallel fiber input that is widely distributed and a climbing fiber input that is highly localized. All models, both verbal-logical and computational, have stressed this point, and those that focus on learning and memory have universally hypothesized that the mossy fiber–granule cell–parallel fiber system is the learning input, and the climbing fiber input is the teaching input (Albus, 1971; Brindley, 1964; Eccles, 1977; Gilbert, 1974; Grossberg, 1969; Ito, 1974; Marr, 1969).

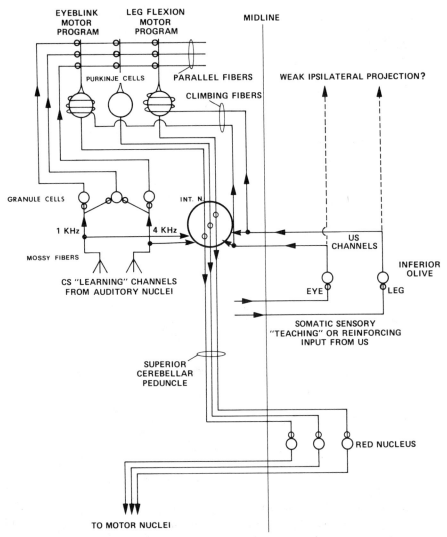

**Fig. 5.** Schema of a hypothetical memory trace system for associative learning of discrete, adaptive, somatic-motor responses to deal with aversive USs. Most interneurons are omitted. It is assumed that the site of the memory trace is at the Purkinje cells shown in the upper left under "motor programs" and/or at associated interneurons. The locus of the memory trace is shown as cerebellar cortex, and the basic notion is very similar to earlier theories of cerebellar plasticity (Albus, Marr, Eccles, Ito), but traces could also or alternatively be formed in the interpositus nucleus (int. n.), we assume by an analogous circuitry. A given CS (1 KHz) activates a subset of parallel fibers that in turn activate weakly all Purkinje cells shown. A different tone also activates all Purkinje cells but by a partially different group of parallel fibers. The US pathway is assumed to be via the inferior olive and climbing fibers. A

In our schema, it is assumed that the site of the memory trace is at the principal neurons (Purkinje cells) shown in the upper left and/or in associated interneurons in the cerebellar cortex (not shown), and/or in the interpositus nucleus. A given CS (1 KHz) is assumed to activate a subset of granule cells and parallel fibers that in turn activate weakly all principal cells. A different tone also activates all principal cells but by a partially different group of parallel fibers. The US pathway is assumed to be via the inferior olive and climbing fibers. A given US is assumed to activate only a limited group of principal cells, coding the motor program for the defensive response that is specific for the US (e.g., eyelid closure, leg flexion). When parallel fiber activation occurs at the appropriate time just prior to climbing fiber activation, the connections of the parallel fibers to the principal cells activated by the particular US are strengthened (or weakened). The efferent pathway from principal cells to motor neurons is by way of the superior cerebellar peduncle and red nucleus. The schema accounts for stimulus specificity (for example, the fact that CRs show a stimulus generalization gradient), for response specificity of learned responses, for transfer, and for lesion-transfer effects (e.g., training one eye and then the other before or after cerebellar lesion), and is consistent with all our evidence to date. Although much of this circuit was hypothetical, insofar as it being a substrate for the formation of memories is concerned, each aspect and assumption is testable. Indeed, current work in our laboratory is providing strong new evidence favoring such a schema.

B.  The Inferior Olive: The Necessary and Sufficient Teaching
    Input for the Learning of Discrete Behavioral Responses

A major afferent system that projects to the cerebellum is the inferior olive (IO)–climbing fiber system (Fig. 6). The dorsal accessory olive (DAO) has a clear somatotopic organization that is maintained in its projection to the interpositus (Gellman, Houk, & Gibson, 1983). In recent work we have found that lesions of the appropriate region of the IO (rostromedial DAO) do not abolish the CR but instead lead to relatively normal *extinction* with continued paired CS-US training (Fig. 7; McCormick, Steinmetz, & Thompson, 1985). Lesions of all other regions of the

---

given US is assumed to activate only a limited group of Purkinje cells, coding the motor program for the defensive response that is specific for the US (eyelid closure, leg flexion). When parallel fiber activation occurs at the appropriate time just prior to climbing fiber activation, the connections of the parallel fibers to the Purkinje cells activated by the particular US are strengthened. The efferent pathway from Purkinje cells to motor neurons is by way of the interpositus nucleus, superior cerebellar peduncle, and red nucleus. Modified from Thompson *et al.* (1986); reproduced by permission.

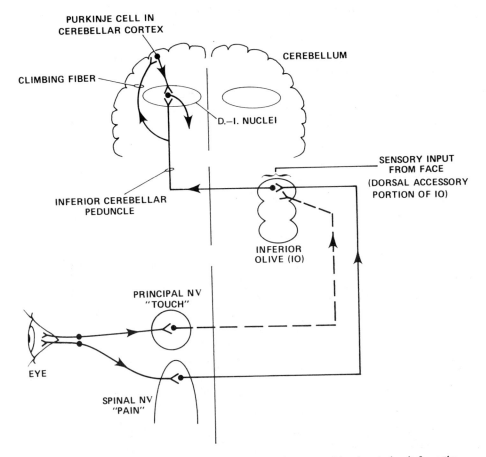

**Fig. 6.** Our hypothesis of the effective US reinforcing or teaching input circuit from the cornea of the eye to the cerebellum. The critical region of the inferior olive is the dorsal accessory olive.

IO do not affect the CR. The DAO appears to be the essential afferent limb for the reinforcing or "teaching" input from the US. The fact that lesions of the DAO do not immediately abolish the CR but instead lead to its eventual extinction argues that the essential memory trace cannot be there.

In current work we find that electrical microstimulation of the DAO can elicit a variety of behavioral responses, including eyelid closure, the nature of the threshold response being determined by the exact location of the stimulating electrode (latency from DAO stimulation ~35 ms). If this is now used as the US/UR and paired with a tone CS, the *exact response*

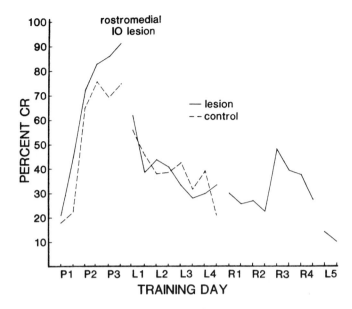

**Fig. 7.** Effect of lesion of the rostromedial inferior olive on the percentage of trials in which conditioned responses were performed. The animals were first trained (P1–P3) and then received either a lesion which included the rostromedial IO (lesion) or disconnection of the airpuff (control), followed by four days of paired trials to the same eye (L1–L4) for the lesion group or tone-alone trials for the control group. Subsequent training to the contralateral eye in the lesion group (R1–R4) gave indications of learning, but the percentage of responses never rose above 50. One final day of training on the left (L5) was then performed. Each data point represents the average of one-half day of training. From McCormick *et al.* (1985); reproduced by permission.

elicited by DAO stimulation is learned to the tone as a CR rapidly and with all the properties of a normal CR (Fig. 8; Mauk & Thompson, 1984; Mauk, Steinmetz, & Thompson, 1986). Lesion of the critical interpositus region abolishes this IO-established CR *and* abolishes the response elicited by IO stimulation (Mauk & Thompson, unpublished observations). Control stimulation 1–2 mm dorsal to the DAO in the reticular formation can also elicit movements, presumably by activation of descending reticular pathways, but these elicited movements cannot be trained to a CS. These IO results strengthen the argument that the IO and its climbing fiber input to the cerebellum is the essential US teaching input and that the trace is localized to the cerebellum (Fig. 6). They are also the first clear empirical evidence supporting the pioneering hypothesis and network models of Albus, Eccles, Ito, Marr, and others that the IO–climbing fiber system is the "teaching" input for behavioral learning in

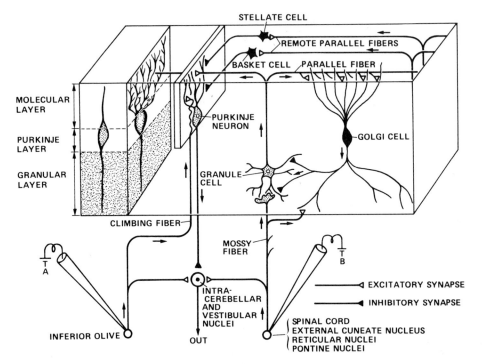

**Fig. 8.** Synaptic organization of the cerebellar cortex. Purkinje cells are excited directly by climbing fibers and indirectly (via parallel fibers from the granule cells) by the mossy fibers. Stellate and basket cells, which are excited by parallel fibers, act as inhibitory interneurons. The Golgi cells act on the granule cells with feedback inhibition (when excited by parallel fibers) and feedforward inhibition (when excited by climbing and mossy fiber collaterals). The output of the Purkinje cell is inhibitory upon the cells of the intracerebellar and vestibular nuclei. Modified from Kandel, E. R. and Schwartz, J. H. (1987). *Principles of Neural Science*. New York, Elsevier, Figure 30.3 p. 338. Reproduced by permission. In normal behavioral training, a tone is used as the CS, and a corneal airpuff, that elicits an eyeblink, is used as the US. However, electrical microstimulation of a portion of the IO–climbing fiber projection to the cerebellum (see TA) can also elicit an eyeblink response and serves as a very effective US in place of the corneal airpuff. Similarly, electrical microstimulation of the mossy fiber projection to the cerebellum (see TB) can serve as a very effective CS in place of tone or light. Finally, joint stimulation of climbing fibers as the US and mossy fibers as the CS produces normal learning of discrete behavioral responses.

the cerebellum. Ito (1984) has developed analogous findings in the context of plasticity of the vestibulo-ocular reflex, and Llinas, Walton, Hillman, and Sotelo (1975) report a similar role for the IO–climbing fiber system in recovery from postural abnormalities following vestibular damage.

## C. Creation of a Known CS Pathway: Mossy Fiber Projections to the Cerebellum

The major remaining unknown portion of the essential memory trace circuit concerns how CS information is projected from primary sensory pathways to the essential cerebellar circuit. But we have succeeded in creating a known CS pathway by using electrical microstimulation of mossy fiber projections to the cerebellum as the CS (Fig. 8; Steinmetz, Lavond, & Thompson, 1985b). Animals rapidly learn normal behavioral CR to this CS (e.g., eyeblink CR with corneal airpuff US). To date we have successfully used stimulation of mossy fibers from the dorsolateral pontine nucleus and the lateral reticular nucleus as CSs (Steinmetz, Rosen, Chapman, Lavond, & Thompson, 1986; Steinmetz, Rosen, Woodruff-Pak, Lavond, & Thompson, in press).

Finally, in current work we find that normal behavioral CRs are learned with electrical stimulation of mossy fibers as the CS and DAO–climbing fibers as the US, thus creating a "reduced" preparation within the intact, behaving animal (Fig. 8; Steinmetz, Lavond, & Thompson, 1985a). This preparation promises much in terms of fine-grained localization of the memory traces and analysis of mechanisms.

We suggest as a working hypothesis that under normal conditions of learning with peripheral stimuli: (a) The essential CS information is projected to the cerebellum via mossy fibers; (b) the essential teaching or reinforcing information from the US is projected to the cerebellum via climbing fibers from the IO; and (c) memory traces are established in highly localized regions in the cerebellar cortex (and interpositus nucleus ?) at loci of convergence of the critical mossy and climbing fiber projections, perhaps at parallel fiber synapses on Purkinje cell dendrites. If this is indeed the case, then it could be hypothesized that training induces either increased (the Marr, 1969, hypothesis) or decreased (the Albus, 1971, hypothesis) responsiveness to the CS in those Purkinje cells projecting to critical interpositus neurons. Ito (1984; Ito, Sakurai, & Tongroach, 1982) has reported that conjunctive stimulation of mossy fibers (vestibular nerve) and climbing fibers (IO) in the high-decerebrate rabbit causes a persisting decrease in excitability of Purkinje cells in the flocculus activated by stimulation of the vestibular nerve, due apparently to a change in parallel fiber–Purkinje cell synapses.

## IV. Conclusions

In more general terms, our results have demonstrated quite clearly that the essential memory trace circuits in the brain for the basic category of associative learning we have studied are highly localized, and all our evidence to date points to discrete regions of the cerebellum as the locus of memory storage for discrete, adaptive behavioral responses learned associatively to deal with aversive events. The overriding fact is that the cerebellum is essential for the learning and memory of all such tasks.

The effects of cerebellar damage in humans are to impair movements, particularly skilled movements. Most movements that humans make are to a significant degree learned, that is, skilled. In this context, Eccles (1977) has proposed the following:

> We can say that normally our most complex muscle movements are carried out subconsciously and with consummate skill. The more subconscious you are in a golf stroke, the better it is, and the same with tennis, skiing, skating, or any other skill. In all these performances we do not have any appreciation of the complexity of muscle contractions and joint movements. All that we are conscious of is a general directive given by what we may call our voluntary command system. It is my thesis that the cerebellum is concerned in this enormously complex organization and control of movement, and that throughout life, *particularly in the early years* [italics added], we are engaged in an incessant teaching program for the cerebellum. As a consequence, it can carry out all of these remarkable tasks that we set it to do in the whole repertoire of our skilled movements in games, in techniques, in musical performances, in speech, dance, song, and so on. (p. 328)

If the cerebellum is in fact the locus of storage for memories of skilled movements, then the postnatal development of the cerebellum and its interaction with movement experience and the development of basic skills like walking and talking becomes a critically important aspect of human development. Indeed, Floater and Greenough (1979) have shown pronounced anatomic changes in the cerebellar cortex of monkeys raised in movement-enriched environments relative to controls. A great deal is known about the embryologic and postnatal development of the cerebellum (Jacobson, 1978). Thus, in terms of width of layers, the chick has a basically adult cerebellum at hatching, the rat at about 20 days after birth, the dog at about 60 days, and humans not until about a year after birth. A significant period of postnatal neuronal development occurs in the cerebellum in mammals. Now that we have a specific category of learning for which the cerebellum is essential, it should permit a detailed neural-behavioral analysis of the ontogeny of basic associative learning and memory.

To take just one recent example, Little, Lipsitt, and Rovee-Collier (1984) conditioned the eyelid response in groups of human infants ages 10, 20, and 30 days postnatal. All of the groups learned poorly compared to adults. But the most striking result was in terms of retention. All groups were retrained 10 days later. In contrast to the older infants, those 10 days of age at first training showed no sign of retention! From our basic work on the rabbit, we predict dramatic changes in the development of parallel fiber and/or climbing fiber synapses, most probably the former, on Purkinje cells in the human cerebellum between 10 and 20 days after birth.

One of the most striking features of the cerebellum is the high degree of regularity in the anatomic organization of the cortex over its extent and over species. It is highly and regularly organized; indeed, hardwired. If a major function of this structure is to code the associative learning of discrete, adaptive movements, and more generally skilled movements, then the basic neural circuitry for such learning preexists. No new "long" pathways are formed. Instead, the memory traces must involve changes in the fine structure of synaptic organization and processes.

The general possibility that learning circuits are hardwired in the mammalian brain is consistent with all we know about the high degree of anatomic organization of the brain and not inconsistent with all we know about learning and memory. Even the most complex form of human learning and memory, language, appears to have differentiated anatomic substrates in the cerebral cortex and uniformities in the "deep structure" of language itself across all languages (e.g., Damasio & Geschwind, 1984). In terms of mechanisms, the possibility that memory circuits are hardwired does not exclude anatomic substrates for memories in terms of the growth or alteration of the microstructure, that is, change in the size and properties of synapses and the development of new synapses (e.g., Greenough, 1984).

As we understand more deeply how memory traces are formed in the adult cerebellum, it will be possible to address fundamental questions of how the developing brain learns; how it is modified and shaped by experience (chap. 9, this volume); and how its organization in turn shapes experience and behavior.

## Acknowledgments

Supported in part by research grants from the National Science Foundation (BNS 81-17115), the Office of Naval Research (N00014-85-K-0238), the McKnight Foundation, and the Sloan Foundation.

## References

Albus, J. S. (1971). A theory of cerebellar function. *Mathematical Biosciences, 10,* 25–61.

Alkon, D. L. (1980). Membrane depolarization accumulates during acquisition of an associative behavioral change. *Science. 210,* 1375–1376.

Amsel, A., & Stanton, M. (1980). Ontogeny and phylogeny of paradoxical reward effects. In J. S. Rosenblatt, R. A. Hind, C. G. Beer, & M. C. Busnel (Eds.), *Advances in the study of behavior* (Vol. II, pp. 227–274). New York: Academic Press.

Berger, T. W., Rinaldi, P., Weisz, D. J., & Thompson, R. F. (1983). Single unit analysis of different hippocampal cell types during classical conditioning of the rabbit nictitating membrane response. *Journal of Neurophysiology, 50,* 1197–1219.

Berger, T. W., & Thompson, R. F. (1978a). Identification of pyramidal cells as the critical elements in hippocampal neuronal plasticity during learning. *Proceedings of the National Academy of Sciences, 75,* 1572–1576.

Berger, T. W., & Thompson, R. F. (1978b). Neuronal plasticity in the limbic system during classical conditioning of the rabbit nictitating membrane response: I. The hippocampus. *Brain Research, 145,* 323–346.

Berger, T. W., & Thompson, R. F. (1978c). Neuronal plasticity in the limbic system during classical conditioning of the rabbit nictitating membrane response: II. Septum and mamillary bodies. *Brain Research, 156,* 293–314.

Brindley, G. S. (1964). The use made by the cerebellum of the information that it receives from sense organs. *International Brain Research Organization Bulletin, 3,* 30.

Cegavske, C. F., Patterson, M. M., & Thompson, R. F. (1979). Neuronal unit activity in the abducens nucleus during classical conditioning of the nictitating membrane response in the rabbit (Oryctolagus cuniculus). *Journal of Comparative and Physiological Psychology, 93,* 595–609.

Cegavske, C. F., Thompson, R. F., Patterson, M. M., & Gormezano, I. (1976). Mechanisms of efferent neuronal control of the reflex nictitating membrane response in the rabbit. *Journal of Comparative and Physiological Psychology, 90,* 411–423.

Chang, J. J., & Gelperin, A. (1980). Rapid taste aversion learning by an isolated molluscan central nervous system. *Proceedings of the National Academy of Sciences, 77,* 6204.

Clark, G. A., McCormick, D. A., Lavond, D. G., Baxter, K., Gray, W. J., & Thompson, R. F. (1982). Effects of electrolytic lesions of cerebellar nuclei on conditioned behavioral and hippocampal neuronal responses. *Neuroscience Abstracts, 8,* 22.

Clark, G. A., McCormick, D. A., Lavond, D. G., & Thompson, R. F. (1984). Effects of lesions of cerebellar nuclei on conditioned behavioral and hippocampal neuronal responses. *Brain Research, 291,* 125–136.

Cohen, D. H. (1980). The functional neuroanatomy of a conditioned response. In R. F. Thompson, L. H. Hicks, & V. B. Shvyrkov (Eds.), *Neural mechanisms of goal-directed behavior and learning* (pp. 283–302). New York: Academic Press.

Damasio, A. R., & Geschwind, N. (1984). The neural basis of language. *Annual Review of Neuroscience, 7,* 127–147.

Davis, W. J., & Gillette, R. (1978). Neural correlates of behavioral plasticity in command neurons of Pleurobranchaea. *Science, 99,* 801–804.

Deaux, E. G., & Gormezano, I. (1963). Eyeball retraction: Classical conditioning and extinction in the albino rabbit. *Science, 141,* 630–631.

Donegan, N. H., Lowry, R. W., & Thompson, R. F. (1983). Effects of lesioning cerebellar nuclei on conditioned leg-flexion responses. *Neuroscience Abstracts, 9,* 331.

Eccles, J. C. (1977). An instruction-selection theory of learning in the cerebellar cortex. *Brain Research, 127,* 327–352.

Esner, D. (1976). Unpublished doctoral dissertation, University of Iowa.

Floater, M. K., & Greenough, W. T. (1979). Cerebellar plasticity: Modification of Purkinje cell structure by differential rearing in monkeys. *Science, 206,* 227–229.

Gellman, R., Houk, J. C., & Gibson, A. R. (1983). Somatosensory properties of the inferior olive of the cat. *Journal of Comparative Neurology, 215,* 228–243.

Gilbert, P. F. C. (1974). A theory of memory that explains the function and structure of the cerebellum. *Brain Research, 70,* 1–18.

Gormezano, I., Schneiderman, N., Deaux, E. G., & Fuentes, I. (1962). Nictitating membrane: Classical conditioning and extinction in the albino rabbit. *Science, 138,* 33–34.

Greenough, W. T. (1984). Structural correlates of information storage. *Trends in Neuroscience, 7,* 229–233.

Grossberg, S. (1969). On learning of spatiotemporal patterns by networks with ordered sensory and motor components: I. Excitatory components of the cerebellum. *Studies in Applied Mathematics, 48,* 105–132.

Haley, D. A., Lavond, D. G., & Thompson, R. F. (1983). Effects of contralateral red nuclear lesions on retention of the classically conditioned nictitating membrane/eyelid response in the rabbit. *Neuroscience Abstracts, 9,* 643.

Hilgard, E. R., & Marquis, D. G. (1940). *Conditioning and learning.* New York: Appleton-Century.

Hoyle, G. (1980). Learning, using natural reinforcements, in insect preparations that permit cellular neuronal analysis. *Journal of Neurobiology, 11,* 323–354.

Ito, M. (1974). The control mechanisms of cerebellar motor system. In F. O. Schmitt & R. G. Worden (Eds.), *The neurosciences, third study program* (pp. 293–303). Cambridge: MIT Press.

Ito, M. (1982). Cerebellar control of the vestibulo-ocular reflex: Around the flocculus hypothesis. *Annual Review of Neuroscience, 5,* 275–296.

Ito, M. (1984). *The cerebellum and neural control.* New York: Raven.

Ito, M., Sakurai, M., & Tongroach, P. (1982). Climbing fibre induced depression of both mossy fibre responsiveness and glutamate sensitivity of cerebellar Purkinje cells. *Journal of Physiology, 324,* 113–134.

Jacobson, M. (1978). *Developmental neurobiology* (2nd ed.). New York: Plenum.

Kandel, E. R. (1976). *Cellular basis of behavior: An introduction to behavioral neurobiology.* San Francisco: W. H. Freeman.

Kandel, E. R., & Schwartz, J. H. (Eds.). (1981). *Principles of neural science.* New York: Elsevier North-Holland.

Kandel, E. R., & Spencer, W. A. (1968). Cellular neurophysiological approaches in the study of learning. *Physiological Reviews, 58,* 65–134.

Kapp, B. S., Gallagher, M., Applegate, C. D., & Fysinger, R. C. (1982). The amygdala central nucleus: Contributions to conditioned cardiovascular responding during aversive Pavlovian conditioning in the rabbit. In C. D. Woody (Ed.), *Conditioning: Representation of involved neural functions* (pp. 581–600). New York: Plenum.

Krasne, F. B. (1969). Excitation and habituation of the crayfish escape reflex: The depolarizing response in lateral giant fibers of the isolated abdomen. *Journal of Experimental Biology, 50,* 29–46.

Lashley, K. S. (1950). In search of the engram. In *Symposium of the Society for Experimental Biology* (No. 4, pp. 454–482). New York: Cambridge University Press.

Lavond, D. G., Hembree, T. L., & Thompson, R. F. (1985). Effect of kainic acid lesions of the cerebellar interpositus nucleus on eyelid conditioning in the rabbit. *Brain Research, 326,* 179–182.

Lavond, D. G., McCormick, D. A., Clark, G. A., Holmes, D. T., & Thompson, R. F. (1981). Effects of ipsilateral rostral pontine reticular lesions on retention of classically conditioned nictitating membrane and eyelid responses. *Physiological Psychology, 9,* 335–339.

Lincoln, J. S., McCormick, D. A., & Thompson, R. F. (1982). Ipsilateral cerebellar lesions prevent learning of the classically conditioned nictitating membrane/eyelid response. *Brain Research, 242,* 190–193.

Little, A. H., Lipsitt, L. P., & Rovee-Collier, C. (1984). Classical conditioning and retention of the infant's eyelid response: Effects of age and intertrial interval. *Journal of Experimental Child Psychology, 37,* 512–524.

Llinas, R., Walton, K., Hillman, D. E., & Sotelo, C. (1975). Inferior olive: Its role in motor learning. *Science, 190,* 1230–1231.

Madden, J., IV, Haley, D. A., Barchas, J. D., & Thompson, R. F. (1983). Microinfusion of picrotoxin into the caudal red nucleus selectively abolishes the classically conditioned nictitating membrane/eyelid response in the rabbit. *Neuroscience Abstracts, 9,* 830.

Marr, D. (1969). A theory of cerebellar cortex. *Journal of Physiology* (London), *202,* 437–470.

Mauk, M. D., Steinmetz, J. E., & Thompson, R. F. (1986). Classical conditioning using stimulation of the inferior olive as the unconditioned stimulus. *Proceedings of the National Academy of Sciences, 83,* 5349–5353.

Mauk, M. D., & Thompson, R. F. (1984). Classical conditioning using stimulation of the inferior olive as the unconditioned stimulus. *Neuroscience Abstracts, 10,* 122 (Abstract No. 36.5).

Mauk, M. D., & Thompson, R. F. (in press). Retention of classically conditioned eyelid responses following acute decerebration. *Brain Research.*

McCormick, D. A., Clark, G. A., Lavond, D. G., & Thompson, R. F. (1982). Initial localization of the memory trace for a basic form of learning. *Proceedings of the National Academy of Sciences, 79,* 2731–2742.

McCormick, D. A., Guyer, P. E., & Thompson, R. F. (1982). Superior cerebellar peduncle lesions selectively abolish the ipsilateral classically conditioned nictitating membrane/eyelid response of the rabbit. *Brain Research, 244,* 347–350.

McCormick, D. A., Lavond, D. G., Clark, G. A., Kettner, R. E., Rising, C. E., & Thompson, R. F. (1981). The engram found? Role of the cerebellum in classical conditioning of nictitating membrane and eyelid responses. *Bulletin of the Psychonomic Society, 18*(3), 103–105.

McCormick, D. A., Lavond, D. G., & Thompson, R. F. (1982). Concomitant classical conditioning of the rabbit nictitating membrane and eyelid responses: Correlations and implications. *Physiology and Behavior, 28,* 769–775.

McCormick, D. A., Lavond, D. G., & Thompson, R. F. (1983). Neuronal responses of the rabbit brainstem during performance of the classically conditioned nictitating membrane (NM)/eyelid response. *Brain Research, 271,* 73–88.

McCormick, D. A., Steinmetz, J. E., & Thompson, R. F. (1985). Lesions of the inferior olivary complex cause extinction of the classically conditioned eyeblink response. *Brain Research, 359,* 120–130.

McCormick, D. A., & Thompson, R. F. (1984a). Cerebellum: Essential involvement in the classically conditioned eyelid response. *Science, 223,* 296–299.

McCormick, D. A., & Thompson, R. F. (1984b). Neuronal responses of the rabbit cerebellum during acquisition and performance of a classically conditioned nictitating membrane-eyelid response. *Journal of Neuroscience, 4,* 2811–2822.

Norman, R. J., Buchwald, J. S., & Villablanca, J. R. (1977). Classical conditioning with auditory discrimination of the eyeblink in decerebrate cats. *Science, 196,* 551–553.

Oakley, D. A., & Russell, I. S. (1972). Neocortical lesions and classical conditioning. *Physiology and Behavior, 8,* 915–926.

Oakley, D. A., & Russell, I. S. (1977). Subcortical storage of Pavlovian conditioning in the rabbit. *Physiology and Behavior, 18,* 931–937.

Sahley, C. L., Rudy, J. W., & Gelperin, A. (1981). An analysis of associative learning in the terrestrial mollusk: I. Higher-order conditioning, blocking, and a US-preexposure effect. *Journal of Comparative Physiology, 144,* 1–8.

Schneiderman, N., Fuentes, I., & Gormezano, I. (1962). Acquisition and extinction of the classically conditioned eyelid response in the albino rabbit. *Science, 136,* 650–652.

Smotherman, W. P., & Robinson, S. R. (in press). The uterus as environment: The ecology of fetal experience. In E. M. Blass (Ed.), *Handbook of behavioral neurobiology: Vol. 9. Developmental psychobiology and behavioral ecology.* New York: Plenum.

Solomon, P. R., & Moore, J. W. (1975). Latent inhibition and stimulus generalization of the classically conditioned nictitating membrane response in rabbits (Oryctolagus cuniculus) following dorsal hippocampal ablation. *Journal of Comparative Physiological Psychology, 89,* 1192–1203.

Steinmetz, J. E., Lavond, D. G., & Thompson, R. F. (1985a). Classical conditioning of skeletal muscle responses with mossy fiber stimulation CS and climbing fiber stimulation US. *Neuroscience Abstracts, 11,* 982 (Abstract No. 290.6).

Steinmetz, J. E., Lavond, D. G., & Thompson, R. F. (1985b). Classical conditioning of the rabbit eyelid response with mossy fiber stimulation as the conditioned stimulus. *Bulletin of the Psychonomic Society, 23*(3), 245–248.

Steinmetz, J. E., Rosen, D. J., Chapman, P. F., Lavond, D. G., & Thompson, R. F. (1986). Classical conditioning of the rabbit eyelid response with a mossy fiber stimulation CS: I. Pontine nuclei and middle cerebellar peduncle stimulation. *Behavioral Neuroscience, 100,* 871–880.

Steinmetz, J. E., Rosen, D. J., Woodruff-Pak, D. S., Lavond, D. G., & Thompson, R. F. (in press). Rapid transfer of training occurs when direct mossy fiber stimulation is used as a conditioned stimulus for classical eyelid conditioning. *Neuroscience Research.*

Thompson, R. F. (1983). Neuronal substrates of simple associative learning: Classical conditioning. *Trends in Neuroscience, 6*(7), 270–275.

Thompson, R. F. (1986). The neurobiology of learning and memory. *Science, 233,* 941–947.

Thompson, R. F., Berger, T. W., Cegavske, C. F., Patterson, M. M., Roemer, R. A., Teyler, T. J., & Young, R. A. (1976). The search for the engram. *American Psychologist, 31,* 209–227.

Thompson, R. F., Berger, T. W., & Madden, J., IV. (1983). Cellular processes of learning and memory in the mammalian CNS. *Annual Review of Neuroscience, 6,* 447–491.

Thompson, R. F., McCormick, D. A., & Lavond, D. G. (1986). Localization of the essential memory trace system for a basic form of associative learning in the mammalian brain. In S. H. Hulse and B. F. Green, Jr. (Eds.), *One hundred years of psychological research in America* (pp. 125–171). Baltimore: Johns Hopkins University Press.

Thompson, R. F., McCormick, D. A., Lavond, D. G., Clark, G. A., Kettner, R. E., & Mauk, M. D. (1983). The engram Found? Initial localization of the memory trace for a basic form of associative learning. In J. M. Sprague & A. N. Epstein (Eds.), *Progress in psychobiology and physiological psychology* Vol. 10 (pp. 167–196). New York: Academic Press.

Thompson, R. F., & Spencer, W. A. (1966). Habituation: A model phenomenon for the study of neuronal substrates of behavior. *Psychological Review, 173,* 16–43.

Tsukahara, N. (1981). Synaptic plasticity in the mammalian central nervous system. *Annual Review of Neuroscience, 4,* 351–379.

Woody, C. D. (Ed.). (1982). *Conditioning: Representation of involved neural functions.* New York: Plenum.

# IV

## PARENT–INFANT
## INTERACTION

# 11

# Shaping Forces within Early Social Relationships

MYRON A. HOFER
*Department of Psychiatry*
*Columbia University College of Physicians and Surgeons*
*and Department of Developmental Psychobiology*
*New York State Psychiatric Institute*
*New York, New York 10032*

## I. Introduction

For the mammalian infant, the mother provides the major source of environmental interaction during a considerable period after birth as well as in the prenatal period. Thus, if we are interested in how development is shaped by experience, we must find ways to discover and analyze the processes within the parent–infant interaction that are capable of producing changes in the development of the young. These processes are hidden within the deceptively simple behavioral interaction that can be observed. Somehow, we must find a way to take the relationship apart, so to speak, in order to see how it works.

### A. Multiple Regulators in Maternal Separation and in Normal Development

A strategy that has proved useful evolved from my initial interest in maternal separation. We first separated 2-week-old infant rats from their mothers and found that this produced widespread changes in behavioral and physiological systems. Then, by focusing on one system at a time, different elements of the maternal interaction were replaced singly or in selective combination in a series of experiments aimed at reversing and/or

Perinatal Development:
A Psychobiological Perspective

**251**

preventing the altered function in the chosen system of the infant. When we found that the level of one function in the infant after separation could be controlled by one aspect of the broad range of stimulation provided by the mother–infant interaction, I began to refer to such a process as a *hidden regulator* within the relationship (Hofer, 1978). And, after we found several different individual regulators operating independently on different physiological and behavioral systems of the infant, the phrase *multiple regulators* seemed appropriate.

This conceptualization was not invented de novo but rather grew out of our being forced to abandon a former assumption: that the pattern of changes in the infant following maternal separation was a unitary syndrome. We had initially supposed that changes in autonomic physiology, hormones, sleep–wake state organization, and behavior following maternal separation were produced as an integrated physiological response pattern set in motion by a signaled discrepancy (absence of the mother) when this was perceived by the infant. (This may indeed be the case for older infants and for species with more highly evolved integrative capacities.) But, when we found that one aspect of the mother–infant interaction (e.g., certain kinds of tactile or olfactory stimulation) could reverse one of the separation-induced functional changes without affecting others, then we had to question the unitary nature of the observed pattern. It seemed possible that following separation, a predictable pattern of changes, with a predictable time course, occurred only because all the different forms of stimulation were withdrawn at once when the young were separated from their mother, giving the appearance of a unitary separation response pattern.

The properties of these regulatory processes have interesting implications for normal development as well as for understanding individual variability in separation responses. The changes in function following withdrawal of these multiple maternal regulators give us an estimate of their significance during maintenance of the interaction. For example, if an infant's resting cardiac rate falls 40%—or its behavioral response to a novel test arena increases 200%—during 18 hr of maternal absence, we can infer that the infant's normal levels of these functions are maintained by action of the maternal regulators. This is at variance with the traditional view that absence of the mother elicits unique responses. It has the advantage of bringing together normative and separation-induced processes, for our evidence suggests that the mother is shaping development in her infants' behavioral systems by maintaining certain levels of functioning: in these instances, by up-regulating cardiac rate and down-regulating neural systems responsible for behavioral activity. It seems likely that mothers having different levels of interaction with their infants would maintain their infants' systems at different levels. Thus variations in mother–infant interactions may have different shaping effects on development of the young. These in turn may account for some of the differences between individuals at maturity.

Similarly, individual differences between infants in their responses to separation may be traced to different levels maintained by the mother in the prior interaction. Thus, instead of regarding the loss as a stress in itself, we would ask, "Precisely what has been lost?"

## B.   Relationship to Attachment Processes

It is significant, from an evolutionary point of view, that behavioral systems for assuring proximity between mother and infants during an appreciable postnatal period are so widespread among mammals. A variety of processes have been described that maintain rat infants near their home nests, near their littermates, and near their mothers for the first 3–4 weeks of postnatal life. This arrangement tends to assure that the developmental effects of the multiple regulators described above will be available to infants. Indeed, the evolution of attachment processes may have allowed these regulators to evolve into their present form. The relationship between attachment systems and the multiple maternal regulators thus becomes a particularly interesting question.

The response times characteristic of infant attachment systems are much more rapid than those that we have traced to the withdrawal of multiple regulators: seconds as opposed to hours. These different latencies of response to separation have been described in human and monkey infants; they are currently referred to as *protest* (immediate) and *despair* (delayed) stages of the separation response. It has been assumed that both stages are part of the same integrated psychophysiological response, albeit a complex, sequential one. Our evidence suggests instead that the delayed responses are the result of withdrawal of multiple regulators and not a delayed response to interruption of the attachment. In fact, we have shown that the delayed responses occur following separation from the mother even when the immediate protest response is prevented by the presence of siblings and home cage nest cues. This raises the question of whether the immediate and the delayed responses to separation are not mediated by fundamentally different processes.

## II.   Hidden Regulators

In Table I, I have summarized the work done in our laboratory and in some others that have established the existence of hidden maternal regulators. This work owes much to my colleagues Herbert Weiner, Sigurd

**Table I**

Regulators Hidden within the Mother–Infant Interaction

| Infant systems | Direction | Maternal regulators |
| --- | --- | --- |
| *Behavioral* | | |
| Activity level | Increased | Body warmth |
|  | Decreased | Tactile and olfactory |
| Sucking | | |
| Nutritive | Decreased | Milk (distention) |
| Nonnutritive | Decreased | Tactile (perioral) |
| *Neurochemical (CNS)* | | |
| NE, DA | Increased | Body warmth |
| ODC | Increased | Tactile (dorsal) |
| *Metabolic* | | |
| Oxygen consumption | Increased | Milk (sugar) |
| *Sleep–wake states* | | |
| REM sleep | Increased | Periodicity, milk and tactile |
| Arousals | Decreased | Periodicity, milk and tactile |
| *Cardiovascular* | | |
| Heart rate ($\beta$-adrenergic) | Increased | Milk (interoreceptors) |
| Resistance ($\alpha$-adrenergic) | Decreased | Milk (interoreceptors) |
| *Endocrine* | | |
| Growth hormone | Increased | Tactile (dorsal) |

*Note.* For references giving evidence for individual regulators, see Hofer, 1984b. NE, norepinephrine; DA, dopamine; ODC, ornithine decarboxylase (enzyme important for tissue growth processes). Reprinted by permission of Elsevier Science Publishing Co., Inc. from "Relationships as Regulators: A Psychobiologic Perspective on Bereavement," by M. A. Hofer, *Psychosomatic Medicine, 46,* 183–197. Copyright 1984 by The American Psychosomatic Society, Inc.

Ackerman, Stephen Brake, and Harry Shair in my laboratory and to Saul Schanberg and Cynthia Kuhn at Duke University. On the left are listed the biologic and behavioral systems that show the slow-developing changes after separation, and on the right, opposite each functional change, are shown the specific aspects of the mother–infant interaction that ordinarily maintain normal levels of that function. The infant's homeostatic system appears to be relatively open to external control; thus, biologic regulation is dependent in part on the mother, even in 2-week-old pups able to survive on their own (Hofer, 1975).

Each of these regulators within the normal mother–infant interaction has its own dynamics and its own physiological mechanisms, which we are beginning to explore. Certain interactions with the mother serve to maintain functions at a relatively high level during normal conditions (for example, heart rate and oxygen consumption); others normally down-regulate systems (for example, systems underlying behavioral reactivity, arousals during sleep, and sucking). Brake and colleagues (Brake, Sager, Sullivan, & Hofer, 1982) have shown the degree of specificity that can exist with these regulators even within one system: intraoral stimulation by the mother's teat governs nonnutritive sucking levels when no milk is provided, whereas when milk is available, gastric fill regulates the pups' sucking levels.

A great deal more must be learned about how these regulators work and how the infant adapts to their withdrawal. Nevertheless, the realization that they exist has already had implications for our understanding of developmental processes (Hofer, 1978, 1981, 1984b). These biologic regulators, hidden within the mother–infant relationship, may constitute an early stage in the development of psychological regulation (e.g., of affect expression) as infants get older and as species evolve (see chaps. 16 and 17).

## III. Slowly Developing Behavioral Responses: Withdrawal of Regulators

Every day, infant rats experience about 17 short periods of maternal absence. These range in average length from 5 to 10 min for the newborn to 2 hr or more for 3-week-olds. At the age we are considering (2 weeks), these absences are 45 min–1 hr, and the mothers' visits with her pups last 15–20 min, during which all nursing takes place (Grota & Ader, 1969). Thus, a regular cycle of interaction and withdrawal is provided by the mother. This pattern, characteristic of the rat, is actually more like the schedule of human mother–infant interaction in most civilized countries than is the nonhuman primate and primitive human pattern of holding the infant in nearly continuous physical contact throughout the day and night.

If the mother is removed from the cage by the experimenter during one of her periodic absences, the litter is denied several of these intermittent behavioral interactions. At the end of a period of separation, the pups can then be tested for their behavioral responses to being placed in an unfamiliar test box. We found that after 18 hr of maternal absence, heart rates were markedly lowered. This was true whether the infants were left in their home cage without additional heat (resulting in a 3°C fall in body temperature over this time period) or whether their temperatures were maintained at 35°C by a regulated heating pad under the cage floor. But whether they were warmed or left at room temperature made a dramatic difference in their behavior when they were placed alone in an unfamiliar test box for observation at the end of the experiment. The cool pups showed fewer characteristic behavioral responses than their normally mothered littermates, whereas the warm pups were very hyperactive on the same measures of locomotion, rearing, and self-grooming (Hofer, 1973a).

This picture is quite different from the usual integrated psychophysiological response to stressful stimulation. Here animals with the same very low resting heart rate could be either hyperactive or less than normally active, depending on the temperature conditions during separation. The role of the mother as a source of thermal input and its importance for behavior regulation is illustrated here. We can have either "agitation" or "apathy" as a response to maternal deprivation, depending on whether the separated infant has had the regulating effect of the mother's body heat withdrawn or whether this aspect of the relationship has been provided artificially. The heart rate is not affected by this thermal regulation of behavior but is regulated by a separate and different mechanism involving nutrient supply to gastrointestinal interceptors (Hofer, 1984a).

A further understanding of the behavioral changes following maternal separation has been provided in neurochemical studies by Stone, Bonnet, and Hofer (1976). Tissue growth, brain DNA and RNA, as well as brain catecholamines were measured in 12–15-day-old pups after 3 days of maternal deprivation either at nest temperature or at room temperature (20°C). Maturation rates of body tissues were generally temperature dependent. Catecholamines showed the most striking differences. For the pups separated at room temperature, brain catecholamines fell below the levels of normally reared agemates, whereas the warm separated pups showed an increased rate of accumulation of norepinephrine and dopamine compared to normally mothered littermates.

These data suggested that the motor deficit of cool pups resulted from reduced levels of central catecholamines, whereas the hyperactivity of warm, separated pups might have resulted from increased availability of these neurotransmitters at central adrenergic terminals. In support of this hypothesis, pretreatment with reserpine at the time of separation (which prevents accumulation of amines at nerve terminals) prevented the development of behavioral hyperactivity in separated, warm infants at a low dose that had no effects on normally mothered pups at the time of behavior testing 24 hr later (Hofer, 1980).

Next we asked how the loss of the mother produces the hyperactivity we found when nest temperature was maintained. We had determined that this response takes time to develop. Only after more than 4 hr was there any change. What was it about the increasing length of separation to which the infants were responding? An obvious candidate was the increasing nutritional deficit, since 18-hr separated pups do not eat well for the next 2 or 3 days. To test this idea, separated infants were fed continuously by an indwelling stomach catheter. Regardless of how much milk they received, they behaved no differently than separated pups that were not fed (Hofer, 1973c). On the other hand, if the mother was left with them to provide behavioral interaction, but with her mammary ducts ligated, the hyperactivity was almost entirely prevented (Hofer, 1973b).

Two hypotheses compete for explanation of these results. The hyperactivity could be viewed in the framework of the attachment hypothesis, as a prolonged protest response to rupture of an inferred psychological bond between infant and mother. Or, it could be the result of withdrawal of regulatory processes that had been acting to reduce levels of activity while the social relationship was intact. It is difficult to rule out an explanation based on an attachment theory, but several predictions of that model failed to be substantiated (Hofer, 1975). First, the hyperactivity was slow to develop (between 4 and 8 hr after separation), which is not at all characteristic of the hyperactivity of separation distress. Second, the maternally separated infants in these experiments were housed in the familiar home cage with seven littermates during separation. Housing them alone and in an unfamiliar environment failed to accentuate the hyperactivity, as predicted by the hypothesis. Thus, this form of behavioral hyperactivity did not meet our criteria for separation distress.

## A. The Roles of Tactile and Vestibular Stimulation

Can we frame and test a hypothesis of separation that depends on simpler processes than those inferred to operate in attachment and social bond formation? We should first recognize that the mother is a source of highly effective environmental stimulation acting upon the infants' developing sensory systems. As one watches a litter of rat pups responding to their mother's approach, one is immediately struck by their response. The infants become remarkably agitated, scrambling over each other to initiate suckling. There is a good deal of audible squealing, as they dislodge each other from the mother's teats. These bursts of activity are repeated many times during a nursing period. If a pup remains asleep through all this, the mother may grip it in her teeth, step on it, or lick it vigorously, which will immediately rouse it to a high level of activity. Nursing is often done with the pup in the supine position, belly up, feet in the air. At any other time, this position evokes vigorous righting reflexes.

I have tried to convey the impression of how effective the mother is as a stimulus to the pups. And yet, the finding is that pups that are normally mothered are less active than separated littermates when placed in an unfamiliar test box. Could it be that although the mother acts to increase arousal levels acutely, the cumulative effect of repeated stimulation by the mother is to maintain behavioral responsiveness at a relatively low level? By this logic, the heightened arousal of separated infants might be viewed as the result of withdrawal of the mother's modulating action (for example, by reducing the availability of central catecholamines, as suggested above).

To test this idea, we designed studies (Hofer, 1975) that would tell us if such a relationship between repeated stimulation and behavioral responsiveness would hold true for simple kinds of stimulation that could be controlled and administered experimentally. The timing and duration of this stimulation should be as similar as possible to the timing of the events in the naturally occurring nursing cycle. Each litter was divided at 9 am, and all infants were separated from the mother for the duration of the 8-hr experiment. One half of the litter was placed in an apparatus, and stimulation was delivered at irregular intervals. Littermate controls were placed in an identical apparatus without stimulation. The stimulation was given intermittently during 15- or 50-min periods, which alternated with 30-min– 1-hr periods without stimulation. Following 8 hr of separation and 45 min after the last stimulation, both groups were tested in novel test boxes for 10 min, during which we observed the number of squares crossed, self-grooming, defecation/urination, and an automated activity count. The 45 min between the last stimulation and testing corresponds to the time allowed to elapse between normal mothering and testing of the mothered control group.

This design allowed us to administer stimulation over a variety of sensory pathways with a time patterning similar to the mother's periodic stimulation. The various modalities of stimulation could then be compared with normal mothering for their capacity to prevent the development of the behavioral changes of separation (see Fig. 1). The first form of stimulation used was mild electrical current (0.05 mA) delivered through the grid floor of a small chamber. This current intensity was found to be the least that would continue to elicit a clear-cut behavioral response in a group of four 2-week-old rats when presented intermittently for 30 min and was undetectable when delivered to the tip of a human finger. The immediate behavioral response elicited was an arousal from inactivity, scrambling over each other, and some audible vocalization. The behavior was very similar in quality and intensity to that observed in a litter of pups with their mother. Three densities of stimulation were tested: 5 s every 15 s, 5s/30s, and 2s/30s. This intermittent stimulation was given only during the periods defined by the periodic visiting schedule of the mother (see above). Control animals were housed in an identical grid box without

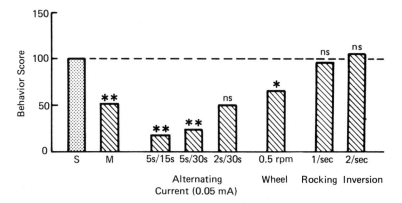

**Fig. 1.**   Behavior scores for infants provided with various types of sensory stimulation over an 8-hr period of maternal absence. Separated (S) and normally mothered (M) infants are represented in the first two bars for comparison. In each of the other bars, the stimulated pups' scores are given as a percentage of the score for nonstimulated, separated littermates, arbitrarily set at 100%, and are compared with them statistically (* = $p < .05$; ** = $p < .02$). Reprinted by permission of Elsevier Science Publishing Co., Inc. from "Studies on How Early Maternal Separation Produces Behavioral Change in Young Rats," by M. A. Hofer, *Psychosomatic Medicine, 37,* 245–264. Copyright 1975 by The American Psychosomatic Society, Inc.

electrical connections. In the highest shock-density group, all four behavioral measures were each significantly reduced, the behavioral score represented in Fig. 1 being a summation of these measures.

These experiments show that intermittent sensory stimulation over an 8-hr period can reduce levels of behavior elicited when the infant is tested 40 min after the last stimulation and can reproduce the same pattern among individual behaviors as is seen after normal mothering.

Since electric current is an artificial form of stimulation, other modalities were also studied. Infants were placed in hamster running wheels ("wheel" in Fig. 1) 15 cm in diameter and 10 cm wide that could be power driven by a motor with reduction drive. One of the wheels was slowly rotated at 0.5 rpm, and the other was fixed. Every 30 s, the infants in the rotating wheel were carried up 90° from the lowest point of the circle and, unless they changed position, were rolled back over their littermates. This procedure in fact elicited considerable activity, consisting of crawling down over littermates plus tactile and vestibular stimulation similar to that seen in normal mothering, and with approximately similar timing. The revolving wheel was driven only for the 15–30-min stimulation periods described above, and the pups were tested as before after 8 hr. A similar behavioral effect was produced by this form of stimulation that was qualitatively very different from electrical current (see Fig. 1).

Since vestibular stimulation is a common feature in most situations that elicit activity and is particularly present in the nursing position frequently adopted by pups of this age (on their back), this modality was tested in two different experiments. In the first, infants were rocked in a small swinging cage at about once per second during the defined stimulation periods ("rocking," Fig. 1). In the second experiment, infants were pressed lightly against the floor of a plastic box by a pad of sponge rubber. Then box and pad, with pups sandwiched between, were inverted and pups held on their backs for 5 out of every 30 s during stimulation periods ("inversion," Fig. 1). Simultaneously, the control groups were lightly pressed with an identical sponge rubber pad. As can be seen in Fig. 1, neither of these procedures for vestibular stimulation had any effect on the behavior score of the stimulated infants. None of the individual behaviors showed any promising trends.

The results of this group of experiments demonstrate that certain forms of artificial stimulation, when repeated at intervals similar to those occurring with the mother, lead to maintenance of a level of behavioral responsiveness that is similar in pattern and intensity to that seen after normal mothering. Of course we cannot be sure that these forms of stimulation act to maintain normal levels of behavioral arousal through processes identical to those involved in normal mothering; a similar end result does not ensure similar means. However, the results tend to support the hypothesized relationship between levels of stimulation and levels of behavioral responsiveness. If the effects of the mother are mediated by the same kind of processes, then the increase in behavioral responsiveness growing out of her absence may be looked upon as a *release phenomenon*, a release from the down-regulating effect of the intermittent stimulation provided to the infants by their interaction with her. We need to know more about the effects of the specific forms of sensory stimulation that are known to make up the mother–infant behavioral interaction. The preceding experiments investigated thermal, nutritional, tactile, and vestibular pathways, but auditory and olfactory systems remained to be explored.

## B.   Olfactory Processes

Leon and Moltz (1972) have shown that young rats of 14–27 days of age detect their mother by a scent or pheromone, emitted in her feces, which elicits approach from considerable distance. It is the pup's olfactory system that mediates the infant-initiated contact found in pups between 2 and 4 weeks of age. Singh, Tucker, and Hofer (1976) have demonstrated that if the olfactory system of infant rats is ablated centrally by bulbectomy or if receptor cells are destroyed peripherally by zinc sulfate ($ZnSO_4$) nasal perfusion, the anosmic pups spend increased time wandering about the cage away from their mothers, lose weight, and show markedly increased mortality. We found that 2-week-old infants made acutely anosmic by $ZnSO_4$ showed a reduced behavioral responsiveness to an anesthetized mother, failed to attach and nurse in this test situation, and tended to respond to their immobile mother as if she were an inanimate object. Saline-control infants oriented to the abdomen of the anesthetized mother and became behaviorally aroused, showing vigorous scrambling until they attached and were suckling.

To explore the contribution of maternal stimulation over olfactory pathways to the regulation of behavior of her offspring, we conducted the following experiments. First, we divided a series of six litters of 2-week-old pups and housed both groups under shallow boxes made of two layers of wire mesh. One half of the litter was provided with the mother, separated from her pups by this barrier in all but olfactory and auditory stimulation. The mother spent her time either on or beside the box, within 3–4 cm of the litter. The other half of the litter was housed in an empty cage. Both halves were provided with home cage shavings. Thermoregulated heat was supplied to both groups as before. After 18 hr, the two halves of the litters were tested as in the previous experiments.

The results, summarized in Fig. 2A, showed that the presence of the mother behind the wire mesh significantly reduced the behavioral score of those infants to levels close to 50% of separated infants. To test whether this effect was due to olfactory or auditory stimuli, the experiment was repeated with both groups having been made anosmic by $ZnSO_4$ nasal perfusion at the beginning of the 18-hr separation period. The results were that the previously described difference was obliterated (Fig. 2B). This

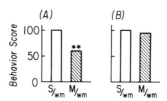

Fig. 2.   Behavior scores for (A) normal and (B) 18-hr anosmic infants confined in double-layer wire mesh (wm) boxes during 18 hr in the home cage. Abbreviations: S/wm, separated entirely from mother; M/wm, mother situated on the other side of the wire mesh. ** = $p <$ .02. Reprinted by permission of Elsevier Science Publishing Co., Inc. from "Studies on How Early Maternal Separation Produces Behavioral Change in Young Rats," by M. A. Hofer, *Psychosomatic Medicine, 37,* 245–264. Copyright 1975 by The American Psychosomatic Society, Inc.

indicates that the effect was most likely due to olfactory rather than auditory stimuli.

If olfactory stimulation is an important pathway mediating the effects of the mother–infant interaction, then infants acutely deprived of this sensory pathway should show some of the effects of separation, even though they remained with their mothers. And indeed, we found that anosmic pups left with their mothers closely resembled their littermates which had been separated for 18 hr. Among the individual measures, neither locomotor, self-grooming, nor total activity count served individually to differentiate the two groups, whereas all three had done so when pups were intact.

One measure within the overall behavioral score did continue to differentiate the mothered from the separated anosmic infants: defecation/urination ($p < .05$) (Fig. 3). The fact that this measure continued to show significant effects of mothering indicates that it must be mediated by some sensory system other than olfactory, probably tactile. Anogenital licking is a regular part of the normal mothering still provided infants of this age, although in much reduced amounts compared to younger offspring.

Alterations are produced by the zinc sulfate treatment in pups' ability to locate nipples (Singh *et al.,* 1976) so that milk intake of the anosmic infants is deficient, despite the presence of their mothers. If we had done only this last experiment, we could not say whether the anosmia had had its effect on the behavior indirectly through the apparent interference to nursing and food intake or directly over the olfactory sensory pathways. The previous experiments with the wire screen, however, show a similar effect without this ambiguity being a factor. Furthermore, experiments

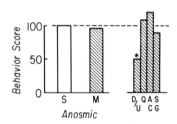

**Fig. 3.** Behavior scores for 2-week-old infants made anosmic and then either separated (S) or replaced with their mothers (M) for 18 hr. The levels of individual behaviors for the anosmic mothered infants are represented on the right. Abbreviations: D/U, defecation and/or urination; Q, quadrants occupied (locomotion); AC, activity count; and SG, self-grooming. * = $p < .05$. Reprinted by permission of Elsevier Science Publishing Co., Inc. from "Studies on How Early Maternal Separation Produces Behavioral Change in Young Rats," by M. A. Hofer, *Psychosomatic Medicine, 37,* 245–264. Copyright 1975 by The American Psychosomatic Society, Inc.

previously performed (Hofer, 1973c) had shown that wide differences in nutritional state have little influence on the behavioral effects of separation. Therefore, we can conclude that it is the sensory deficit rather than the secondary nutritional deficit that obliterates the behavioral differences between mothered and separated infants.

But, does the anosmia obliterate the difference by making the mothered infants resemble intact separated infants? Or does $ZnSO_4$ anosmia create abnormal levels of behavior by all pups in the observation box? If the latter were true, this treatment could be overriding the differences produced by separation rather than demonstrating the effect of a selective sensory deficit. We did not think that $ZnSO_4$ was toxic when absorbed because we had previously found that infants whose oral cavities and stomachs were irrigated with the $ZnSO_4$ solution in even greater amounts showed normal weight gain, orientation, attachment, nursing, and survival (Singh *et al.*, 1976). To further explore the two questions, we have compared data across several experiments reported above (see Fig. 4). It is apparent that anosmic mothered pups are behaviorally much more like intact separated infants than intact mothered ones. Anosmic mothered, intact separated, and anosmic separated groups did not differ significantly, whereas intact mothered pups had much lower behavior ratings than any of the three other groups. When the individual behavioral measures were examined separately, they supported the findings shown for the overall ratings. Mothered infants that were anosmic showed levels of locomotor behavior, self-grooming, and defecation/urination nearly identical to separated intact infants. Finally, we may ask, is there any evidence on the extent to which $ZnSO_4$ anosmia alters the infants' behavioral

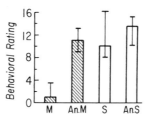

**Fig. 4.** Behavioral ratings (median of locomotor, self-grooming, and defecation/urination measures) for normally mothered (M), anosmic mothered (An.M), separated (S), and anosmic separated (An.S) infants after 18 hr. Brackets represent midquartile ranges. The mothered group is statistically different from other groups ($p < .02$). Reprinted by permission of Elsevier Science Publishing Co., Inc. from "Studies on How Early Maternal Separation Produces Behavioral Change in Young Rats," by M. A. Hofer, *Psychosomatic Medicine 37*, 245–264. Copyright 1975 by The American Psychosomatic Society, Inc.

response to the testing situation itself? A comparison of separated anosmic and separated intact infants shows that the anosmic separated group was entirely comparable in median behavioral rating level to the intact separated infants, and the two groups could not be distinguished in comparisons of individual behaviors.

In conclusion, these experiments demonstrate first that olfactory sensory stimulation of the pups by the mother prevents the development of the behavioral arousal characteristic of separation. Second, an intact olfactory system is necessary for the infants' interaction with its mother to be effective in maintaining the behavioral responses characteristic of mothered infants. Anosmic pups behave as if they were separated, despite the continued presence of the mother. Apparently, without the input from olfactory receptors, the infants fail to derive from their mother whatever it is that regulates their behavior and that maintains their arousal at relatively low levels. The data from the work on tactile stimulation suggests that the level of stimulation itself is the factor. The implication is that levels of olfactory and tactile stimulation by the mother interact synergistically in the organization and regulation of the infants' behavior at this developmental age. Separation from the mother constitutes loss of this sensory input and removal of its hypothesized modulating effect. The ensuing increase in behavioral arousal may be the expression of an underlying response potential, previously held in check by the repeated stimulation from the mother over tactile and olfactory pathways.

## IV. Immediate Behavioral Responses: Attachment in the Rat?

We have found that rat pups of the same age as those in the previously described experiments (2 weeks) also show an immediate behavioral response to isolation and that tactile and olfactory modalities are critically involved in the alleviation of this isolation distress by mother or littermates. These results suggest that a simple form of attachment seems to have developed between 2-week-old pups and their familiar social companions.

Psychological attachment is usually inferred from the strong tendency of the infant to maintain proximity to familiar social companions and from the infant's immediate responses to separation, which generally consist of an intensification of attachment behaviors accompanied by emotional behaviors indicative of distress. Clinging and huddling are the most proximal attachment behaviors, whereas following, intermittent vocalization, and locomotor search are the more distal forms. The behavior most consistently reported as an index of emotional distress after separation, across mammalian species, is vocalization, with aimless locomotion, self-grooming, rocking, or apathetic withdrawal less consistently found. Characteristically, the vocalization of separation distress is rapidly alleviated by reunion with the object of attachment, the social companion. In the infant rat, vocalizations are in the ultrasonic range (35–45 kHz) but can be observed and recorded with a Holgate bat detector (Sales & Pye, 1974).

First, we wanted to know whether 2-week-old rats responded by vocalizing to the periodic maternal absences that normally occur in this species and whether the mother returns to her young because of an increase in their vocalization after a lengthy absence. We found that ultrasonic vocalizations (USV) increased more than fourfold immediately after the mother left the nest but that these levels dropped to basal rates within 4 min and did not increase again until after the mother returned, when they showed the same pattern of a sharp rise and decrement (Hofer & Shair, 1978). Pups observed in a group in the home cage for as long as 24 hr after maternal separation showed no increase in USV beyond the transient disturbance response described above.

Next, we asked whether sudden separation of the infant from *all* social companions would elicit increased vocalization if the infant remained undisturbed in the home cage nest area. We found that sleeping pups usually sensed their isolation within a minute or two and began an outcry with much higher rates than observed in the previous litter situation. Pups maintained USV levels steadily on the average throughout a 30–min observation period when isolated in their home cages with a mean rate of 12 USV/min. In addition to vocalizing, isolated pups spent more than one half the time either locomoting or self-grooming. Rates of USV were highest during locomotion.

These experiments demonstrated that young rats responded to separation from familiar social companions with high levels of USV, locomotion, and self-grooming, even in their own home cage. Would their response to isolation in an unfamiliar place be even greater, as has been found in monkeys and humans? And if so, would interaction with mother or littermates be sufficient to reduce USV significantly? We found that a single pup placed in an unfamiliar test area vocalized at twice the home cage isolation rate (25 pulses/min) during 80–100% of the 6-min observation period and often moved ceaselessly about the enclosure, whereas when allowed access to an anesthetized mother, or when groups of four pups were placed in the same situation, they became virtually silent within 2 min, as they huddled together with their companions. Using a long-term measure of locomotor activity, Randall and Campbell (1976) found similar effects of novelty and of presence of conspecifics on this measure.

Our results showed that an unfamiliar environment intensified the USV response to isolation. These findings led us to an extensive inquiry into the properties of the social companion critical to the alleviation of the high-intensity vocalization produced by separation in an unfamiliar area (Hofer & Shair, 1980). An active behavioral interaction was not found to be necessary, for a single anesthetized pup was as effective as an awake one. The mother, anesthetized, was more effective than a single litter-mate, whereas a plastic object in the shape and size of a littermate and warmed to body temperature did not influence vocalization rate at all.

## A.   Texture and Other Sensory Properties of Surrogates

A series of surrogates were then designed to present tactile, olfactory, and other sensory cues ordinarily possessed by a passive littermate. In some cases, a single cue or modality was presented alone (e.g., home cage odor or furry texture), and in others, only one or two modalities were removed from the complex array of the littermates (e.g., odor, respiratory sounds, and movement). The results for USV are presented in Fig. 5, together with a table showing an analysis of the modalities presented by each surrogate.

The only two conditions that did not consistently reduce USV were the smooth, warm model which lacked odor or texture, and the presence of home cage nest-shavings odor in the absence of any other cue. Texture (artificial fur laid flat on the bottom of the test area) was the only cue that was effective when presented without other cues. But the response was not as great as that to more complex surrogates that presented other modalities as well. Pups do not respond maximally to a single cue but instead give a graded response to several sensory modalities in a cumulative fashion. An artificial surrogate as effective as a littermate in reducing USV could be constructed by wrapping a piece of fur that had previously become impregnated with home cage odor around a warmed flashlight battery (Model, furry, warm, odor [nest], Fig. 5). However, none of the surrogates were very effective in reducing most other behaviors elicited by the novel test box. The fur (flat) condition did significantly reduce rises, however, and both the fur (flat) and the dead warm littermate reduced the activity counts significantly.

The duration of body contact elicited by the different surrogates bore a clear relation to the amount by which each surrogate reduced the USV of the pup in the test box with them. Figure 6 displays this relation graphically. Those combinations of features most effective in reducing USV were also most effective in maintaining body contact between the test pup and the surrogate. This relation did not apply to individual animals, how-

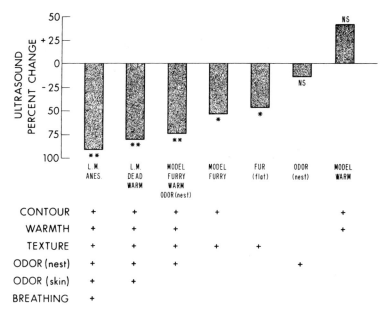

**Fig. 5.** Percentage change in ultrasonic vocalization between tests in isolation and those in experimental conditions, as a function of the modalities presented by the various stimulus objects. L.M. = littermate. (* = *p* < .05 and ** = *p* < .01, Wilcoxon-White paired samples test.) From Hofer & Shair (1980), the *Journal of Comparative and Physiological Psychology,* 1980, *94,* 271–279, Arlington, VA. Copyright 1980 by the American Psychological Association. Reprinted by permission of the publisher.

ever, in that some pups showed marked reduction in vocalization despite little body contact, and others vocalized incessantly despite constant body contact.

Pups do not appear to respond to a single cue from their passive companion but instead are influenced by combinations of sensory modalities which become more effective as their number is increased. Warmth, contour, and smell appear to be ineffective unless combined with a fur-textured surface but are capable of adding to the effect of texture, which by itself is only minimally effective in reducing USV. The odor of home cage shavings in these experiments was provided without a localized source and did not emanate from the surface underlying the pups (as in Conely & Bell, 1978). Possibly these differences account for the lack of agreement of the present results with those of Oswalt and Meier (1975) and Conely and Bell (1978), who found effects of odor in younger pups. The role of olfaction is studied further in the next series of experiments.

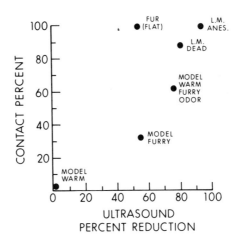

**Fig. 6.** Percentage of the 6-min test time during which the pup was in contact with the stimulus object as a function of the percentage reduction in ultrasonic vocalization. (There are no contact figures for the odor (nest) condition.) Spearman $r = +.94$, $p < .01$. From Hofer & Shair (1980), the *Journal of Comparative and Physiological Psychology*, 1980, *94*, 271–279, Arlington, VA. Copyright 1980 by the American Psychological Association. Reprinted by permission of the publisher.

## B. The Role of Olfaction

The role of pup odor was not individually assessed in the previous experiments, and the contribution of the infant rats' olfactory system to the isolation-induced vocalization was not explored. We did find that the odor of home cage shavings was not sufficient and that specific nest odors were not necessary for reduction of USV. But how would an animal behave if it could not smell at all? In other words, we are asking the question: What is the relation between loss of sensory cues and loss of the sensory system to perceive them?

In the first experiment, saline control and $ZnSO_4$-treated pups were compared on their behavioral responses to being placed in the empty test box. Both groups showed almost identical levels of USV (Fig. 7A), and no significant differences were observed for the other behaviors except that anosmic pups were more generally active (Hofer & Shair, 1980). Since anosmia did not interfere with the USV induced by testing in the empty box, would it interfere with the process by which this vocalization was reduced in the presence of a passive companion? In a second experiment we found that anosmia entirely prevented the reduction in USV normally elicited by the presence of a passive companion (Fig. 7B). But the anosmic pups were not unresponsive to the anesthetized littermate. They reduced their locomotor behavior and maintained a high percentage of

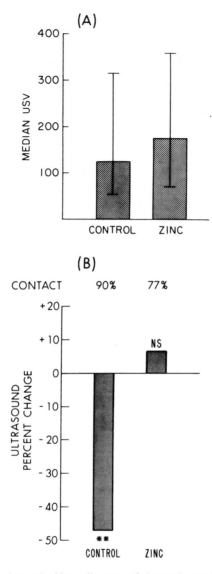

**Fig. 7.** (A) Median number and midquartile range of ultrasonic vocalizations (USV) during 6 min alone in the unfamiliar test box for pups made anosmic by ZnSO₄ olfactory deafferentation (Zinc) and for saline-treated controls. (B) Percentage change in USV between alone and littermate conditions for anosmic pups (Zinc) and controls. Percentage of time during which body contact with the littermate was maintained by the two groups is given at the top of this panel. From Hofer & Shair (1980), the *Journal of Comparative and Physiological Psychology*, 1980, *94*, 271–279, Arlington, VA. Copyright 1980 by the American Psychological Association. Reprinted by permission of the publisher.

time in contact with their passive companion (77%). On neither of these measures did they differ from intact pups, and they did not differ on the other behavioral measures with the exception of vocalization.

Thus, loss of sensory capacity in the main olfactory system eliminated the capacity of the pup to reduce USV in the presence of a social companion, without altering its rate of USV in the empty test box and without significantly altering its tendency to maintain body contact with its companion. These results can be accounted for in several ways. One possibility is that the anesthetized littermate possesses a special odor, secreted by glands in its skin, which is an important property eliciting the reduction in USV by its active companion. But we found no evidence for an independent odor effect: neither removal of odors by sequential solvent washing nor presentation of the pup encased in screen mesh (odor without other cues) revealed any modification of USV levels. These results are puzzling and suggest that odor may be effective only in association with another cue (e.g., texture) or that olfactory sensory processing must be intact for an animal to respond to other cues.

## V.  Neonatal Tactile and Olfactory Associations

What the foregoing experiments have shown is that tactile and olfactory stimulation within the litter situation appear to play important roles in the regulation of levels of behavioral reactivity, USV, and body contact in 2-week-old rat pups. Anosmic pups respond behaviorally as if they had been maternally deprived, even though housed with their normal mother and littermates. And they fail to respond with decreased vocalizations when provided with a familiar social companion during acute isolation. Olfactory stimulation, particularly in combination with tactile stimulation, can substitute for social companions in the long-term regulation of behavioral activity levels and in the short-term regulation of USV in a novel environment. Tactile stimulation by itself is effective to varying degrees in both these forms of regulation.

How did these two forms of stimulation come to acquire these properties? Is there any evidence that experience earlier in postnatal life may have played a role in the development of these sensory regulatory processes that we have found hidden within the early social interactions of the infant rat? Michael Leon's chapter in this volume (Chap. 7) describes how an odor comes to elicit special responses in the olfactory system of adult rats as a result of having been associated with tactile stimulation during their infancy. Recently published studies by Regina Sullivan and Stephen Brake in our laboratories (Sullivan, Hofer, & Brake, 1986; Sullivan, Brake, Hofer, & Williams, 1986) have described a novel process, occurring during the first postnatal week, by which novel odors acquire the capacity to attract infant rats, to enhance olfactory-guided orientation, and to increase huddling as a result of having been presented in temporal contiguity with activating tactile stimulation. This work begins to explore a novel associative process, present (exclusively ?) in the neonatal period and capable of linking activation, elicited by a fairly wide range of stimuli, with novel odors. Individual olfactory stimuli may thus acquire the capacity to activate a range of useful behaviors, their specific form being determined by immediate sensory cues in the environment. In this way, odors may gain a "permissive" role in the operation of other forms of sensory control present later in development.

Such an associative process could underlie transfer of the general property of incentive from one cue to another in early development (Rosenblatt, 1983) and become the basis for later olfactory-based social behavior. For example, in the studies described in this chapter, the long-term regulatory effects of prolonged olfactory and repeated tactile stimulation on activity levels and the short-term effects of texture and odor on USV and contact maintenance in isolated 2-week-old infants may have been forged during the neonatal period by the frequent associations between tactile and olfactory stimulation taking place in the early mother–infant interactions. In the same way, the disruptive effects of acute olfactory deafferentation on both forms of behavioral regulation in 2-week-olds may possibly be understood as a reflection of the importance of olfactory processes acquired by associative experience in the first postnatal week. For in those experiments, loss of olfaction by $ZnSO_4$ anosmia seemed to deprive the infants of the capacity to be influenced by their social companions: In the first case they developed high levels of activity despite having been housed with their mothers, and in the second case they maintained high levels of USV despite the presence of a normal littermate in the novel test arena and despite maintaining contact with that littermate. Apparently olfactory stimulation had become "permissive" in that the regulatory effects of tactile stimulation were rendered inoperative by the absence of olfactory input.

## VI. Implications and Perspectives

The experiments described in this chapter most probably give us only a hint of the delicate interweaving of sensory-based processes upon which the mammalian parent–infant relationship is based. Even in this relatively "simple" mammal, these processes are surprisingly complex and subtle (see also Alberts, 1981; Rosenblatt, 1983). In studying more highly evolved mammals, where we are quick to infer complex psychological processes as determining how parents and infants behave together, it may be well to bear in mind some of the simpler sensorimotor processes uncovered in these experiments with infant rats. By analyzing how the mother–infant relationship is organized at the level of the relatively simple processes I have begun to describe in this chapter, we may begin to understand the forces underlying the way in which early social relationships shape development of the infant's physiological and behavioral systems (Hofer, 1981).

In terms of future directions, our approach is not one of cataloging the variety of developmental consequences of early separation but rather of attempting to understand, in representative physiological and behavioral systems, *how* the experience exerts its effects. This focus is based on reasoning that there is already enough evidence, in a variety of species, that early maternal deprivation can have widespread and severe effects on development. What is needed is some understanding of the factors responsible, so that eventually we will know how to intervene helpfully. A global approach toward restoring good parenting is often not possible, and in fact we know little about what elements of parent–infant interaction are essential for development.

The mother appears from our studies to function as a regulator of physiological and behavioral function in her developing offspring, even at an age when the young are able to survive without her. Separation appears to exert some of its effects on the infant through the sudden withdrawal of these regulatory influences. Released from this external regulation, new rhythms and levels of function are revealed. Thus, it may be useful to think about some of the changes following separation as *release phenomena,* or responses to loss as distinct from responses to separation.

This view may be complementary to the concept of attachment and the data in other species supporting it. Attachment behavior maintains close proximity and ensures that the mother–infant interaction can have its important regulatory action on development. The importance of the mother as a regulator, even after the infant can survive on its own, may explain why vigorous and persistent attachment behavior, on both infants' and mothers' part, has been selected by evolutionary pressures in such a broad range of mammalian species. The relative importance of attachment and release from maternal regulation, in the production of a given separation effect, may well be a function of the maturity of the infant and the nature of the mother–infant relationship at the time of separation. By our current formulation, distress elicited by failure of attachment behaviors to maintain proximity is the first response to separation, but this process is soon overridden by slower developing shifts in internal regulation.

We have chosen to study early maternal separation because the mother is the most pervasive, powerful, and least well understood source of early experience for the mammalian infant. In addition to studying the impact of early separation as an experience, we have found that knowledge about the processes involved can tell us unexpected things about how the mother regulates the physiology and behavior of her infants. Thus, separation of an infant from its mother can be regarded as a means of finding out what role the mother normally plays in the regulation of the infants' functioning at that developmental age. This approach has the potential of disclosing processes hidden within the observable events of the early mother–infant interaction, processes which may play major roles in shaping the infants' development under conditions which do not involve separation. In this way, separation studies can illuminate the fundamental developmental role of the parent–infant interaction.

## Acknowledgments

The research described in this paper was supported by a Research Scientist Award and a Project Grant from the National Institutes of Mental Health.

## References

Alberts, J. R. (1981). Ontogeny of olfaction: Reciprocal roles of sensation and behavior in the development of perception. In R. N. Aslin, J. R. Alberts & M. R. Petersen (Eds.), *Development of perception: Vol. 1. Audition, somatic perception and the chemical senses* (pp. 322–347). New York: Academic Press.

Brake, S. C., Sager, D. J., Sullivan, R., & Hofer, M. A. (1982). The role of intraoral and gastrointestinal cues in the control of sucking and milk consumption in rat pups. *Developmental Psychobiology, 15*, 529–541.

Conely, L., & Bell, R. W. (1978). Neonatal ultrasounds elicited by odor cues. *Developmental Psychobiology, 11*, 193–198.

Grota, L. J., & Ader, R. (1969). Continuous recording of maternal behavior in Rattus Norvegicus. *Animal Behavior, 17*, 722–729.

Hofer, M. A. (1973a). The effects of brief maternal separations on behavior and heart rate of two week old rat pups. *Physiology and Behavior, 10*, 423–427.

Hofer, M. A. (1973b). Maternal separation affects infant rats' behavior. *Journal of Behavioral Biology, 9*, 629–633.

Hofer, M. A. (1973c). The role of nutrition in the physiological and behavioral effects of early maternal separation on infant rats. *Psychosomatic Medicine, 35*, 350–359.

Hofer, M. A. (1975). Studies on how early maternal separation produces behavioral change in young rats. *Psychosomatic Medicine, 37*, 245–264.

Hofer, M. A. (1978). Hidden regulatory processes in early social relationships. In P. P. G. Bateson & P. H. Klopfer (Eds.), *Perspectives in Ethology* (Vol. 3, pp. 135–166). New York: Plenum.

Hofer, M. A. (1980). Effects of reserpine and amphetamine on the development of hyperactivity in maternally deprived rat pups. *Psychosomatic Medicine, 42,* 513–520.

Hofer, M. A. (1981). *The roots of human behavior: An introduction to the psychobiology of human development.* San Francisco: W. H. Freeman.

Hofer, M. A. (1984a). Early stages in the organization of cardiovascular control. *Proceedings of the Society of Experimental Biology and Medicine, 175,* 147–157.

Hofer, M. A. (1984b). Relationships as regulators: A psychobiologic perspective on bereavement. *Psychosomatic Medicine, 46,* 183–197.

Hofer, M. A., & Shair, H. (1978). Ultrasonic vocalization during social interaction and isolation in 2-week-old rats. *Developmental Psychobiology, 11,* 495–504.

Hofer, M. A., & Shair, H. (1980). Sensory processes in control of isolation-induced ultrasonic vocalization by 2-week-old rats. *Journal of Comparative and Physiological Psychology, 94,* 271–279.

Leon, M., & Moltz, H. (1972). The development of the pheromonal bond in the albino rat. *Physiology and Behavior, 8,* 683–686.

Oswalt, G. L., & Meier, G. W. (1975). Olfactory, thermal and tactual influences on infantile ultrasonic vocalization in rats. *Developmental Psychobiology, 8,* 129–135.

Randall, P. K., & Campbell, B. A. (1976). Ontogeny of behavior arousal in rats: Effect of maternal and sibling presence. *Journal of Comparative and Physiological Psychology, 90,* 453–459.

Rosenblatt, J. S. (1983). Olfaction mediates developmental transitions in the altricial newborn of selected species of mammals. *Developmental Psychobiology, 16,* 347–376.

Sales, G., & Pye, D. (1974). *Ultrasonic communication by animals.* New York: Wiley.

Singh, P., Tucker, A. M., & Hofer, M. A. (1976). Effects of nasal ZnSO irrigation and olfactory bulbectomy on rat pups. *Physiology and Behavior, 174,* 373–382.

Stone, E., Bonnet, K., & Hofer, M. A. (1976). Survival and development of maternally deprived rats: Role of body temperature. *Psychosomatic Medicine, 38,* 242–249.

Sullivan, R. M., Brake, S. C., Hofer, M. A., & Williams, C. L. (1986). Huddling and independent feeding of neonatal rats can be facilitated by a conditioned change in behavioral state. *Developmental Psychobiology, 19,* 625–636.

Sullivan, R. M., Hofer, M. A., & Brake, S. C. (1986). Olfactory-guided orientation in neonatal rats is enhanced by a conditioned change in behavioral state. *Developmental Psychobiology, 19,* 615–624.

# 12

## Preoptic Area Neural Circuitry Relevant to Maternal Behavior in the Rat

MICHAEL NUMAN
*Department of Psychology*
*Boston College*
*Chestnut Hill, Massachusetts 02167*

## I. Introduction

The purpose of this chapter is to review some of the recent advances in our understanding of the neural basis of maternal behavior in the rat. *Maternal behavior* will be used to refer to those behaviors shown by the mother which increase the probability that her offspring will survive to maturity. Rats give birth to *altricial young;* that is, the young are helpless, essentially immobile, incapable of temperature regulation, and completely dependent on maternal care for their growth and survival. With appropriate care, the young develop behaviorally and physiologically and are usually weaned at between 3 and 4 weeks of age. The major components of maternal behavior in the rat are nursing, nest building, licking, and retrieving. The mother gives birth in a nest which she builds from materials such as paper strips. These materials are carried to the nest site in the female's mouth, and she also uses her mouth (and secondarily, her forepaws) to weave the nest material into a compact structure. The nest serves to insulate the young and, therefore, to keep them warm in the mother's absence. In the nest, the mother can be seen to lick the anogenital region of the young, and this stimulates urination and defecation. If a young pup should become displaced from the nest, or if the mother changes her nesting area, she can be observed to retrieve or transport the

Perinatal Development:
A Psychobiological Perspective

275

young by carrying them with her mouth. Finally, during nursing, the mother crouches over the young in order to expose her mammary region.

Beginning with the initial studies of Fisher (1956), several lines of research have indicated that the medial preoptic area (MPOA) of the basal telencephalon plays a central role in the regulation of maternal behavior in the rat. This chapter will outline these findings and will begin an analysis of how the MPOA fits into a larger neural circuitry underlying maternal behavior. The major points for which evidence will be presented are: (a) The MPOA contains neurons which are specifically involved in the control of maternal behavior; (b) estrogen acts on MPOA neurons in order to facilitate maternal responsiveness; and (c) preoptic projections to the ventral tegmental area (VTA) of the midbrain appear to be essential for maternal behavior, particularly its oral motor components (retrieving and nest building). Since the VTA has connections to motor areas of the brain, the hypothesis will be advanced that preoptic projections to the VTA allow MPOA neurons relevant to maternal behavior to gain access to the motor system, in this way permitting the MPOA to promote the somatic-motor processes underlying maternal behavior.

Concerning the relevancy of these findings to the neural circuitry underlying maternal behavior in humans, we should note that the circuitry mapped out in the rat involves the phylogenetically older parts of the brain. It does not seem unreasonable to consider the possibility that limbic and brainstem structures may be similarly involved in the maternal motivation of rats and primates. Although the specific maternal responses shown by rats and primates differ, it might be the case that in both rats and primates, preoptic projections to the midbrain serve the general function of allowing preoptic "maternal" neurons access to the motor system so that species-appropriate maternal responses (and their underlying emotional states) occur at the proper time. Research, of course, will have to be done on primates in order to test these views. In this regard, it should be noted that although very little research exists on the neural basis of maternal behavior for species other than the rat (see Numan, 1985, in press), there is research which shows that the preoptic region is involved in nonmaternal aspects of reproductive function in a variety of vertebrates, including primates (Morrell & Pfaff, 1978).

One of the major goals of neuroscience research is to define the chemical neuroanatomy of particular behavioral states. That is, to define the neural circuitry underlying particular behaviors and to define the particular neurotransmitters used in such circuits. Given this knowledge, we might better understand the neurobiology of abnormal behavior. With respect to maternal behavior, an understanding of its neural circuitry is a first step toward understanding its chemical neuroanatomy. Such an understanding might eventually lead to therapeutic drug treatments for certain abnormalities associated with the maternal condition, such as the occurrence of certain types of child abuse.

## II.  The MPOA and Maternal Behavior

Figure 1 shows a sagittal and a coronal section of the rat brain at the level of the MPOA. The MPOA lies just rostral to the anterior hypothalamus and just caudal to the diagonal band–septal area. Lateral to the MPOA is the lateral preoptic area (LPOA), and dorsal to the MPOA is the

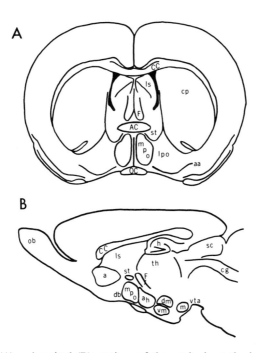

**Fig. 1.**  Frontal (A) and sagittal (B) sections of the rat brain at the level of the medial preoptic area (modified from Konig & Klippel, 1963). Abbreviations: a, nucleus accumbens; aa, anterior amygdaloid area; AC, anterior commissure; ah, anterior hypothalamic area; CC, corpus collosum; cg, central gray; cp, caudate-putamen; db, nucleus of the diagonal band; dm, dorsomedial nucleus of the hypothalamus; F, fornix; h, hippocampus; lpo, lateral preoptic area; ls, lateral septal nucleus; m, mammillary bodies; mpo, medial preoptic area; ob, olfactory bulb; OC, optic chiasm; sc, superior colliculus; st, bed nucleus of the stria terminalis; th, thalamus; vm, ventromedial hypothalamic nucleus; vta, ventral tegmental area. Reproduced from Numan (in press). "Maternal Behavior." In E. Knobil & J. D. Neill (Eds.), *The Physiology of Reproduction*. New York: Raven Press.

medial aspect of the bed nucleus of the stria terminalis, the anterior commissure, and the septal region. Research from several laboratories has
shown that radiofrequency or electrolytic lesions restricted to the MPOA
disrupt maternal behavior in the rat, which includes an interference with
retrieving, nest building, and nursing behavior (Gray & Brooks, 1984;
Jacobson, Terkel, Gorski, & Sawyer, 1980; Numan, 1974; Numan, Rosenblatt, & Komisaruk, 1977). Since radiofrequency and electrolytic lesions are nonselective, destroying all tissue near the lesioning electrode,
an important question is whether the maternal behavior deficits induced
by such lesions are due to damage to MPOA neurons and their efferent
connections or to damage to fibers of passage, that is, axons passing
through the MPOA but having their origins elsewhere. The evidence indicates that damage to MPOA neurons themselves disrupts maternal behavior. Numan, Corodimas, and Factor (1985) studied the effects of N-
methyl-DL-aspartic acid (NMA) lesions of the MPOA on maternal
behavior in the rat. N-Methyl-DL-aspartic acid is an excitotoxic amino
acid which selectively destroys neuronal cell bodies while sparing fibers
of passage (Olney, 1978). Since the design of this experiment is similar to
others which have examined the effects of preoptic damage on maternal
behavior, it will be worthwhile to describe it in some detail. The maternal
behavior of lactating rats was studied preoperatively on postpartum Days
1–4. On Day 4 the following groups were formed: Group NMA-MPOA
received bilateral injections of NMA into the MPOA. Group RF-MPOA
received bilateral radiofrequency lesions of the MPOA. Group NMA-AH
received bilateral injections of NMA into the anterior hypothalamus.
Group PB-MPOA received bilateral injections of phosphate buffer into
the MPOA. Maternal behavior tests resumed on Day 5 postpartum and
continued through Day 12. In comparison to the PB-MPOA group, all
aspects of maternal behavior (retrieving, nest building, and nursing) were
depressed in the groups that received NMA or RF lesions of the MPOA.
Females in the NMA-AH group continued to show normal maternal behavior postoperatively, not differing from the PB-MPOA group. These
results show that destruction of MPOA cell bodies with NMA produces
deficits in maternal behavior similar to those observed after radiofrequency lesions of the MPOA, providing direct evidence for the importance of MPOA neurons for maternal behavior.

  Evidence concerning the MPOA efferents that may be important for
maternal behavior has been gained from studies which have used the
knife-cut technique (Miceli, Fleming, & Malsbury, 1983; Numan, 1974;
Numan & Callahan, 1980; Terkel, Bridges, & Sawyer, 1979). These studies suggest that it is the lateral efferent projections from the MPOA which
are most critical for maternal behavior. The most complete evidence has

been provided by Numan and Callahan (1980). They studied the maternal behavior of female rats that received knife cuts which severed either the lateral, dorsal, anterior, or posterior connections of the MPOA or sham knife cuts. The various cuts are shown in Fig. 2. The basic findings were that females that received knife cuts severing either the lateral or anterior connections of the MPOA showed a severe disruption of maternal behavior, whereas females with knife cuts severing the dorsal or posterior connections of the MPOA showed normal maternal behavior. Therefore, the lateral or the anterior efferents, or both, of the MPOA may be critical for maternal behavior. Because the females with the anterior cuts not only showed a disruption of maternal behavior, but were also hypoactive and lost a large amount of body weight postoperatively, Numan and Callahan (1980) suggested that their maternal deficits may have been the result of an anterior cut-induced general physical debilitation. In contrast, the females with the lateral cuts showed normal activity and body-weight levels. The bulk of the evidence, therefore, indicates the prime importance of the lateral efferents of the MPOA for maternal behavior.

Concerning the nature of the maternal behavior deficits observed after damage to the MPOA or its lateral connections, several studies have indicated that retrieving and nest building are disrupted more severely than nursing behavior (Jacobson et al., 1980; Numan & Callahan, 1980; Terkel et al., 1979). In other words, although all aspects of maternal behavior are depressed by preoptic damage, the oral components are depressed the most (both nest building and retrieving require that an item be manipulated by the mouth). Indeed, preoptic damage completely eliminates retrieval behavior.

An important research goal is to determine which particular preoptic neurons are important for maternal behavior, and a start in this direction has been made by noting the importance of the lateral connections of the MPOA. Another approach to this problem would be to determine whether maternally relevant MPOA neurons are located in a particular place within the MPOA. Because future anatomic findings may indicate a spatial differentiation of particular preoptic efferent and afferent connections (cf. Simerly, Swanson, & Gorski, 1984a, 1984b), research showing that there is a spatial localization of "maternal" neurons within the MPOA will aid in determining the larger neural circuitry within which the MPOA operates to influence maternal behavior. Only three studies have approached the question of whether a particular part of the MPOA is important for maternal behavior, and the results are conflicting and clearly preliminary. Gray and Brooks (1984) have provided evidence that the anterior MPOA is more important for maternal behavior than the posterior MPOA. In contrast, Jacobson et al. (1980) and Terkel et al. (1979)

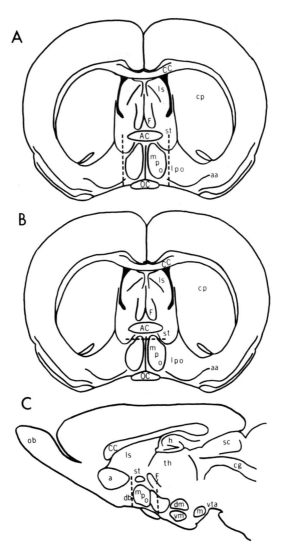

**Fig. 2.** (A) A frontal section through the medial preoptic area showing a knife cut (dashed lines) severing the lateral connections of the medial preoptic area. (B) A frontal section through the medial preoptic area showing a knife cut (dashed line) severing the dorsal connections of the medial preoptic area. (C) A sagittal section through the level of the medial preoptic area showing the placement of a knife cut severing the anterior connections of the medial preoptic area (dashed line between db and mpo) and a knife cut severing the posterior connections of the medial preoptic area (dashed line below F). For abbreviations, see Fig. 1. Reproduced from Numan (in press). "Maternal Behavior." In E. Knobil & J. D. Neill (Eds.), *The Physiology of Reproduction.* New York: Raven Press.

have argued that the dorsocaudal aspect of the MPOA, near its junction with the bed nucleus of the stria terminalis, is particularly important for maternal behavior.

## III.  The Specificity of the Effects of MPOA Damage on Maternal Behavior

Several studies have examined the effects of preoptic damage on maternal behavior and other behaviors and/or regulatory processes in the same animals. The results suggest that the effects of preoptic damage, particularly to its lateral connections, are relatively specific to maternal behavior. Numan and Callahan (1980) have shown that nonmaternal rats with knife cuts severing the lateral connections of the MPOA show normal body-weight regulation and open field activity levels, and Numan (1974) has shown that similar nonmaternal rats show normal female sexual receptivity. Clearly, a general physical debilitation cannot be used to explain the maternal deficits in animals whose lateral MPOA connections have been disrupted. Also, although the oral components of maternal behavior are most severely disrupted by preoptic damage, this cannot be attributed to a general oral motor deficit. Numan and Corodimas (1985) have shown that nonretrieving females with lateral MPOA cuts are capable of hoarding candy that approximates the size and weight of rat pups.

Disturbances in one process have been associated with maternal deficits in preoptic damaged rats: Such animals show a disruption of temperature regulation, and their body temperatures are elevated at normal ambient temperatures (Miceli *et al.,* 1983; Numan & Callahan, 1980). Significantly, there are important relationships between body temperature regulation and maternal behavior: (a) High ambient temperatures have been found to disrupt maternal behavior in rats (Hearnshaw & Wodzicka-Tomaszewska, 1973; Pennycuik, 1964); (b) engaging in nursing behavior raises a lactating rat's body temperature, and nursing bouts are terminated by the mother once her temperature rises above some critical level (Leon, Croskerry, & Smith, 1978); and (c) direct heating of the MPOA causes a nursing female to terminate her nursing bout (Woodside, Pelchat, & Leon, 1980). These findings can be interpreted as indicating that high body temperatures depress maternal responsiveness. Since the MPOA has long been known to be involved in temperature regulation (Boulant, 1980), it could be argued that the absence of maternal behavior after preoptic damage is secondary to a lesion-produced hyperthermia. Although worthy of continued investigation, the current evidence suggests that such a hypothesis is incorrect: (a) Rats with preoptic damage show a transient hyperthermia which recovers, while the maternal behavior deficits persist (Numan & Callahan, 1980); (b) if maternal deficits are secondary to a preoptic lesion-induced disruption of temperature regulation, then one would expect peoptic damage to cause nursing deficits greater than or equal to any resultant retrieval deficit because nursing raises body temperature, whereas in fact, however, the retrieval deficit is greater than the nursing deficit; and (c) rats with preoptic damage that have also had their fur shaved off are normothermic but still show an absence of maternal behavior (Miceli et al., 1983).

A final issue concerns whether rats with preoptic damage can recover from the lesion-induced maternal deficits. In most studies examining the effects of preoptic damage on maternal behavior, the tests for maternal responsiveness have begun within 24 hr after the infliction of the brain damage and have continued for 1 or 2 weeks (Jacobson et al., 1980; Miceli et al., 1983; Numan, 1974; Numan & Callahan, 1980; Terkel et al., 1979). This raises the question of whether a longer interval between lesion production and behavioral testing would result in the same maternal deficits as occur when maternal behavior is tested soon after lesion production. A recent study by Numan (1983) examined this question. Female rats received knife cuts which severed the lateral connections of the MPOA or sham knife cuts. After a 2-week postoperative recovery period, these rats were mated. Following a 22-day pregnancy, the rats gave birth and their maternal behavior was studied for 2 weeks. The females with preoptic knife cuts showed severe deficits in maternal behavior, and retrieving behavior was completely eliminated. These results indicate the permanency of preoptic lesion-induced maternal deficits.

Although the MPOA contains neuronal systems that are involved in more than one function, the evidence cited in this section suggests that there are neurons within the MPOA that are specifically related to maternal behavior.

## IV. Hormonal Basis of Maternal Behavior: The Neural Site of Hormone Action

At the time of parturition, a female rat shows immediate maternal attention toward her young, or toward foster young presented at this time (Moltz, Robbins, & Parks, 1966), and research has shown that this immediate onset of maternal behavior has an endocrine basis. Research has stressed the importance of the near-term decline in progesterone levels and rise in estrogen and prolactin levels as the critical endocrine factors which trigger maternal behavior at parturition (see chap. 14, this volume).

Rosenblatt and Siegel (1975) and Siegel and Rosenblatt (1975) have developed a valuable preparation for studying hormonal mechanisms underlying maternal behavior. They note that female rats on Day 16 of a 22-day pregnancy are not immediately responsive to foster test pups but that pregnancy termination by hysterectomy stimulates maternal behavior in such females. They provide evidence that the hysterectomy prematurely causes a decline in blood levels of progesterone and a subsequent rise in estrogen and that this facilitates maternal behavior. Importantly, if the ovaries are removed when the pregnant rats are hysterectomized, the facilitation of maternal behavior fails to appear. If estrogen is administered to such females, then the inhibitory effect of the ovariectomy is reversed, and maternal behavior is again facilitated. This shows the importance of estrogen for maternal behavior.

Since the MPOA contains a high concentration of estrogen-binding neurons (Pfaff & Keiner, 1973; Rainbow, Parsons, MacLusky, & McEwen, 1982), it might be the site where estrogen acts to affect the onset of maternal behavior. Convincing evidence for this has been presented by Numan et al. (1977). They found that implants of estradiol benzoate into the MPOA facilitated the maternal behavior of rats that were hysterectomized and ovariectomized on Day 16 of pregnancy, while estradiol implants into other neural regions or cholesterol implants into the MPOA were without effect.

## V.  Sensory Factors, the MPOA, and Maternal Behavior

Virgin female rats do not show immediate maternal responsiveness toward foster test pups. Recent work indicates that olfactory input, presumably from the test pups, inhibits maternal responsiveness in virgins (Fleming & Rosenblatt, 1974; Mayer & Rosenblatt, 1977). These studies have shown that peripheral anosmia induced by intranasal $ZnSO_4$ administration facilitates the maternal responsiveness of virgin females toward young, so that they respond more like females exposed to the hormonal events associated with pregnancy termination. This has led to the suggestion that hormones might act to facilitate maternal behavior in the rat by altering the females' perception and/or reaction to olfactory input (see Numan, 1985). The MPOA may be one of the central neural sites where such an interaction between sensory input and hormonal events occurs. Olfactory input from the vomeronasal organ has been shown to depress maternal responsiveness in virgins (Fleming, Vaccarino, Tambosso, & Chee, 1979), and such input is capable of reaching the MPOA. The accesory olfactory bulb, which receives vomeronasal input, projects to the medial amygdala and to the bed nucleus of the stria terminalis (Scalia & Winans, 1975), and both of these structures have anatomic connections with the MPOA (De Olmos & Ingram, 1972; Krettek & Price, 1978; Swanson & Cowan, 1979). Perhaps one of the functions of estrogen action on the MPOA in its facilitation of maternal behavior is to alter the female rat's response to vomeronasal input.

## VI. The Neural Circuitry within Which the MPOA Operates to Influence Maternal Behavior

The research already reviewed indicates that the MPOA and its lateral efferents are directly involved in the control of maternal behavior and that the MPOA may be the site where hormonal and vomeronasal inputs act to affect maternal responsiveness. Concerning the output of the MPOA, its lateral efferents have been shown to project to the LPOA, amygdala, septum, lateral hypothalamus, medial hypothalamic nuclei posterior to the MPOA, ventral tegmental area of the midbrain, midbrain reticular formation, and midbrain central gray (Barone, Wayner, Scharoun, Guevara-Aguilar, & Aguilar-Baturoni, 1981; Conrad & Pfaff, 1976b; Millhouse, 1969; Swanson, 1976). An important research problem is to determine which of these neural connections is (or are) important for maternal behavior. Recent research has examined the possibility that MPOA projections which influence the ventral tegmental area (VTA) are critical for maternal behavior. Before describing this research, the neuroanatomy of the MPOA-to-VTA projection system, and the rationale for singling out this system for investigation, will be presented.

Figure 3 shows the two major routes through which the lateral efferents of the MPOA can reach the VTA (Barone et al., 1981; Conrad & Pfaff, 1976b; Millhouse, 1969; Phillipson, 1979; Swanson, 1976). First, there is a direct MPOA-to-VTA projection. Second, the MPOA projects to the LPOA, which then projects to the VTA. Both MPOA and LPOA efferents pass through the lateral hypothalamus (LH) on their descent to the VTA. It can be seen that severing the lateral connections of the MPOA would interfere with both the MPOA-to-VTA and the MPOA-to-LPOA-to-VTA circuit. Lesions of the LH would also interfere with both circuits, and therefore, it is interesting to note that Avar and Monos (1969) have found that LH lesions disrupt maternal behavior in rats and that the deficits are similar to those observed after severing the lateral connections of the MPOA.

The VTA has diverse ascending and descending projections (Beckstead, Domesick, & Nauta, 1979; Fallon & Moore, 1978; Simon, Le Moal,

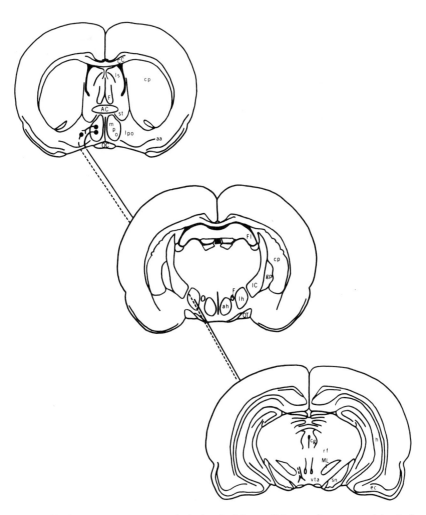

**Fig. 3.**   Frontal plane sections through the level of the medial preoptic area, caudal anterior hypothalamic area, and ventral tegmental area showing the two major routes through which the lateral efferents of the medial preoptic area can reach the ventral tegmental area. For clarity the pathways are only shown on one side of the brain. Medial preoptic axons are shown as a solid line. Lateral preoptic axons are shown as a dashed line. Abbreviations: ec, entorhinal cortex; FI, fimbria; gp, globus pallidus; IC, internal capsule; lh, lateral hypothalamus; ML, medial lemniscus; OT, optic tract; rf, reticular formation; sn, substantia nigra. For additional abbreviations, see Fig. 1. Reproduced from Numan (in press). "Maternal Behavior." In E. Knobil & J. D. Neill (Eds.), *The Physiology of Reproduction*. New York: Raven Press.

& Calas, 1979; Swanson, 1982). Importantly, some of the ascending projections of the VTA reach the striatum (nucleus accumbens and medial caudate-putamen). Striatal structures make up an important part of the extrapyramidal motor system and have influences on both cortical and brainstem motor mechanisms (Conrad & Pfaff, 1976a; Heimer, Switzer, & Van Hoesen, 1982; Mogenson, Swanson, & Wu, 1983; Nauta, Smith, Faull, & Domesick, 1978; Swanson, Mogenson, Gerfen, & Robinson, 1984). Therefore, an MPOA-to-VTA or an MPOA-to-LPOA-to-VTA circuit might allow MPOA neurons relevant to maternal behavior to gain access to the motor system, in this way allowing the MPOA to promote the somatic-motor processes underlying maternal behavior.

Numan and Smith (1984) have provided evidence consistent with the idea that preoptic projections to the VTA are important for maternal behavior (also see Gaffori & Le Moal, 1979; Numan & Nagle, 1983). The maternal behavior of lactating rats was studied preoperatively over postpartum Days 1–4. On Day 4 the surgical procedures were performed, and the maternal behavior of the rats was then studied postoperatively for postpartum Days 5–14. In their first experiment, Numan and Smith found that bilateral electrolytic lesions of the VTA severely disrupted maternal behavior. In their second, and critical, experiment, an asymmetrical lesion design was used, and the various groups that were formed are shown in Fig. 4 (compare to Fig. 3). The maternal behavior of rats that received a unilateral knife cut severing the lateral connections of the MPOA and a contralateral electrolytic lesion of the VTA (C-ML-VTA group) was compared with that of females that received one of the following treatments: (a) sham lesions (SH-C-ML-VTA); (b) a unilateral knife cut severing the lateral connections of the MPOA and an ipsilateral lesion of the VTA (I-ML-VTA); (c) a unilateral knife cut severing the lateral connections of the MPOA paired with a contralateral lesion of the medial hypothalamus posterior to the MPOA (C-ML-MH); (d) a unilateral parasagittal knife cut placed lateral to the LPOA paired with a contralateral lesion of the VTA (C-FL-VTA). It was predicted that the group that received the MPOA lateral cut and the VTA lesion on opposite sides of the brain would show the most severe maternal behavior deficits because only in this group would preoptic projections to the VTA be interfered with bilaterally. The three remaining lesion groups would receive only unilateral damage to this projection route. This prediction was based on the facts that (a) the descending projections of the preoptic region are ipsilateral (Conrad & Pfaff, 1976b; Swanson, 1976) and (b) the effects of unilateral lesions are less severe than those of bilateral lesions (Hendricks & Scheetz, 1973).

The results supported the prediction. The C-ML-VTA group showed the largest postoperative retrieval deficits, differing significantly from each of the remaining groups. Postoperatively, the C-ML-VTA group also showed inferior nest building when compared to each of the remaining groups. Although nursing was depressed postoperatively in the C-ML-VTA females, this measure did not distinguish these females from those in the I-ML-VTA group. These findings are consistent with the suggestion that preoptic projections to the VTA are particularly important for the oral components of maternal behavior.

If preoptic projections to the VTA are critical for maternal behavior, then which projection route, MPOA-to-VTA or MPOA-to-LPOA-to-VTA, is important? Recent data have been provided by Numan, Morrell, and Pfaff (1985) which are relevant to this issue. They studied the maternal behavior of postpartum rats that received coronal knife cuts through either the dorsal or the ventral lateral hypothalamus. The knife used to make the cuts was coated with horseradish peroxidase (HRP) (after Scouten, Harley, & Malsbury, 1982), which would be taken up by damaged axons and transported back to their cell bodies. The logic of this design is based on the spatial segregation of descending hypothalamic and limbic efferents within the LH (Pfaff, 1980; Veening, Swanson, Cowan, Nieuwenhuys, & Geeraedts, 1982). In particular, MPOA efferents which descend to the midbrain via the LH are concentrated within the ventral LH. Therefore, if an MPOA-to-VTA projection is critical for maternal behavior, then the ventral LH cuts should disrupt maternal behavior, and this should be correlated with HRP labeling of MPOA neurons.

The behavioral results indicated that it was the dorsal LH cuts, rather than the ventral LH cuts, which disrupted maternal behavior. Retrieving was eliminated in six of nine females with dorsal LH cuts, while all nine females that received ventral LH cuts continued to retrieve their young postoperatively. The dorsal-cut females also showed inferior nursing and nest building when compared to the ventral-cut females.

The histological findings are shown in Figs. 5 and 6, which show the distribution of HRP-labeled cells in a representative dorsal-cut and ventral-cut brain. As predicted, the ventral LH cuts labeled many MPOA neurons with HRP. Such cuts also labeled many neurons in the septal area. In contrast, the dorsal LH cuts labeled few cells in the septal area and MPOA with HRP, but such cuts did heavily label neurons in a variety of other areas, which included the LPOA. A quantitative analysis based on the distribution of HRP-labeled cells in selected nuclear regions of all of the brains indicated that the ventral cuts labeled more cells with HRP than did the dorsal cuts in the MPOA and septal area. The dorsal cuts labeled more cells with HRP than did the ventral cuts in the LPOA, bed nucleus of the stria terminalis, VTA, substantia nigra, and central gray.

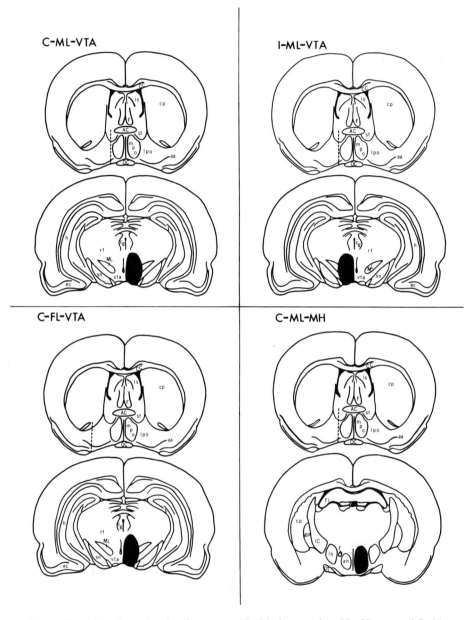

**Fig. 4.** Frontal sections showing the asymmetrical lesions produced by Numan and Smith (1984). C-ML-VTA: A unilateral knife cut severing the lateral connections of the medial preoptic area (dashed line) paired with a contralateral lesion of the ventral tegmental area (solid black). I-ML-VTA: A unilateral knife cut severing the lateral connections of the

These results suggest that a direct MPOA-to-VTA projection is not important for maternal behavior because the ventral cuts severed most of the descending MPOA axons within the LH but did not disrupt maternal behavior. The results are more consistent with the view that an MPOA-to-LPOA-to-VTA circuit is important for maternal behavior because the dorsal LH cuts heavily labeled LPOA cell bodies with HRP, suggesting that such cuts may have disrupted maternal behavior by damaging the LPOA-to-VTA link of the MPOA-to-LPOA-to-VTA circuit. These findings are valuable because they have focused attention on the possible importance of the LPOA. However, their correlational nature should be noted. The dorsal LH cuts label neurons with HRP in a variety of areas, and interference with the efferents from any one of these regions may have been involved in the disruption of maternal behavior.

In contrast to the findings of Numan, Morrell, and Pfaff (1985), recent findings by Fahrbach, Morrell, and Pfaff (1986) have provided anatomic evidence consistent with a view favoring the importance of a direct MPOA-to-VTA circuit for maternal behavior. Combining the methods of retrograde neuroanatomic tracing with steriod autoradiography, it was shown that many MPOA neurons both concentrate estrogen and send their axons directly to the VTA. Although many LPOA neurons projected to the VTA, only a few of these also concentrated estrogen. Fahrbach *et al.* (1986) suggest that estrogen may act to facilitate maternal behavior by binding to MPOA neurons which project directly to the midbrain. Anatomic evidence, however, is only suggestive, and it should be noted that many estrogen-binding MPOA neurons did not project to the midbrain. Perhaps some of these estrogen-binding neurons project to the LPOA and form the first leg of an MPOA-to-LPOA-to-VTA circuit important for maternal behavior.

Clearly, much more research is needed in order to determine whether preoptic projections to the VTA are indeed important for maternal behavior. Although all the research reviewed is consistent with the possible importance of such a projection, many problems remain. The correlational nature of the HRP findings of Numan, Morrell, and Pfaff (1985) has already been noted. In addition, the interpretation of the finding that

medial preoptic area paired with an ipsilateral lesion of the ventral tegmental area. C-FL-VTA: A unilateral knife cut lateral to the lateral preoptic area paired with a contralateral lesion of the ventral tegmental area. C-ML-MH: A unilateral knife cut severing the lateral connections of the medial preoptic area paired with a contralateral lesion of the medial hypothalamus posterior to the medial preoptic area. For abbreviations, see Figs. 1 and 3. Reproduced from Numan (in press). "Maternal Behavior." In E. Knobil & J. D. Neill (Eds.), *The Physiology of Reproduction*. New York: Raven Press.

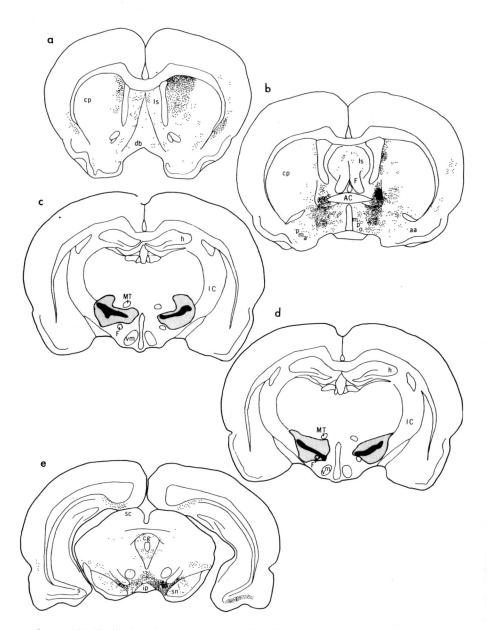

**Fig. 5.** The distribution of neurons labeled with HRP at septal (a), preoptic (b), and midbrain (e) levels in a representative brain from the dorsal-cut group. Each dot represents a labeled cell. Sections c and d show the knife cuts through the dorsal lateral hypothalamus (solid black) and the HRP deposit sites (stipple). Abbreviations: ip, interpeduncular nucleus; MT, mammillothalamic tract; pma, magnocellular preoptic nucleus; s, subiculum. For additional abbreviations, see Figs. 1 and 3. Data from Numan, Morrell, and Pfaff (1985). Copyright © 1985 by Alan R. Liss, Inc.

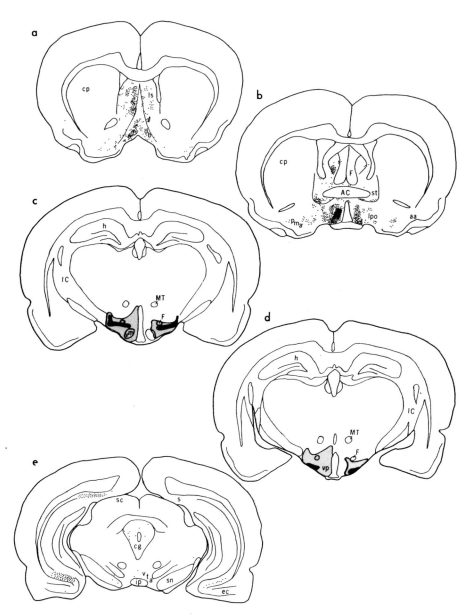

**Fig. 6.** The distribution of neurons labeled with HRP at septal (a), preoptic (b), and mid-brain (e) levels in a representative brain from the ventral-cut group. Each dot represents a labeled cell. Sections c and d show the knife cuts through the ventral lateral hypothalamus (solid black) and the HRP deposit sites (stipple). Abbreviations: vp, ventral premammillary nucleus. For additional abbreviations, see Fig. 5. Data from Numan, Morrell, and Pfaff (1985). Copyright © 1985 by Alan R. Liss, Inc.

females with C-ML-VTA asymmetrical lesions show a disruption of maternal behavior (Numan & Smith, 1984) is hindered by the nonselective nature of the lesioning techniques used (knife cuts and electrolytic lesions), which destroyed efferents, afferents, and fibers of passage of the neural structures involved. All that can be concluded with confidence from the findings of Numan and Smith is that a neural pathway which travels between the preoptic region and the VTA is important for maternal behavior. Although research with the excitotoxic amino acid NMA indicates that MPOA efferents are critical for maternal behavior (Numan, Corodimas, & Factor, 1985), as yet no evidence is available with respect to the question of whether LPOA neurons and VTA neurons, rather than fibers of passage through these regions, are critical for maternal behavior. Research is currently underway in the author's laboratory exploring these issues.

## VII.  Proposed Neural Circuitry: Two Alternative Models

The research already reviewed indicates that we are beginning to uncover certain aspects of the neural circuitry underlying maternal behavior. If it becomes established that preoptic projections to the VTA are important for maternal behavior, then research should examine the structure(s) to which the VTA projects in order to influence maternal behavior. The VTA has diverse ascending (striatum, amygdala, septum, frontal cortex) and descending (locus ceruleus, parabrachial nuclei) neural connections (Beckstead et al., 1979; Fallon & Moore, 1978; Simon et al., 1979; Swanson, 1982), and any one of these might be important for maternal behavior.

To stimulate and direct future research, two alternative hypothetical neural circuits which may underly maternal behavior will be presented. These models are based on the assumption that preoptic projections to the VTA are important for maternal behavior. In devising these circuits, consideration was given to the fact that disruption of the pathway extending between the preoptic area and the VTA appears to interfere primarily with the oral components of maternal behavior. Therefore, if an MPOA-to-LPOA-to-VTA circuit were to underly maternal behavior, then a mechanism by which the output of this circuit could act to influence the somatic-motor processes underlying retrieving and nest building should be clear.

The two proposed neural circuits are shown in Fig. 7. In the first circuit we have MPOA-to-LPOA-to-VTA-to-striatum. This is the pathway that Numan and Smith (1984) originally proposed as possibly being important

**A**

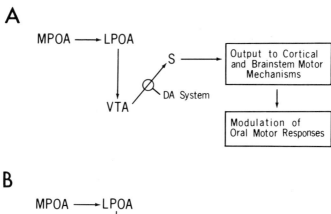

**B**

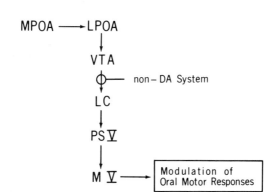

**Fig. 7.** Two alternative hypothetical neural circuits which may underly maternal behavior. Abbreviations: MPOA, medial preoptic area; LPOA, lateral preoptic area; VTA, ventral tegmental area; DA, dopamine; S, striatum; LC, locus ceruleus; PSV, principal sensory nucleus of the trigeminal nerve; MV, motor nucleus of the trigeminal nerve. That VTA projections to the striatum are primarily dopaminergic and those to the locus ceruleus are primarily nondopaminergic is taken from the work of Swanson (1982).

for maternal behavior, and the evidence in favor of the MPOA-to-LPOA-to-VTA part of the circuit has already been described in this chapter. Because evidence exists that the VTA-to-striatum circuit has influences over oral motor responses (Jones & Mogenson, 1979; Kelley & Stinus, 1985), preoptic projections to this circuit may provide the route over which the preoptic region influences retrieving and nest building.

The second of the proposed circuits shown in Fig. 7 emphasizes the possible importance of the descending projections of the VTA for maternal behavior. The circuit shows MPOA-to-LPOA-to-VTA-to-locus ceruleus (LC)-to-principal sensory nucleus of the trigeminal nerve (PSV)-to-motor nucleus of the trigeminal nerve (MV). The PSV receives somatic sensory input from oral and perioral regions, and the MV innervates the muscles which control jaw opening and closing (Contreras, Beckstead, & Norgren, 1982; Jacquin, Rhoades, Enfiejian, & Egger, 1983; Jacquin & Zeigler, 1983; Zeigler, 1983). The LC, PSV, and MV are located in the pons. This interesting pathway suggests that the MPOA may exert its effects on the oral components of maternal behavior by a fairly direct projection to the motor neurons controlling mouth movements. There is anatomic evidence in support of a VTA-to-LC connection (Beckstead *et al.*, 1979; Simon *et al.*, 1979; Swanson, 1982), a LC-to-PSV connection (Levitt & Moore, 1979; McBride & Sutin, 1984; Vornov & Sutin, 1983), and a PSV-to-MV connection (Travers & Norgren, 1983; Vornov & Sutin, 1983).

Although the validity of each of these hypothesized circuits awaits experimental analysis, the fact that we have been able to propose such circuits indicates that we are beginning to understand how "motivational centers" might exert their influences over particular behaviors.

## Acknowledgments

The research from the author's laboratory was supported, in part, by National Institutes of Health grants HD10395, HD06377, and HD18904.

## References

Avar, Z., & Monos, E. (1969). Biological role of lateral hypothalamic structures participating in the control of maternal behavior in the rat. *Acta Physiologica Academiae Scientiarum Hungaricae, 35,* 285–294.

Barone, F. C., Wayner, M. J., Scharoun, S. L., Guevara-Aguilar, R., & Aguilar-Baturoni, H. U. (1981). Afferent connections of the lateral hypothalamus: A horseradish peroxidase study in the rat. *Brain Research Bulletin, 7,* 75–88.

Beckstead, R. M., Domesick, V. B., & Nauta, W. J. H. (1979). Efferent connections of the substantia nigra and ventral tegmental area in the rat. *Brain Research, 175,* 191–217.

Boulant, J. A. (1980). Hypothalamic control of thermoregulation. In P. J. Morgane & J. Panksepp (Eds.), *Handbook of the hypothalamus: Vol. 3, Part A. Behavioral studies of the hypothalamus* (pp. 1–82). New York: Dekker.

Conrad, L. C. A., & Pfaff, D. W. (1976a). Autoradiographic tracing of nucleus accumbens efferents in the rat. *Brain Research, 113,* 589–596.

Conrad, L. C. A., & Pfaff, D. W. (1976b). Efferents from medial basal forebrain and hypothalamus in the rat: I. Medial preoptic area. *Journal of Comparative Neurology, 169,* 185–220.

Contreras, R. J., Beckstead, R. M., & Norgren, R. (1982). The central projections of the trigeminal, facial, glossopharyngeal and vagus nerves: An autoradiographic study in the rat. *Journal of the Autonomic Nervous System, 6,* 303–322.

De Olmos, J. S., & Ingram, W. R. (1972). The projection field of the stria terminalis in rat brain: An experimental study. *Journal of Comparative Neurology, 146,* 303–334.

Fahrbach, S. E., Morrell, J. I., and Pfaff, D. W. (1986). Identification of medial preoptic neurons that concentrate estradiol and project to the midbrain in the rat. *Journal of Comparative Neurology, 247,* 364–382.

Fallon, J. H., & Moore, R. Y. (1978). Catecholamine innervation of the basal forebrain. *Journal of Comparative Neurology, 180,* 545–580.

Fisher, A. E. (1956). Maternal and sexual behavior induced by intracranial chemical stimulation. *Science, 124,* 228–229.

Fleming, A. S., & Rosenblatt, J. S. (1974). Olfactory regulation of maternal behavior in rats: II. Effects of peripherally induced anosmia and lesions of the lateral olfactory tract in pup-induced virgins. *Journal of Comparative and Physiological Psychology, 86,* 233–246.

Fleming, A. S., Vaccarino, F., Tambosso, L., & Chee, P. (1979). Vomeronasal and olfactory system modulation of maternal behavior in the rat. *Science, 203,* 372–374.

Gaffori, O., & Le Moal, M. (1979). Disruption of maternal behavior and appearance of cannibalism after ventral mesencephalic tegmentum lesions. *Physiology and Behavior, 23,* 317–323.

Gray, P., & Brooks, P. J. (1984). Effect of lesion location within the medial preoptic–anterior hypothalamic continuum on maternal and male sexual behaviors in female rats. *Behavioral Neuroscience, 98,* 703–711.

Hearnshaw, H., & Wodzicka-Tomaszewska, M. (1973). Effect of high temperature in early and late lactation on litter growth and survival in rats. *Australian Journal of Biological Science, 26,* 1171–1178.

Heimer, L., Switzer, R. D., & Van Hoesen, G. W. (1982). Ventral striatum and ventral pallidum—components of the motor system? *Trends in Neuroscience, 5,* 83–87.

Hendricks, S. E., & Scheetz, H. A. (1973). Interaction of hypothalamic structures in the mediation of male sexual behavior. *Physiology and Behavior, 8,* 595–598.

Jacobson, C. D., Terkel, J., Gorski, R. A., & Sawyer, C. H. (1980). Effects of small medial preoptic area lesions on maternal behavior: Retrieving and nest building in the rat. *Brain Research, 194,* 471–478.

Jacquin, M. F., Rhoades, R. W., Enfiejian, H. L., & Egger, M. D. (1983). Organization and morphology of masticatory neurons in the rat: A retrograde HRP study. *Journal of Comparative Neurology, 218,* 239–256.

Jacquin, M. F., & Zeigler, H. P. (1983). Trigeminal orosensation and ingestive behavior in the rat. *Behavioral Neuroscience, 97,* 62–97.

Jones, D. L., & Mogenson, G. J. (1979). Oral motor performance following central dopamine receptor blockade. *European Journal of Pharmacology, 59,* 11–21.

Kelley, A. E., & Stinus, L. (1985). Disappearance of hoarding behavior after 6-hydroxydopamine lesions of the mesolimbic dopamine neurons and its reinstatement with L-dopa. *Behavioral Neuroscience, 99,* 531–545.

Konig, J. F. R., & Klippel, R. A. (1963). *The rat brain.* Baltimore: Williams & Wilkins.

Krettek, J. E., & Price, J. L. (1978). Amygdaloid projections to subcortical structures within the basal forebrain and brainstem in the rat and cat. *Journal of Comparative Neurology, 178,* 225–254.

Leon, M., Croskerry, P. G., & Smith, G. K. (1978). Thermal control of mother–young contact in rats. *Physiology and Behavior, 21,* 793–811.

Levitt, P., & Moore, R. Y. (1979). Origin and organization of brainstem catecholamine innervation in the rat. *Journal of Comparative Neurology, 186,* 505–528.

Mayer, A. D., & Rosenblatt, J. S. (1977). Effects of intranasal zinc sulfate on open field and maternal behavior in female rats. *Physiology and Behavior, 18,* 101–109.

McBride, R. L., & Sutin, J. (1984). Noradrenergic hyperinnervation of the trigeminal sensory nuclei. *Brain Research, 324,* 211–221.

Miceli, M. O., Fleming, A. S., & Malsbury, C. W. (1983). Disruption of maternal behaviour in virgin and postparturient rats following sagittal plane knife cuts in the preoptic area–hypothalamus. *Behavioural Brain Research, 9,* 337–360.

Millhouse, O. E. (1969). A Golgi study of the descending medial forebrain bundle. *Brain Research, 15,* 341–363.

Mogenson, G. J., Swanson, L. W., & Wu, M. (1983). Neural projections from nucleus accumbens to globus pallidus, substantia innominata, and lateral preoptic–lateral hypothalamic area: An anatomical and electrophysiological investigation in the rat. *Neuroscience, 3,* 189–202.

Moltz, H., Robbins, D., & Parks, M. (1966). Caesarean delivery and the maternal behavior of primiparous and multiparous rats. *Journal of Comparative and Physiological Psychology, 61,* 455–460.

Morrell, J. I., & Pfaff, D. W. (1978). A neuroendocrine approach to brain function: Localization of sex steroid concentrating cells in vertebrate brains. *American Zoologist, 18,* 447–460.

Nauta, W. J. H., Smith, G. P., Faull, R. L. M., & Domesick, V. B. (1978). Efferent connections and nigral afferents of the nucleus accumbens septi in the rat. *Neuroscience, 3,* 385–401.

Numan, M. (1974). Medial preoptic area and maternal behavior in the female rat. *Journal of Comparative and Physiological Psychology, 87,* 746–759.

Numan, M. (1983). *Further studies on the lateral connections of the medial preoptic area in relation to maternal behavior in the rat.* Paper presented at the Conference on Reproductive Behavior, Medford, MA.

Numan, M. (1985). Brain mechanisms and parental behavior. In N. Adler, D. W. Pfaff, & R. W. Goy (Eds.), *Handbook of behavioral neurobiology: Vol. 7, Reproduction* (pp. 537–605). New York: Plenum.

Numan, M. (in press). Maternal behavior. In E. Knobil & J. D. Neill (Eds.), *The physiology of reproduction.* New York: Raven.

Numan, M., & Callahan, E. C. (1980). The connections of the medial preoptic region and maternal behavior in the rat. *Physiology and Behavior, 25,* 653–665.

Numan, M., & Corodimas, K. P. (1985). The effects of paraventricular hypothalamic lesions on maternal behavior in rats. *Physiology and Behavior, 35,* 417–425.

Numan, M., Corodimas, K. P., & Factor, E. M. (1985). *Effects of N-methyl-DL-aspartic acid lesions of the medial preoptic area on the maternal behavior of rats.* Paper presented at the Conference on Reproductive Behavior, Asilomar, CA.

Numan, M., Morrell, J. I., & Pfaff, D. W. (1985). Anatomical identification of neurons in selected brain regions associated with maternal behavior deficits induced by knife cuts of the lateral hypothalamus in rats. *Journal of Comparative Neurology, 237,* 552–564.

Numan, M., & Nagle, D. S. (1983). Preoptic area and substantia nigra interact in the control of maternal behavior in the rat. *Behavioral Neuroscience, 97,* 120–139.

Numan, M., Rosenblatt, J. S., & Komisaruk, B. R. (1977). Medial preoptic area and onset of maternal behavior in the rat. *Journal of Comparative and Physiological Psychology, 91,* 146–164.

Numan, M., & Smith, H. G. (1984). Maternal behavior in rats: Evidence for the involvement of preoptic projections to the ventral tegmental area. *Behavioral Neuroscience, 98,* 712–727.

Olney, J. W. (1978). Neurotoxicity of excitatory amino acids. In E. G. McGeer, J. W. Olney, & P. C. McGeer (Eds.), *Kainic acid as a tool in neurobiology* (pp. 95–121). New York: Raven.

Pennycuik, P. R. (1964). The effects on rats of chronic exposure to 34°C: IV. Reproduction. *Australian Journal of Biological Sciences, 17,* 245–260.

Pfaff, D. W. (1980). *Estrogens and brain function.* New York: Springer-Verlag.

Pfaff, D. W., & Keiner, M. (1973). Atlas of estradiol-concentrating cells in the central nervous system of the female rat. *Journal of Comparative Neurology, 151,* 121–158.

Phillipson, O. T. (1979). Afferent projections to the ventral tegmental area of Tsai and interfascicular nucleus: A horseradish peroxidase study in the rat. *Journal of Comparative Neurology, 187,* 117–144.

Rainbow, T. C., Parsons, B., MacLusky, N. J., & McEwen, B. S. (1982). Estradiol receptor levels in rat hypothalamic and limbic nuclei. *Journal of Neuroscience, 2,* 1439–1445.

Rosenblatt, J. S., & Siegel, H. I. (1975). Hysterectomy-induced maternal behavior during pregnancy in the rat. *Journal of Comparative and Physiological Psychology, 89,* 685–700.

Scalia, F., & Winans, S. S. (1975). The differential projections of the olfactory bulb and accessory olfactory bulb in mammals. *Journal of Comparative Neurology, 161,* 31–55.

Scouten, C. W., Harley, C. W., & Malsbury, C. W. (1982). Labeling knife cuts: A new method for revealing the functional anatomy of the CNS demonstrated on the noradrenergic dorsal bundle. *Brain Research Bulletin, 8,* 229–232.

Siegel, H. I., & Rosenblatt, J. S. (1975). Hormonal basis of hysterectomy induced maternal behavior during pregnancy in the rat. *Hormones and Behavior, 6,* 211–222.

Simerly, R. B., Swanson, L. W., & Gorski, R. A. (1984a). The cells of origin of a sexually dimorphic serotonergic input to the medial preoptic nucleus of the rat. *Brain Research, 324,* 185–189.

Simerly, R. B., Swanson, L. W., & Gorski, R. A. (1984b). Demonstration of a sexual dimorphism in the distribution of serotonin-immunoreactive fibers in the medial preoptic nucleus of the rat. *Journal of Comparative Neurology, 225,* 151–166.

Simon, H., Le Moal, M., & Calas, A. (1979). Efferents and afferents of the ventral tegmental-A10 region studied after local injections of $^3$H leucine and horseradish peroxidase. *Brain Research, 178,* 17–40.

Swanson, L. W. (1976). An autoradiographic study of the efferent connections of the preoptic region in the rat. *Journal of Comparative Neurology, 167,* 227–256.

Swanson, L. W. (1982). The projections of the ventral tegmental area and adjacent regions: A combined fluorescent retrograde tracer and immunofluorescence study in the rat. *Brain Research Bulletin, 9,* 321–353.

Swanson, L. W., & Cowan, W. M. (1979). The connections of the septal region in the rat. *Journal of Comparative Neurology, 186,* 621–656.

Swanson, L. W., Mogenson, G. J., Gerfen, C. R., & Robinson, P. (1984). Evidence for a projection from the lateral preoptic area and substantia innominata to the mesencephalic locomotor region in the rat. *Brain Research, 295,* 161–178.

Terkel, J., Bridges, R. S., & Sawyer, C. H. (1979). Effects of transecting lateral neural connections of the medial preoptic area on maternal behavior in the rat: Nest building, pup retrieval and prolactin secretion. *Brain Research, 169,* 369–380.

Travers, J. B., & Norgren, R. (1983). Afferent projections to the oral motor nuclei in the rat. *Journal of Comparative Neurology, 220,* 280–298.

Veening, J. G., Swanson, L. W., Cowan, W. M., Nieuwenhuys, R., & Geeraedts, L. M. G. (1982). The medial forebrain bundle of the rat: II. An autoradiographic study of the topography of the major descending and ascending components. *Journal of Comparative Neurology, 206,* 82–108.

Vornov, J. J., & Sutin, J. (1983). Brainstem projections to the normal and noradrenergically hyperinnervated trigeminal motor nucleus. *Journal of Comparative Neurology, 214,* 198–208.

Woodside, B., Pelchat, R., & Leon, M. (1980). Acute elevation of the heat load of mother rats curtails maternal nest bouts. *Journal of Comparative and Physiological Psychology, 94,* 61–68.

Zeigler, H. P. (1983). The trigeminal system and ingestive behavior. In E. Satinoff & P. Teitelbaum (Eds.), *The handbook of behavioral neurobiology: Motivation* (pp. 265–327). New York: Plenum.

# 13

## Evidence That Central Oxytocin Plays a Role in the Activation of Maternal Behavior

CORT A. PEDERSEN and ARTHUR J. PRANGE, JR.
*Department of Psychiatry*
*Biological Sciences Research Center*
*and Neurobiology Curriculum*
*University of North Caroline School of Medicine*
*Chapel Hill, North Carolina 27514*

## I. Introduction

In this chapter we review evidence that the nonapeptide oxytocin (OXY) may play a physiologically relevant role within the CNS in the activation of maternal behavior (MB) in rats. Oxytocin, long considered a hormone released solely into blood and having only peripheral effects, has recently been shown to be widely distributed and released within the CNS. We describe how this evolution in our understanding of the localization of distribution, release, and action of OXY has influenced investigations of MB effects of this peptide. Findings from our laboratory and others concerning the influence of central administration of OXY on the onset of MB are presented. Investigations of the role of endogenous OXY in ovarian steroid–induced MB are described as well as investigations of the influence of central administration of OXY on reemergent MB in experienced rat mothers. Important methodological issues in the investigation of OXY-induced MB are summarized. Where appropriate we discuss the implications of findings for the understanding of brain mechanisms organizing MB and point out future directions that this research may take.

Perinatal Development:
A Psychobiological Perspective

**299**

## II. Oxytocin: A Peripheral Hormone *and* a Neuropeptide

Oxytocin is a nonapeptide that has been known for decades to cause milk ejection and uterine contraction. Oxytocin is synthesized as part of a much larger precursor molecule in nuclei of the anterior hypothalamus. During transport along the neurohypophysial pathway to the posterior pituitary, the precursor is cleared to form OXY and its associated neurophysin (White & McKelvy, 1985). Stimulation of the vagina/cervix or stimulation of the nipples activate diffuse neuronal pathways within the CNS that increase the firing rate of oxytocinergic neurons in the neurohypophysial pathway leading to release of OXY into blood (Cross & Dyball, 1974; Lincoln & Russell, 1985). Oxytocin release is essential for milk ejection during nursing (Mena, Clapp, Martinez-Escalera, Pachero, & Grosvenor, 1985). While OXY release does occur during expulsion of the fetus (Fuchs, 1985), the initiation of parturition may result from increased OXY-receptor binding occurring in the uterus (Soloff, 1985).

Application of immunohistochemical techniques over the past decade has revealed that fibers immunostaining for OXY are widely distributed within the CNS (Buijs, DeVries, Van Leeuwen, & Swaab, 1983; Sofroniew, 1983; Swanson & Sawchenko, 1983). Evidence has accumulated that OXY is released within the CNS independently of peripheral release (Dogterom, Van Wimersma Greidanus, & Swaab, 1977; Jones, Robinson, & Harris, 1983). Contributing to the impression that central release of OXY may play a physiologically relevant role in many neural systems are numerous reports of behavioral and homeostatic effects produced by central administration of this nonapeptide (Dyball & Paterson, 1983; Meisenberg & Simmons, 1983).

## III. Oxytocin and Mothering Behavior: Early Hypothesis, Experiments, and Observations Concerning the Role of Peripheral Oxytocin

Klopfer (1971) was the first investigator to hypothesize that OXY release during labor may precipitate the onset of MB. He noted that the surge of OXY release during second-stage labor was ideally timed to trigger a maternal response toward the emerging offspring. Hemmes (1969), a student of Klopfer, found that mechanical vaginal distention, a well-established stimulus for release of OXY (Roberts & Share, 1968), precipitated MB in nulliparous goats. However, intravenous (IV) administration of a single bolus of OXY failed to induce MB. Rosenblatt (1969) reported that IV injection of OXY failed to prevent the normal decline in rat mothers' MB response to older pups occurring prior to weaning. Herrenkohl and Rosenberg (1974) found that deafferentation of the medial basal hypothalamus that severed the neurohypophysial pathway prevented milk ejection but failed to disrupt the onset of postpartum MB. A number of studies of the milk ejection reflex have involved lesioning of the neurohypophysial pathway at various levels (Cross & Dyball, 1974). Although none of these studies included measurement of the MB of the lesioned animals, at least one report (Yokoyama, Halasz, & Sawyer, 1967) commented that maternal response continued unabated after lesioning. Yokoyama and Ota (1959) made large bilateral electrolytic lesions at various sites in the hypothalami of postpartum rats. These investigators specifically noted that MB was completely absent (and in many cases cannibalism of pups ensued) in all rats with bilateral destruction of the paraventricular nucleus (PVN). The MB of rats with lesions that spared the PVN was unaffected even though milk ejection was abolished.

A number of earlier behavioral observations also suggested that the reflexive release of OXY during labor and nursing is not necessary for normal maternal response in rats. Moltz, Robbins, and Parks (1966) reported that cesarean section delivery of primigestational animals on Day 22 of gestation before the onset of labor did not significantly disrupt the onset of MB. Slotnick, Carpenter, and Fusco (1973) and more recently Mayer and Rosenblatt (1984) observed that primiparturient animals often became maternally responsive hours before delivery of pups and the rise of OXY in blood that occurs with expulsion of fetuses (Fuchs, 1985). Others have demonstrated (Moltz, Gesler, & Levin, 1967) that total mammectomy prior to impregnation produced no deficits in the onset or maintenance of postpartum MB. These observations taken together suggested that peripheral release of OXY plays no significant role in the postpartum activation of MB. However, the induction of MB by vaginal stimulation (Hemmes, 1969) and the abolition of MB following lesioning of the PVN (Yokoyama & Ota, 1959) remained to be explained.

It should be emphasized that the design and interpretation of the experiments described above were influenced by the concept that OXY was solely a peripheral hormone. If OXY was indeed distributed only to the posterior pituitary along the neurohypophysial pathway and released only into the bloodstream, the studies described above would have been adequate to rule out OXY as a significant factor in the activation of MB. However, the more recent evidence that OXY is widely distributed and released *within the CNS* by pathways other than the neurohypophysial pathway but still originating from the vicinity of the PVN leads to a quite different interpretation of the results of these earlier investigations. Clearly, experiments designed to simulate or block peripheral release of

OXY were not adequate to test possible MB effects of OXY within the
CNS. Peripheral administration of OXY in a single bolus may not have
significantly increased the levels of OXY in MB-mediating areas of the
brain. Destruction of the PVN may have eliminated MB because this
nucleus may be the origin of pathways releasing OXY within the brain,
and lesioning of the neurohypophysial pathway may have had no effect on
MB because only peripheral release of OXY was affected. Vaginal stimulation may have induced MB by producing central as well as peripheral
release of OXY. These considerations led us to test the effects of central
administration of OXY on the onset of MB.

## IV.  The Effects of Central Administration of Oxytocin on the Onset of Maternal Behavior in Nulliparous Rats

In our initial investigation (Pedersen & Prange, 1979), we tested the
effects of intracerebroventricular (ICV) administration of OXY on the
response of intact virgin female Sprague-Dawley rats from Zivic Miller
Laboratories (ZMSDs). In the first 2 hr after introduction of young rat
pups, which occurred immediately after ICV infusion, 38% of rats receiving 400 ng of OXY displayed full maternal behavior (FMB; for a description of how behavior was scored and a definition of FMB, see Pedersen &
Prange, 1985), while none of the rats receiving an equimolar dose of
arginine vasopressin (AVP) or normal saline (NS) vehicle displayed FMB.
In rats receiving OXY, a strong association was noted between estrous
state at the time of ICV infusion and FMB response. With one exception,
all rats that became fully maternal after ICV administration of OXY were
in diestrus, proestrus, or estrus on the day of testing. Because these
stages of the estrous cycle are associated with rising, elevated, or recently
elevated secretion of estrogen from the ovaries (Shaikh, 1971), we speculated that the facilitating effect of OXY on the onset of MB was estrogen
dependent. Further investigation confirmed this hypothesis (Pedersen &
Prange, 1979). Immediately after ovariectomy (OVX), ZMSDs were given
a single SC injection containing either 100 μg/kg estradiol benzoate (EB)
or corn oil vehicle alone. After 48 hr rats received ICV either OXY (400
ng) or NS and were then given pups. As depicted in Fig. 1, estrogen-
primed animals infused with OXY responded at a very high rate of FMB
in the first 2 hr of pup contact, whereas none of the corn oil–primed rats
displayed FMB after OXY.

Using the OVXed, EB-primed ZMSD model described above, we investigated the dose–response relationships and the specificity of OXY
induction of MB (Pedersen, Ascher, Monroe, & Prange, 1982). Increasing

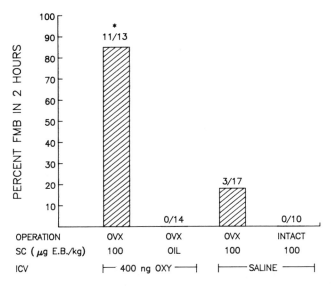

**Fig. 1.** The incidence of FMB following ICV administration of OXY or normal saline in ovariectomized or intact rats primed with estrogen or corn oil. Abbreviations: EB, estradiol benzoate; FMB, full maternal behavior; ICV, intracerebroventricular; OVX, ovariectomy; OXY, oxytocin; SC, subcutaneous. * $p < .002$, Fisher's exact probability test. From "Oxytocin and Mothering Behavior in the Rat" by Cort A. Pedersen and Arthur J. Prange, Jr., *Pharmacology and Therapeutics*, 1985, *28*, 287–302. Copyright 1985 by Pergamon Press Ltd, publisher. Reprinted by permission.

ICV doses of OXY (between 100 and 400 ng) produced increasing incidences of FMB, suggesting a linear dose–response relationship. Various peptides, ovarian steroids, and prostaglandins (PGs) were administered ICV at doses equimolar to 400 ng of OXY (see Table I). The incidence of FMB was determined for the 1st, the 2nd, and (for many rats) the 5th hr after introduction of pups. Oxytocin produced a significant incidence of FMB in the 1st hr of observation that persisted through the 5th hr of observation. Tocinoic acid (the ring structure of the OXY molecule) had significant potency in inducing FMB while Pro-Leu-Gly-NH2 (the tail structure of the OXY molecule) was ineffective. Arginine vasopressin, which is structurally similar to OXY, had a more delayed but significantly facilitating effect on the incidence of FMB. No other substances tested produced a significant increase in the incidence of FMB. However, a significant number of rats receiving $PGF_{2\alpha}$ (but not $PGE_2$) displayed several components of MB but not FMB in the 1st hr of observation after ICV infusions. Thus $PGF_{2\alpha}$ produced transient partial MB. It is of interest to note that administration of $PGF_{2\alpha}$ into the third cerebral ventricle of

**Table I**

The Incidence of FMB over Various Time Periods after ICV
Administration of OXY (400 ng) or Equimolar Doses of Other
Substances in Ovariectomized Estrogen-primed (100 $\mu$g EB/kg) Rats

|  |  | Percentage of animals fully maternal | | |
| --- | --- | --- | --- | --- |
| Substance | $N$ | 0 to 60 minutes | 60 to 120 minutes | 240 to 300 minutes |
| Oxytocin | 107 | 72* | 72* | 72* ($N = 58$)† |
| Tocinoic acid | 24 | 50‡ | 50‡ | 54‡ |
| $\beta$-Endorphin | 11 | 27 | 27 | |
| Luteinizing hormone-releasing hormone | 23 | 26 | 26 | |
| Thyrotropin-releasing hormone | 12 | 25 | 25 | |
| Pro-Leu-Gly-NH$_2$ | 12 | 25 | 25 | |
| Prolactin | 12 | 25 | 25 | |
| 17$\beta$-Estradiol | 12 | 25 | 25 | |
| Progesterone | 12 | 25 | 25 | |
| Prostaglandin E$_2$ | 14 | 21 | 21 | 36 |
| Lysine vasopressin | 29 | 21 | 24 | 24 |
| Pressinoic acid | 15 | 20 | 20 | 20 |
| Bradykinin | 10 | 20 | 20 | |
| Arginine vasotocin | 11 | 18 | 27 | |
| Saline | 51 | 18 | 18 | 19 ($N = 26$)† |
| Prostaglandin F$_{2\alpha}$ | 19 | 16 | 16 | 21 |
| Arginine vasopressin | 31 | 16 | 42§ | 55‡ |
| No ICV injection | 20 | 15 | 15 | 15 |
| Substance P | 17 | 12 | 12 | |
| Neurotensin | 11 | 9 | 9 | |

*Note.* From "Oxytocin Induces Maternal Behavior in Virgin Female Rats" by Cort A.
Pedersen, John A. Ascher, Yvonne L. Monroe, and Arthur J. Prange, Jr., *Science,* 1982,
*216,* 648–650. Copyright 1982 by American Association for the Advancement of Science,
publisher. Reprinted by permission.
  * $p < .001$. † $N$ shows the number of animals observed during the third observation
period added part way through the experiment. ‡ $p < .01$. § $p < .05$ compared to the group
treated with saline (Fisher's exact probability test).

rats has been reported to selectively increase the electrical activity of
oxytocinergic neurons in the PVN (Akaishi & Negoro, 1979).

Since our original reports (Pedersen & Prange, 1979; Pedersen *et al.*,
1982), several investigators have conducted their own studies of the effects of OXY administration on the onset of MB. Rubin, Menniti, and
Bridges (1983) and Bolwerk and Swanson (1984) reported that in their

laboratories OXY failed to increase the incidence of MB in the first several hours after ICV administration. These experiments, however, differed from those of Pedersen and Prange (1979) and Pedersen *et al.* (1982) in strains or substrains of rats used, sources of OXY, period of habituation to observation cages, timing of OVX and ovarian steroid treatments, doses of ovarian steroids, and/or doses of OXY. (See "Methodological Issues" below for a discussion of these parameters.) In contrast, Fahrbach, Morrell, and Pfaff (1984) employed methods and procedures almost identical to those of Pedersen and Prange (1979) to test the effects of central administration of OXY on the onset of MB. They observed an incidence of FMB very similar to that reported by Pedersen *et al.* (1982). Fahrbach *et al.* (1984) also reported data confirming the estrogen dependence of OXY induction of MB.

Hernandez, Guerra, and Hancke (unpublished observations) studied the effects of hypophysectomy (HPX) on OXY-induced maternal response. In intact, nulliparous Wistar-Holtzmann rats, they observed that ICV infusion of 40 ng of OXY on the morning of diestrus produced a significant increase in the incidence of FMB (using the scoring method of Pedersen and Prange) within 2 hr after administration (see Fig. 2). Oxytocin, however, had no effect in animals HPXed 4 weeks prior to ICV infusion and behavioral testing. Hypophysectomy may have inhibited OXY induction of MB by disrupting release of gonadotropins and, therefore, ovarian steroids.

McCarthy, Bare, and vom Saal (1986) have studied the effects of SC administration of OXY in nulliparous and late-gestational wild female mice (that spontaneously kill pups at the rates of 60% and 90% respectively). In both conditions OXY significantly inhibited infanticide and increased MB. Also, in agreement with the results of specificity studies reported by Pedersen *et al.* (1982), McCarthy *et al.* observed that SC administration of $PGF_{2\alpha}$ significantly diminished infanticide in late-gestational wild mice. It is not clear from these experiments whether OXY and $PGF_{2\alpha}$ influenced behavior toward pups by peripheral or central action. However, administration of the very large doses used in these experiments probably resulted in some penetration of these substances into the CNS. Thus, the original report by Pedersen and Prange (1979) that OXY administration induced a significant incidence of MB has gained considerable experimental support from a number of investigators. Keverne, Levy, Poindron, and Lindsay (1982) reported that vaginal stimulation, a potent releaser of OXY (Roberts & Share, 1968) produced immediate onset MB in estrogen- and progesterone-primed sheep. These results and the unpublished findings of Hemmes (1969) in goats that vaginal stimula-

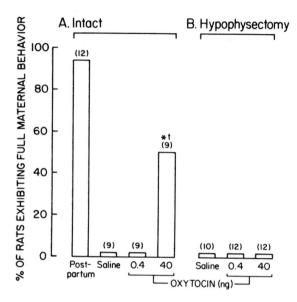

**Fig. 2.** The incidence of full maternal behavior occurring in intact postparturient rats (A, left bar), intact estrous-cycling virgin rats in diestrus (A, three bars at right), or hypophysectomized virgin female rats (B) in the first 2 hr after presentation of pups. Virgin rats (A and B) received either saline vehicle (10 $\mu$l) or oxytocin (0.4 or 40.0 ng) ICV just prior to introduction of pups. * $p < .01$ versus saline-treated rats; † = $p < .01$ versus postpartum rats (Fisher's exact probability test).

tion produces rapid-onset MB (see above) suggest that OXY may promote the onset of MB in mammalian species other than rodents.

Lesion studies have implicated a number of brain regions (olfactory bulbs, amygdala, hippocampus, septum, MPOA, VTA, stria terminalis) in the regulation of MB (for reviews see Numan, 1985 and chap. 12, this volume). Many of these regions are either terminal fields for OXY pathways (olfactory bulbs, amygdala, hippocampus, septum) or contain cell bodies or axons of passage from OXY-synthesizing neurons (MPOA, VTA, stria terminalis; see Buijs et al., 1983; Rhodes, Morrell, & Pfaff, 1981; Sofroniew, 1983; Swanson & Sawchenko, 1983). Oxytocin pathways project to other brain areas where lesions have no effect on MB or where the effect of lesioning has not been tested in MB (mesencephalic central gray, nucleus parabrachialis, nucleus tractus solitarius; see Swanson & Sawchenko, 1983). Recently, Fahrbach, Morrell, and Pfaff (1985b) have begun to investigate which of these regions may mediate the MB effects of centrally administered OXY in OVXed EB-primed ZMSDs. Infusion of 200 ng OXY into the mesencephalic central gray or the VTA produced a significant increase in FMB, whereas infusion into the medial amygdala had no enhancing effect. Clearly these observations require confirmation, and other brain sites require investigation.

## V.  The Role of CNS Oxytocin in the Onset of Ovarian Steroid-Induced Maternal Behavior

Estrogen levels rise gradually in the rat over the last 5–7 days of gestation, and progesterone levels fall rapidly over the 2–3 days prior to parturition (Bridges, 1984). Considerable evidence suggests that these ovarian steroid changes, especially the rise in estrogen, facilitate the initial onset of MB after the first parturition in rats. Moltz and Wiener (1966) reported that OVX of primigestational animals on Day 20 of pregnancy significantly diminished the incidence of MB after delivery of pups by cesarean section on Day 22. Others found that treatment of OVXed nulliparous rats for approximately 2 weeks with $17\beta$-estradiol ($E_2$) markedly shortened the mean latency of onset of MB (Bridges, 1984; Rosenblatt, chap. 14, this volume). The potency of $E_2$ in facilitating the onset of MB appeared to be increased by progesterone (P) withdrawal; that is, doses of $E_2$ that by themselves would not decrease latency of onset of MB became very effective in shortening latency when given concomitantly with P treatment and withdrawal (Bridges, 1984). Treatment with P followed by withdrawal in the absence of $E_2$ had no effect on the onset of MB in nulliparous rats (Bridges, 1984). Hysterectomy (H) in the last half of gestation in the rat significantly shortened the latency of onset of MB in primigestational rats. This effect was abolished by OVX at the time of H (HO). Estrogen treatment after HO produced an even more rapid onset of MB than H alone in late primigestational rats. Progesterone treatment prevented the rapid onset of MB in HOed primigestational rats treated with one dose of estrogen. These results (Rosenblatt, chap. 14, this volume) have led to the conclusion that estrogen is essential to the rapid onset of MB occurring after the first parturition in rats. Progesterone withdrawal appears to play a secondary role by increasing sensitivity to the MB effects of estrogen.

Estrogen treatment has been reported to release OXY from the posterior pituitary and to increase the frequency of action potentials in oxytocinergic cells within the PVN (Negoro, Visessuwan, & Holland, 1973; Yamaguchi, Akaishi, & Negora, 1979). Also, the ovarian steroid changes at the end of pregnancy have been associated with a dramatic increase in OXY binding in the uterus occurring several hours prior to the onset of labor (Soloff, 1985). We (Pedersen, Caldwell, Johnson, Fort, & Prange, 1985) as well as Fahrbach et al. (1985a, 1985b) have hypothesized that

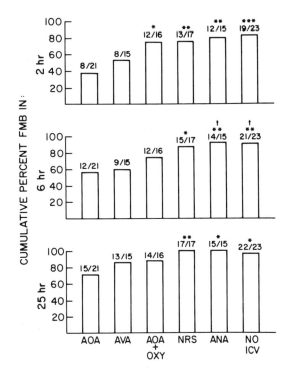

**Fig. 3.** The effect of ICV administration of AOA or other serums on the cumulative incidence of FMB in ovarian steroid–primed rats at various times after introduction of pups. Abbreviations: ANA, antineurotensin antiserum; AOA, antioxytocin antiserum; AVA, anti-arginine vasopressin antiserum; FMB, full maternal behavior; no ICV, no intracerebroventricular infusion; NRS, normal rabbit serum; OXY, oxytocin. * $p < .05$, ** $p < .02$, *** $p < .005$ (Fisher's exact probability test; comparisons with AOA); † $p < .05$ (comparisons with AVA). From "Oxytocin Antiserum Delays Onset of Ovarian Steroid–induced Maternal Behavior" by C. A. Pedersen, J. D. Caldwell, M. F. Johnson, S. A. Fort, and A. J. Prange, Jr. *Neuropeptides*, 1985, *6*, 175–182. Copyright 1985 by Churchill Livingstone, publisher. Reprinted by permission.

ovarian steroid treatments that accelerate the onset of MB may do so by releasing OXY and increasing binding of OXY within the CNS. Each group has conducted experiments using a different model of ovarian steroid–induced MB to test this hypothesis. In these experiments, we have both taken advantage of the considerably greater sensitivity of ZMSDs to ovarian steroid induction of MB compared to other substrains of Sprague-Dawley rats (see "Methodological Issues" below).

In our experiments (Pedersen *et al.*, 1985), ZMSDs were OVXed and treated for a 2-week period by SC placement of one Silastic capsule containing 4 mg E$_2$ (4 mm in length) and three capsules each containing 40 mg P (each 30 mm in length). Progesterone capsules were removed 24 hr prior to behavioral testing. One hour before introduction of pups, rats were infused ICV with 10 μl of undiluted antioxytocin antiserum (AOA) or various other serums, or they received no ICV infusion. Behavioral observations were conducted over the first 6 hr after introduction of pups and then for a 1-hr period every 24 hr. New pups were exchanged for old every 24 hr before the daily observation period. Results are summarized in Fig. 3.

Rats receiving AOA displayed a significantly lower incidence of FMB over the first 2, 6, and 25 hr of pup contact compared to rats receiving normal rabbit serum (NRS), antineurotensin antiserum (ANA), or no ICV infusion. Addition of OXY (250 ng) prior to ICV infusion significantly reversed the inhibitory effect of AOA on the onset of FMB over the first 2 hr of observation. Infusion of antiarginine vasopressin antiserum (AVA) significantly inhibited the onset of FMB compared to infusion of ANA or no ICV infusion over the first 6 hr of observation but not over any other observation period. Our results with AVA complement our earlier findings after ICV administration of AVP in OVXed EB-primed nullipara. Antiarginine vasopressin antiserum produced a delayed inhibitory effect on the onset of ovarian steroid–induced FMB, while AVP produced a delayed increase in the incidence of FMB (Table I; Pedersen et al., 1982).

Fahrbach et al. (1985a, 1985b) observed that HO followed by administration of 100 μg EB/kg SC in a single dose in 16-day primigestational ZMSDs produced a 100% incidence of FMB within 2 hr following introduction of pups 48 hr after surgery. Using this model of estrogen-induced MB, Fahrbach and her colleagues determined the effects of ICV administration of antiserum directed against OXY (anti-OXY) or an antagonist analogue of OXY, d(CH$_2$)$_5$-8-ornithine-vasotocin (OXY-antag), on the rate of onset of MB. Some rats received either 2 μl of dilute (10 : 1) anti-OXY, antiserum directed against AVP, (anti-ADH), or NRS three times per day beginning on Day 15 of gestation (prior to HO and EB). A final 5-μl infusion of each of these substances was delivered ICV 30 min prior to introduction of pups. Other rats received 800 ng of OXY-antag in 10 μl NS both 2 hr and several minutes prior to introduction of pups. Both anti-OXY and OXY-antag significantly inhibited the incidence of MB (see Fig. 4) and the quality of nest building over the first 5 hr of pup contact and significantly increased the latency of MB response over a 5-day period of pup contact. Anti-ADH or NRS had not significant effect on the rate of onset of MB.

Our results (Pedersen et al., 1985) and those of Fahrbach et al. (1985a, 1985b) summarized above strongly support the hypothesis that ovarian steroid acceleration of the onset of MB in rats is mediated by a mecha-

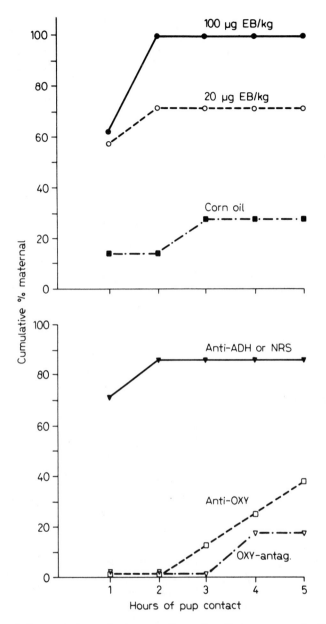

**Fig. 4.** Cumulative percentages of rats responding maternally to pups over the first 5 hr of pup contact beginning 48 hr after hysterectomy and ovariectomy on Day 16 of gestation. Animals receiving Anti-OXY, OXY-antag, Anti-ADH, or NRS received 100 μg EB/kg at the time of surgery. Over 1 and 5 hr of pup contact, there was no difference in cumulative incidences of maternal behavior between groups receiving EB alone and groups receiving EB and NRS or anti-ADH. Also, there was no difference between the group receiving corn oil and the groups receiving Anti-OXY or OXY-antag (Fisher's exact probability test, one-

nism involving OXY within the brain. While our experiments do not delineate what those mechanisms may be, the enhancing effect of estrogen on peripheral release and binding of OXY (Negoro *et al.,* 1973; Soloff, 1985; Yamaguchi *et al.,* 1979) suggests that estrogen (especially in combination with P withdrawal) may increase release and binding of OXY in discrete brain regions. Thus, ovarian steroid changes similar to those at the end of gestation appear to mobilize sufficient OXY within the brain to successfully induce MB. The reflexive release of OXY that occurs during labor (Fuchs, 1985) may not be necessary, therefore, for the onset of MB. Ovarian steroid activation of MB-inducing OXY mechanisms in the brain may, in part, explain why maternal responses to pups appear in many primigestational rats hours before delivery of pups (Mayer & Rosenblatt, 1984; Slotnick *et al.,* 1973).

## VI.  The Effects of Intracerebroventricular Administration of Oxytocin on the Reemergence of Maternal Behavior

Most primiparturient Sprague-Dawley rats from Charles River Breeders (CRSDs) allowed some postpartum mothering experience and then separated from pups for approximately 1 month will begin to display MB within 48 hr after reintroduction of young pups (Bridges, 1975, 1977, 1978). The latency of reemergence of MB is more rapid than the latency of onset of MB observed in naive nullipara kept in continuous contact with young pups. If, however, pups are taken from primiparturient rats shortly after birth, preventing the full expression of maternal response, latencies of onset of MB after 1 month of separation from pups are not significantly different from the latencies of naive nullipara (Bridges, 1977). Thus, in parturient rats, postpartum mothering experience appears to be necessary to produce persistent rapid reemergence of MB toward young pups. The relatively rapid rate of reemergence of MB is not inhibited by alteration of the ovarian steroid environment (Bridges, 1978).

We hypothesized that the rapid reemergence of MB seen in experienced rat mothers may in part be mediated by sensitivity to the MB effects of OXY. To test this hypothesis, we allowed primiparous CRSDs

tailed, † = .05). Abbreviations: Anti-ADH, antiarginine vasopressin antiserum; Anti-OXY, antioxytocin antiserum; EB, estradiol benzoate; NRS, normal rabbit serum; OXY, oxytocin; OXY-antag, d(CH₂)₅-8-ornithine-vasotocin. From "Possible Role for Endogenous Oxytocin in Estrogen-Facilitated Maternal Behavior in Rats" by S. E. Fahrbach, J. I. Morrell, and D. W. Pfaff, *Neuroendocrinology,* 1985, *40,* 526–532. Copyright 1985 by S. Karger, publisher. Reprinted by permission.

4–24 hr of postpartum mothering experience and then separated them from pups for 30–40 days. Some primiparous rats were OVXed 8–10 days prior to reintroduction of pups. Just before introduction of pups, rats received ICV either OXY (800 ng) or NS vehicle alone or no ICV infusion. Naive nulliparous CRSDs (some intact, others OVXed 8–10 days prior to testing) received the same treatments and were observed at the same times as primipara. Behavior was observed over a 2-hr period, and MB scores were assigned. Results for intact primipara are summarized in Fig. 5. Results in OVXed primipara are similar. Both intact and OVXed primipara that received OXY displayed a significantly increased incidence of reemergent FMB. Nullipara did not respond after OXY (See "Methodological Issues" below for a discussion of conditions under which OXY induces MB in nulliparous CRSDs.) Comparisons between treatment groups of distributions of MB scores revealed the same pattern of significance. Thus, primipara with brief postpartum mothering experience appear to have a persistent sensitivity to the MB-facilitating effects of OXY that is not ovarian steroid dependent.

Other primiparous CRSDs with brief postpartum mothering experience were separated from pups for 12–14 weeks and then given the same treatments as described above just before reintroduction of pups. In the first 2 hr and during the 5th hr of pup contact, rats infused ICV with OXY did not show a significantly increased incidence of FMB. However, the distribution of MB scores over the initial 2 hr and the 5th hr of pup contact were significantly "more maternal" for rats receiving OXY than for rats receiving NS or no ICV infusion. Thus postpartum sensitivity to the MB-facilitating effects of OXY appears to persist at a significant level for at least 12–14 weeks after separation from pups.

## VII. Methodological Issues: The Effects of Rat Strain, Source of Oxytocin, and Period of Pretest Habituation to Observation Cages

Our original observation that ICV administration of 400 ng of OXY produced a significant incidence of FMB was made using intact ZMSDs. When we studied the estrogen dependency of OXY-induced MB, we again used ZMSDs. We found that 400 ng of OXY produced a high incidence of FMB when administered ICV 48 hr after OVX and SC treatment with 100 $\mu$g/kg EB in one dose. Our specificity and dose-response work reported above were all conducted using this OVXed, EB-primed ZMSD model. We and others, however, found that Sprague-Dawleys from other breeders (Charles River Breeders) or other strains (Wistars) that were

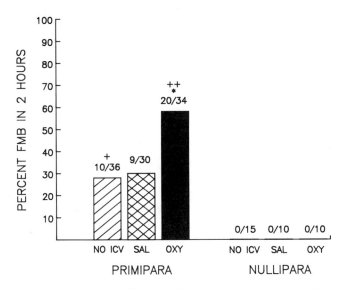

**Fig. 5.**   The incidence of FMB following ICV administration of OXY (800 ng), normal saline, or no ICV treatment in intact primiparous rats separated from pups for 30–40 days or in intact nulliparous rats naive to pups. Abbreviations: FMB, full maternal behavior; no ICV, no intracerebroventricular infusion; OXY, oxytocin; SAL, normal saline. * $p < .02$, Fisher's exact probability test (OXY versus no ICV and OXY versus SAL in primipara). † $p < .02$, ‡ $p < .001$ (primipara versus nullipara). From "Oxytocin and Mothering Behavior in the Rat" by Cort A. Pedersen and Arthur J. Prange, Jr., *Pharmacology and Therapeutics*, 1985, *28*, 287–302. Copyright 1985 by Pergamon Press Ltd, publisher. Reprinted by permission.

OVXed and primed with 100 μg/kg EB did not display an increased incidence of FMB after ICV administration of 400 ng of OXY (Ascher, Pedersen, Hernandez, & Prange, 1982, Bolwerk & Swanson, 1984; Rubin *et al.*, 1983). However, our experiments described above demonstrating increased reemergent MB in experienced rat mothers after central administration of OXY were conducted in CRSDs.

We have found that naive, nulliparous ZMSDs and CRSDs differ in their sensitivities to the MB-facilitating effects of ovarian steroids and in the estrogen treatment regimens required to sensitize animals to the MB effects of OXY. Prolonged treatment with ovarian steroids on a schedule designed to mimic ovarian steroid changes in late pregnancy was found to have significantly different MB effects in ZMSDs compared to CRSDs (Pedersen, Johnson, & Prange, 1983). Nullipara of both substrains were either OVXed or sham-OVXed. Eight days after surgery, each animal received SC one Silastic capsule implant (2 mm in length) containing 2.2. mg of $E_2$ or nothing (blank $E_2$). Ten days after OVX, three Silastic capsules, each 30 mm in length and each containing 40 mg of P or nothing (blank P), were placed SC in each animal. Twenty days after surgery and 24 hr before introduction of pups and the beginning of a 2-hr observation period, all P and blank P implants were removed. Animals were allowed 24 hr of habituation to observation cages prior to behavioral testing. Sham-OVXed ZMSDs implanted with blank capsules displayed a significantly higher incidence of FMB during the observation period than similarly prepared CRSDs (8/20 versus 0/17; $p < .004$, Fisher's exact probability test). Ovariectomized ZMSDs and CRSDs implanted with blank capsules showed low incidences of FMB that were not significantly different. Ovariectomized ZMSDs implanted with $E_2$ and P capsules, however, displayed a significantly higher incidence of FMB than OVXed CRSDs implanted with $E_2$ and P capsules (12/17 versus 5/16; $p < .03$). These results suggest that ZMSD rats are more sensitive to the MB effects of ovarian steroids than CRSDs.

Because CRSDs were less sensitive to ovarian steroids than ZMSDs, we hypothesized that higher doses and/or longer periods of treatment with estrogen that had been used in ZMSDs would sensitize CRSDs to the MB-facilitating effects of OXY. Indeed, we have found this to be true. CRSDs were OVXed and primed SC with one of several doses of EB (100, 150 or 200 $\mu$g/kg) 48 hr prior to ICV infusion of OXY (400 or 800 ng) or NS. As shown in Fig. 6, OXY was effective in increasing the incidence of FMB in CRSDs primed with 150 or 200 $\mu$g/kg EB but not in CRSDs primed with 100 $\mu$g/kg EB. Other OVXed CRSDs were given daily SC injections of 3 $\mu$g EB for 10 days and 24 $\mu$g EB SC 72 and 48 hr prior to ICV infusions of OXY (800 ng) or NS and introduction of young pups. Under these conditions, OXY produced a significantly higher incidence of FMB than NS (18/58 vs 5/40; $p < .03$). These results suggest that Sprague-Dawley rats from sources other than Zivic Miller Laboratories as well as some other strains of rats may simply require more or longer estrogen pretreatment than do ZMSDs to sensitize them to the MB effects of OXY. On the other hand, the observation by Hernandez et al. (see above) that ICV administration of only 40 ng of OXY produced a significant incidence of FMB in intact Wistar-Holtzman rats in diestrus suggests that some strains of rats may be even more sensitive to the MB effects of OXY than are ZMSDs and may require relatively low estrogen conditions for OXY to be effective.

We and others (Ascher et al., 1982; Fahrbach et al., 1984) have found that OXY from various sources differs markedly in its potencies in inducing MB. In our original work (Pedersen & Prange, 1979) we observed that ICV administration of 400 ng of OXY from Lot Number 9721 from Bachem produced over an 80% incidence of FMB in a 2-hr postinfusion observation period in OVXed, EB-primed ZMSDs. When Lot Number 9721 was no longer available, we obtained OXY from Bachem Lot Number R2622. This lot produced no significant incidence of FMB at any dose ICV. We then contacted Dr. Victor Hruby at the University of Arizona, who has since kindly provided us with OXY synthesized in his laboratory. Over a period of several years, we found that a 400-ng dose of Hruby OXY consistently produced an incidence of FMB of around 70% in OVXed EB-primed ZMSDs.

Fahrbach et al. (1984) used Hruby OXY in their investigations and observed an incidence of FMB very similar to what we had reported earlier. They also tested Bachem Lot Number R2622 and found it completely ineffective in inducing FMB. Another lot of OXY from Penninsula, Number 003249, was significantly effective but produced an incidence of FMB somewhat lower than Hruby OXY. Interestingly, at Fahrbach's request, Dr. Wilbur Sawyer tested Lot Number R2622 in the rat uterine strip bioassay and found no deficit in potency. Thus the MB potency of commercial lots of OXY can vary widely and is not necessarily guaranteed by potency in producing uterine contractions. Incidently, we and Fahrbach et al. (1984) have often observed convulsions and barrel rotation after ICV administration of OXY obtained from various commercial sources. We have yet to observe this effect with Hruby OXY.

In our initial investigations of the effects of OXY and other substances on the onset of MB, we placed our ZMSD rats in individual observation cages 1–2 hr prior to ICV infusions and introduction of pups. Fahrbach et al. (1985b) recently published evidence that varying the pretest period of habituation to observation cages alters the efficacy of OXY in the induction of MB. When rats were allowed either no habituation or prolonged (1-week) habituation to observation cages prior to ICV infusions, OXY had no significant MB-facilitating effect. Rats allowed 2 hr of habituation displayed a significant increase in the incidence of FMB in a 1-hr observation period after ICV administration of OXY. These results suggest that OXY is most effective in triggering MB in combination with some, but not total, environmental novelty. Fahrbach et al. (1985b) have suggested that other neuroendocrine factors released when a rat is placed in an unfamiliar environment may interact with OXY to produce high rates of MB. Clearly the role of such interactions requires future investigation.

We have tested the effects of a novel cage environment on the onset of MB in OVXed virgin ZMSDs treated for 2 weeks with Silastic capsules containing $E_2$ and P (Pedersen, Caldwell, & Prange, 1984). Rats allowed 24 hr of pretest habituation to observation cages displayed a 79% incidence of FMB in 2 hr, whereas rats introduced to pups in an unfamiliar cage displayed an incidence of FMB of only 43% (26/33 vs 10/23, $p <$

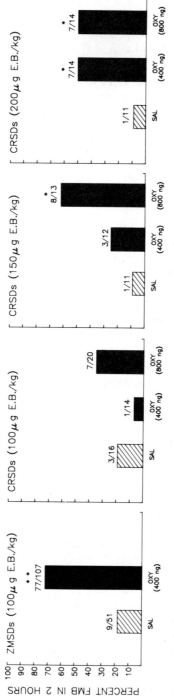

**Fig. 6.** The incidence of FMB following ICV administration of OXY in Sprague-Dawley rats from different breeders primed with varying doses of EB. Abbreviations: CRSDs, Sprague-Dawley rats from Charles River Breeders; EB, estradiol benzoate; FMB, full maternal behavior; OXY, oxytocin; SAL, normal saline; ZMSDs, Sprague-Dawley rats from Zivic Miller Laboratories. * $p < .05$, ** $p < .001$ (Fisher's exact probability test, OXY versus SAL). From "Oxytocin and Mothering Behavior in Rat" by Cort A. Pedersen and Arthur J. Prange, Jr., *Pharmacology and Therapeutics*, 1985, 28, 287–302. Copyright 1985 by Pergamon Press Ltd, publisher. Reprinted by permission.

.005). However, when rats were given OXY (400 ng) or NS ICV just before presentation of pups in an unfamiliar cage, OXY reinstated a high incidence of FMB compared to NS (15/18 vs 7/19, $p < .007$). Thus, ICV administration of OXY reversed novelty inhibition of the onset of ovarian steroid–induced MB. There are two questions raised by these findings that require further investigation. Is central release of OXY suppressed by novelty? It has been reported that release of OXY from the posterior pituitary is inhibited by certain types of stress (Cross & Dyball, 1974). Does OXY have the effect of reversing behavioral inhibition produced by novelty or other stressors? It will be of great interest to determine if OXY ameliorates the inhibitory effects of novelty or other stressors in behavioral situations other than first exposure to young pups.

## VIII. Concluding Remarks

Our investigations and those of Fahrbach *et al.* (1985a, 1985b) strongly support the hypothesis that OXY endogenous to the brain plays a central role in the rapid onset of MB associated with ovarian steroid changes at the end of pregnancy. Our work also suggests that the rapid reemergence of MB displayed by experienced rat mothers may also depend upon central mechanisms involving OXY. It remains to be determined, however, whether binding or competititve inhibition of central OXY will interfere with prepartum or postpartum onset of MB or the maintenance or reemergence of established MB. These fundamental questions will direct future investigations.

### Acknowledgments

We wish to recognize the excellent work of Debra A. Lowery in manuscript preparation. Much of the research described in this chapter was supported by National Institutes of Health Grants HD16159 and HD20640 and National Institute of Mental Health Grant MH22536.

### References

Akaishi, T., & Negoro, H. (1979). Differential effects of prostaglandin F2alpha on oxytocinergic and nonoxytocinergic neurones in the paraventricular nucleus of the lactating rat. *Endocrinologia Japonica, 26,* 725–730.
Ascher, J. A., Pedersen, C. A., Hernandez, D. E., & Prange, A. J., Jr. (1982). Sources of variance in oxytocin-induced maternal behavior. *Society for Neurosciences Abstracts, 8,* 368 (Abstract No. 100.3)

Bolwerk, E. L. M., & Swanson, H. H. (1984). Does oxytocin play a role in the onset of maternal behaviour in the rat? *Journal of Endocrinology, 101,* 353–357.

Bridges, R. S. (1975). Long-term effects of pregnancy and parturition upon maternal responsiveness in the rat. *Physiology and Behavior, 14,* 245–249.

Bridges, R. S. (1977). Parturition: Its role in the long term retention of maternal behavior in the rat. *Physiology and Behavior, 18,* 487–490.

Bridges, R. S. (1978). Retention of rapid onset of maternal behavior during pregnancy in primiparous rats. *Behavioral Biology, 24,* 113–117.

Bridges, R. S. (1984). A quantitative analysis of the roles of dosage, sequence, and duration of estradiol and progesterone exposure in the regulation of maternal behavior in the rat. *Endocrinology, 114,* 930–940.

Buijs, R. M., DeVries, G. J., Van Leeuwen, F. W., & Swaab, D. F. (1983). Vasopressin and oxytocin: Distribution and putative functions in the brain. In B. A. Cross & G. Leng (Eds.), *The neurohypophysis function and control* (pp. 115–122). (Progress in Brain Research, Vol. 60). New York, Amsterdam: Elsevier.

Cross, B. A., & Dyball, R. E. J. (1974). Central pathways for neurohypophysial hormone release. In E. Knobil & W. H. Sawyer (Eds.), *Handbook of physiology* (Sec. 7, Vol. 4, Pt. 1, (pp. 269–286). Baltimore: Williams & Wilkins.

Dogterom, J., Van Wimersma Greidanus, Tj. B., & Swaab, D. F. (1977). Evidence for the release of vasopressin and oxytocin into cerebrospinal fluid: Measurements in plasma and CSF of intact and hypophysectomized rats. *Neuroendocrinology, 24,* 108–118.

Dyball, R. E. J., & Paterson, T. (1983). Neurohypophysial hormones and brain function: The neurophysiological effects of oxytocin and vasopressin. *Pharmacology and Therapeutics, 20,* 419–436.

Fahrbach, S. E., Morrell, J. I., & Pfaff, D. W. (1984). Oxytocin induction of short-latency maternal behavior in nulliparous, estrogen-primed female rats. *Hormones and Behavior, 18,* 267–286.

Fahrbach, S. E., Morrell, J. I., & Pfaff, D. W. (1985a). Possible role for endogenous oxytocin in estrogen-facilitated maternal behavior in rats. *Neuroendocrinology, 40,* 526–532.

Fahrbach, S. E., Morrell, J. I., & Pfaff, D. W. (1985b). Role of oxytocin in the onset of estrogen-facilitated maternal behavior. In J. A. Amico & A. G. Robinson (Eds.), *Oxytocin: Clinical and laboratory studies* (pp. 372–388). Amsterdam: Elsevier/North Holland.

Fuchs, A. R. (1985). Oxytocin in animal parturition. In J. A. Amico & A. G. Robinson (Eds.), *Oxytocin: Clinical and laboratory Studies* (pp. 207–235). Amsterdam: Elsevier/North Holland.

Hemmes, R. B. (1969). *The ontogeny of the maternal–filial bond in the domestic goat.* Unpublished doctoral dissertation, Duke University, Durham, NC.

Herrenkohl, L. R., & Rosenberg, P. A. (1974). Effects of hypothalamic deafferentation late in gestation on lactation and nursing behavior in the rat. *Hormones and Behavior, 5,* 33–41.

Jones, P. M., Robinson, I. C. A. F., & Harris, M. C. (1983). Release of oxytocin into blood and cerebrospinal fluid by electrical stimulation of the hypothalamus or neural lobe in the rat. *Neuroendocrinology, 37,* 454–458.

Keverne, E. B., Levy, F., Poindron, P., & Lindsay, D. R. (1982). Vaginal stimulation: An important determinant of maternal bonding in sheep. *Science, 219,* 81–83.

Klopfer, P. H. (1971). Mother love: What turns it on? *American Scientist, 59,* 404–407.

Lincoln, D. W., & Russell, J. A. The electrophysiology of magnocellular oxytocin neurons. In J. A. Amico & A. G. Robinson (Eds.), *Oxytocin: Clinical and laboratory studies* (pp. 53–76). Amsterdam: Elsevier/North Holland.

Mayer, A. D., & Rosenblatt, J. S. (1984). Prepartum changes in maternal responsiveness and nest defense in *Rattus norvegicus*. *Journal of Comparative Psychology, 98,* 177–188.

McCarthy, M. M., Bare, J. E., & vom Saal, F. S. (1986). Infanticide and parental behavior in wild female mice: Effects of ovariectomy, adrenalectomy, and administration of oxytocin and prostaglandin $F_2$-alpha. *Physiology and Behavior, 36,* 17–24.

Meisenberg, G., & Simmons, W. H. (1983). Centrally mediated effects of neurohypophyseal hormones. *Neuroscience and Biobehavioral Reviews, 7,* 263–280.

Mena, F., Clapp, C., Martinez-Escalera, G., Pachero, P., & Grosvenor, C. E. (1985). Integrative regulation of milk ejection. In J. A. Amico & A. G. Robinson (Eds.), *Oxytocin: Clinical and laboratory studies* (pp. 179–199). Amsterdam: Elsevier/North Holland.

Moltz, H., Gesler, D., and Levin, R. (1967). Maternal behavior in the totally mammectomized rat. *Journal of Comparative and Physiological Psychology, 64,* 225–230.

Moltz, H., Robbins, D., & Parks, M. (1966). Caesarean delivery and the maternal behavior of primiparous and multiparous rats. *Journal of Comparative and Physiological Psychology, 61,* 455–460.

Moltz, H., & Wiener, H. (1966). Effects of ovariectomy on maternal behavior of primiparous and multiparous rats. *Journal of Comparative and Physiological Psychology, 62,* 382–387.

Negoro, H., Visessuwan, S., & Holland, R. C. (1973). Unit activity in the paraventricular nucleus of female rats at different stages of the reproductive cycle and after ovariectomy, with or without estrogen or progesterone treatment. *Journal of Endocrinology, 59,* 545–558.

Numan, M. (1985). Brain mechanisms and parental behavior. In N. Adler, D. W. Pfaff, & R. W. Goy (Eds.), *Handbook of behavioral neurobiology: Vol. 7. Reproduction* (pp. 537–605). New York: Plenum.

Pedersen, C. A., Ascher, J. A., Monroe, Y. L., & Prange, A. J., Jr. (1982). Oxytocin induces maternal behavior in virgin female rats. *Science, 216,* 648–650.

Pedersen, C. A., Caldwell, J. D., Johnson, M. F., Fort, S. A., & Prange, A. J., Jr. (1985). Oxytocin antiserum delays onset of ovarian steroid–induced maternal behavior. *Neuropeptides, 6,* 175–182.

Pedersen, C. A., Caldwell, J. D., & Prange, A. J., Jr. (1984). Oxytocin reverses novelty inhibition of onset of ovarian steroid–induced maternal behavior. *Society for Neurosciences Abstracts, 10,* pg. 170. (Abstract No. 52.7).

Pedersen, C. A., Johnson, M. F., & Prange, A. J., Jr. (1983). Differences in rat substrain sensitivities to the maternal behavioral effects of ovarian steroids and oxytocin. *Society for Neurosciences Abstracts, 9,* 1079. (Abstract No. 315.1).

Pedersen, C. A., & Prange, A. J., Jr. (1979). Induction of maternal behavior in virgin rats after intracerebroventricular administration of oxytocin. *Proceedings of the National Academy of Sciences, 76,* 6661–6665.

Pedersen, C. A., & Prange, A. J., Jr. (1985). Oxytocin and mothering behavior in the rat. *Pharmacology and Therapeutics 28,* 287–302.

Rhodes, C. H., Morrell, J. I., & Pfaff, D. W. (1981). Immunohistochemical analysis of magnocellular elements in rat hypothalamus: Distribution of cells containing neurophysin, oxytocin, and vasopressin. *Journal of Comparative Neurology, 198,* 45–64.

Roberts, J. S., & Share, L. (1968). Oxytocin in plasma of pregnant, lactating and cycling ewes during vaginal stimulation. *Endocrinology, 83,* 272–278.

Rosenblatt, J. S. (1969). The development of maternal responsiveness in the rat. *American Journal of Orthopsychiatry, 39,* 36–56.

Rubin, B. S., Menniti, F. S., & Bridges, R. S. (1983). Intracerebroventricular administration of oxytocin and maternal behavior in rats after prolonged and acute steroid pretreatment. *Hormones and Behavior, 17,* 45–53.

Shaikh, A. A. (1971). Estrone and estradiol levels in the ovarian venous blood from rats during the estrous cycle and pregnancy. *Biology of Reproduction, 5,* 297–307.

Slotnick, B. M., Carpenter, M. L., & Fusco, R. (1973). Initiation of maternal behavior in pregnant nulliparous rats. *Hormones and Behavior, 4,* 53–59.

Sofroniew, M. V. (1983). Morphology of vasopressin and oxytocin neurones and their central and vascular projections. In B. A. Cross & G. Leng (Eds.), *The neurohypophysis function and control* (pp. 101–114). (Progress in Brain Research, Vol. *60*). New York, Amsterdam: Elsevier.

Soloff, M. S. (1985). Oxytocin receptors and mechanisms of oxytocin action. In J. A. Amico, & A. G. Robinson (Eds.), *Oxytocin: Clinical and laboratory studies* (pp. 259–276). Amsterdam: Elsevier/North Holland.

Swanson, L. W., & Sawchenko, P. E. (1983). Hypothalamic integration: Organization of the paraventricular and supraoptic nuclei. *Annual Review of Neuroscience, 6,* 269–324.

White, J. D., & McKelvy, J. F. (1985). Biosynthesis and transport of oxytocin in the central nervous sytem. In J. A. Amico & A. G. Robinson (Eds.), *Oxytocin: Clinical and laboratory studies* (pp. 124–132). Amsterdam: Elsevier/North Holland.

Yamaguchi, K., Akaishi, T., & Negoro, H. (1979). Effect of estrogen treatment on plasma oxytocin and vasopressin in ovariectomized rats. *Endocrinologia Japonica, 26,* 197–205.

Yokoyama, A., Halasz, B., & Sawyer, C. H. (1967). Effect of hypothalamic deafferentation on lactation in rats. *Proceedings of the Society for Experimental Biology and Medicine, 125,* 623–626.

Yokoyama, A., & Ota, K. (1959). The effect of hypothalamic lesions on litter growth in rats. *Endocrinologia Japonica, 6,* 14–20.

# 14

## Biologic and Behavioral Factors Underlying the Onset and Maintenance of Maternal Behavior in the Rat

JAY S. ROSENBLATT
*Institute of Animal Behavior*
*Rutgers University*
*Newark, New Jersey 07102*

Maternal behavior in the rat is discussed most clearly within the framework of our current theory which proposes that there are separate phases in the control and regulation of this interesting behavior pattern. First we must define the term *maternal behavior*. The simplest definition, and perhaps the best, is: Maternal behavior consists of whatever the mother does to foster the care and development of her young. Many of her behaviors are directed toward the young themselves, as for example, when she nurses them; retrieves them should they leave the nest or be dragged from it; licks their body and anogenital regions, the latter eliciting elimination, necessary for pup survival; and remains with them in the nest to warm them because they are unable to regulate their own body temperatures for several weeks after birth. Other behaviors such as nest building and nest defense or maternal aggression are not directed at the young. They are directed at nesting material or at intruding males or females near the nest or predators which the female attacks.

The underlying physiological processes involved in MB provide a basis for the more overt behavioral responses. For example, nursing depends upon milk production (lactogenesis) and release (letdown), and these, in turn, depend upon the suckling stimulation the female receives during nursing (Grosvenor & Mena, 1982). Altered thermogenesis during pregnancy (Wilson & Stricker, 1979) and lactation (Leon, Croskerry, &

Smith, 1978; Woodside & Leon, 1980) regulate the mother's contact with her young in the nest and her licking of their anogenital region, eliciting urination, which serves to maintain her water balance (Friedman, Bruno, & Alberts, 1981; Gubernick & Alberts, 1983). These aspects of MB will not be discussed in this article, but we have reviewed them in a recent treatment of the subject (Rosenblatt, Mayer, & Siegel, 1985).

The organization of MB, as we view it, is depicted in Fig. 1. It shows that there are two main phases, the *pre-* and *postpartum phases,* and an intervening period labeled the *transition period.* Although interest in learning in newborn involves mainly (but not exclusively) the postpartum period of MB when the mother and young interact, for the mother the phase of routine postpartum care of the young is dependent upon what happens prepartum and especially in the short transition period. Maternal behavior is established during the prepartum phase, which serves to prepare the female to behave maternally toward the young when they appear during parturition. In discussing this phase we show that MB arises out of the endocrine processes of pregnancy. At the start of the postpartum phase, the endocrine basis of MB gradually wanes yet MB continues

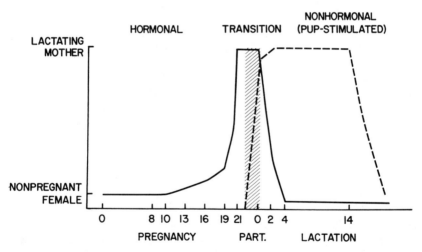

**Fig. 1.** Scheme of the regulation of maternal behavior during the maternal behavior cycle of the female rat. The ordinate shows levels of maternal behavior represented by lactating mothers (high) and nonpregnant females (low), and the abscissa shows three phases: pregnancy, parturition, and lactation. From "Maternal Behavior in the Laboratory Rat" by J. S. Rosenblatt and H. I. Siegel. In R. W. Bell and W. P. Smotherman (Eds.), *Maternal Influences and Early Behavior,* Chapter 7, Figure 1, p. 156. Jamaica, NY: Spectrum Publications, 1980b. Copyright 1980 by Spectrum Publications, Inc. Reprinted by permission of the publisher.

based upon stimulation that the mother receives from the young. Studies have shown that the regulation of MB shifts from a hormonal to a nonhormonal or behavioral basis and that this occurs during the transition period.

Characterizing the prepartum phase as endocrine in nature and the postpartum phase as behavioral is not meant to ignore the fact that each phase has components of the other. There are behavioral components during pregnancy (e.g., changes in self-licking, altered thermoregulation and related behavioral changes, changes in feeding, etc.). Postpartum maternal behavior involves physiological processes that are crucial, involving endocrine secretions and other endogenous neuroactive agents. By making this broad distinction between the two phases, we are attempting to characterize the predominant factors governing MB during each of them.

It is not known yet how general among mammals is the characterization of MB into phases. Of course, in all species there are two principal periods during the cycle of maternal care: the gestation period and the period of MB and lactation. During the former period, the endocrine secretions of pregnancy predominate, and during the latter, the female interacts with the young. However, for many species we do not know whether MB is initiated prepartum, as has been determined in the rat, or is nonhormonally based in the postpartum period or continues to depend upon hormones (Rosenblatt & Siegel, 1981a).

This article will be divided into three principal sections dealing with the pre- and postpartum phases and the intervening transition period. Each section, in turn, will deal with a number of specific issues.

## I.  Prepartum Phase: Onset of Maternal Behavior

### A.  Role of Estrogen and Progesterone

In several strains of rats it has been shown that prepartum females tested with young pups shortly before giving birth display the principal components of MB, namely, nursing behavior, retrieving, licking of the pups, nest building, and nest defense or maternal aggression against conspecifics (Rosenblatt & Siegel, 1981c; Rosenblatt, Siegel, & Mayer, 1979). Timing of the onset depends upon the age of the pups used to test the female: Toward newborn pups (i.e., those less than 2 hr of age), females may exhibit the principal components of MB as early as 24 hr prepartum, and toward slightly older pups, 4–9 days old, as late as $3\frac{1}{2}$ hr prepartum (Mayer & Rosenblatt, 1984). In Sprague-Dawley females, nearly all are responsive to pups before they deliver, whereas only half of Long-Evans females retrieve pups and exhibit other components of MB prepartum (Bridges, Feder, & Rosenblatt, 1977; Slotnick, Carpenter, & Fusco, 1973).

An early conception held by many that parturition played a role in stimulating females to become maternal has been replaced by the conception, quite reasonable when one thinks about it, that females are already capable of exhibiting MB when they begin parturition. Those females that have not exhibited MB before parturition rapidly initiate it once the pups have been delivered. It has been shown, however, that females which initiate it prepartum are more strongly motivated postpartum than those which initiate it postpartum (Slotnick, Carpenter, & Fusco, 1973).

Through a procedure, which has been called "sensitization," in which females are exposed to pups in their cages continuously for several days (the pups are replaced with fresh pups every 24 hrs), if needed, it has been shown that the latencies for the onset of MB gradually are reduced from 3 or 4 days to 1 or 2 days as pregnancy advances (Cosnier & Couturier, 1966; Rosenblatt, 1967; Rosenblatt & Siegel, 1975; Wiesner & Sheard, 1933). At the end of pregnancy, however, this process is accelerated and females may exhibit MB within minutes after pups have been placed in their cages. This suggests that the physiological (endocrine) changes underlying MB also accelerate at the end of pregnancy.

Which of the endocrine changes known to occur at the end of pregnancy (Fig. 2) are responsible for the onset of MB has been studied in various ways. It has been difficult to investigate this question in the late-pregnant female directly, however, because the endocrine changes are intertwined through feedback relationships and hormonal interactions. Therefore, investigators have used various models to study experimentally how the pattern of hormonal secretion by the ovaries under the influence of the placentas and pituitary gland (Fig. 2) can be related to the initiation of MB. In 1933 Weisner and Sheard proposed an hormonal basis for the onset of MB, and we have shown that blood or plasma from a mother injected or transfused into a nonpregnant female is capable of stimulating MB; there is little doubt, therefore, that this behavior is hormonally stimulated (Terkel & Rosenblatt, 1968, 1972).

Two successful treatments, based upon circulating levels of hormones shown in Fig. 2, for inducing MB in ovariectomized nonpregnant rats are shown in Fig. 3 (Moltz, Lubin, Leon, & Numan, 1970; Zarrow, Gandelman, & Denenberg, 1971). The main features of these treatments are the prolonged estradiol benzoate administration and the intervening period of progesterone injections terminating before the administration of prolactin. When pups were introduced at the end of these treatments, females responded maternally either immediately or within 40 hr. It was

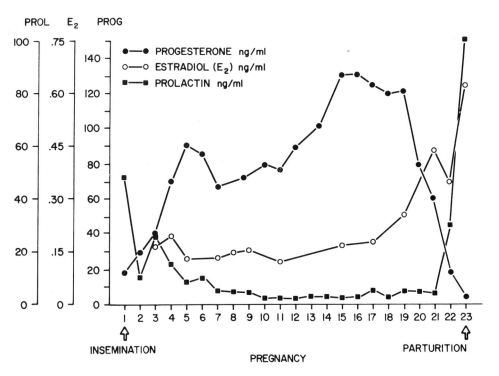

Fig. 2. Circulating levels of estradiol (E₂), progesterone (PROG), and prolactin (PROL) during pregnancy in the rat. Based on Pepe and Rothchild (1974), progesterone; Shaikh (1971), estradiol; Morishige, Pepe, & Rothchild (1974), prolactin. From "Progress in the Study of Maternal Behavior in the Rat: Hormonal, Nonhormonal, Sensory, and Developmental Aspects" by J. S. Rosenblatt, H. I. Siegel, and A. D. Mayer. In J. S. Rosenblatt, R. A. Hinde, C. G. Beer, and M. C. Busnel (Eds.), *Advances in the Study of Behavior* (Vol. 10). New York: Academic Press, 1979. Copyright 1979 by Academic Press, Inc. Reprinted by permission.

not clear, however, which aspects of the treatment were effective in stimulating MB and why they were effective.

Another model, adopted by us, was the use of premature termination of pregnancy by hysterectomy in late-pregnant females, which resulted in a rapid (2- to 3-day latency from surgery) onset of MB (Rosenblatt & Siegel, 1975). When in addition to removal of uteri and fetuses, females were ovariectomized, there was a delay in the rapid onset of MB, indicating that the hormonal stimulus for MB was secreted from the ovaries (Rosenblatt & Siegel, 1975). Later studies enabled us to isolate this factor as ovarian estradiol (Siegel & Rosenblatt, 1975a, 1975b).

During the 4 hr following hysterectomy, there is a rapid decline in ovarian secretion of progesterone and in the circulating levels of this

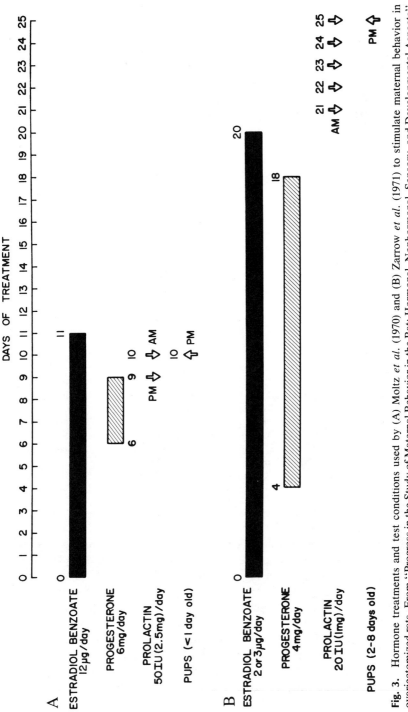

**Fig. 3.** Hormone treatments and test conditions used by (A) Moltz *et al.* (1970) and (B) Zarrow *et al.* (1971) to stimulate maternal behavior in ovariectomized rats. From "Progress in the Study of Maternal Behavior in the Rat: Hormonal, Nonhormonal, Sensory, and Developmental Aspects" by J. S. Rosenblatt, H. I. Siegel, and A. D. Mayer. In J. S. Rosenblatt, R. A. Hinde, C. G. Beer, and M. C. Busnel (Eds.), *Advances in the Study of Behavior* (Vol. 10), New York: Academic Press, 1979. Copyright 1979 by Academic Press, Inc. Reprinted by permission.

hormone, which is then followed by an increase in the secretion of ovarian estradiol (Rosenblatt, Siegel, & Mayer, 1979). At the end of 48 hr, females initiate MB when pups are presented to them in their home cages.

One consequence of these hormonal changes is that we find very high levels of estrogen receptors in nuclei of cells of the preoptic area of the brain, where we believe estrogen acts to stimulate MB (Numan, Rosenblatt, & Komisaruk, 1977; see Numan, chap. 12, this volume). Following hysterectomy, receptor levels decline during the next 12 hr, then begin to increase, reaching peak levels again at 24 hr posthysterectomy. This increase is caused by the increase in ovarian estrogen secretion when pregnancy is terminated. In the absence of the inhibitory effect of high levels of progesterone (Rosenblatt, Siegel, & Mayer, 1979), the estrogen stimulates MB in these females.

Under normal circumstances there is a high level of estradiol in circulation just before parturition (Fig. 2), and recent studies in our laboratory have shown that there is a corresponding high level of nuclear estradiol receptors in the preoptic area that may be instrumental in the prepartum onset of MB.

Further evidence of the role of estrogen in the initiation of MB in the rat comes from several sources in addition to the correlational studies just described. Maternal behavior is reliably elicited from late-pregnant females in which pregnancy is terminated by hysterectomy-ovariectomy and estradiol benzoate is administered at surgery (Siegel & Rosenblatt, 1975b). Nonpregnant females subjected to hysterectomy-ovariectomy also initiate MB when given EB, but higher doses are needed (100 or 200 $\mu$g/kg) than in pregnancy-terminated females (Siegel & Rosenblatt, 1975a). Estrogen implanted directly into the MPOA also elicits MB in late-pregnant, pregnancy-terminated females (Numan, Rosenblatt, & Komisaruk, 1977). Conversely, blocking the action of EB with tamoxifen or CI-628, potent antiestrogens, prevents the onset of MB in estrogen-treated pregnant females subjected to hysterectomy-ovariectomy (Doerr, Siegel, & Rosenblatt, unpublished data).

Normally progesterone levels have declined when circulating levels of estradiol rise at the end of pregnancy. These changes serve as a trigger for parturition and for the initiation of lactation, but the decline in progesterone is also a necessary condition for the initiation of MB. It has been shown in several studies that progesterone inhibits the action of estrogen in stimulating MB (Bridges, Rosenblatt, & Feder, 1978; Siegel & Rosenblatt, 1975c, 1978). Both pregnancy-terminated females and nonpregnant females subjected to hysterectomy-ovariectomy and treated with estrogen fail to exhibit MB if progesterone is given at the same time as the estrogen or within 24 hr (Siegel & Rosenblatt, 1975c, 1978). Also, maintaining high levels of progesterone at parturition when these levels normally fail prevents the normal onset of MB, probably by a direct action on estrogen stimulation (Moltz, Levin, & Leon, 1969). The mechanism underlying progesterone inhibition of MB is not known. However, it cannot be the same mechanism as progesterone inhibition of sexual behavior in female rats, namely, the blocking of later progesterone action, because stimulation of MB does not require the successive action of estrogen and progesterone as sexual behavior does.

Progesterone alone or in combination with estrogen also has a facilitating action with respect to MB, as one might expect considering that during most of pregnancy, circulating progesterone levels are very high (Fig. 2) and there is a low level of estrogen. In several studies, progesterone administered by subcutaneous implant during the first 16–17 days primed estrogen action, and either smaller doses of estrogen were needed to stimulate MB or females exhibited shorter latencies when subsequently administered estrogen (Bridges, 1983; Bridges & Russell, 1981; Doerr, Siegel, & Rosenblatt, 1981). Progesterone paired with estrogen has an even greater effect in shortening latencies for MB.

It is not entirely clear how progesterone facilitates the action of estrogen in stimulating MB, but it may increase either the concentration or the retention of estrogen receptors in cells responsive to this hormone in the preoptic region and thereby facilitate the subsequent rapid uptake and action of this hormone (Lisk & Reuter, 1977).

## B. Oxytocin and Prolactin

The studies on EB or endogenous estrogen stimulation of MB do not rule out the possibility that additional hormones, either as mediators of the estrogen stimulation or synergizing with estrogen, may be involved in the onset of MB. Several studies have, in fact, shown that in ZMSD rats, the neuropeptide OXY introduced directly ICV is capable of stimulating the rapid onset of MB in ovariectomized, estrogen-primed females (Fahrbach, Morrell, & Pfaff, 1984; Pedersen, Ascher, Monroe, & Prange, 1982; Pedersen & Prange, 1979). Oxytocin does not appear to stimulate MB in other strains of rats (Wistar, Long-Evans) or even in Sprague-Dawley rats from other breeders (CRSD) (Bolwerk & Swanson, 1984; Rosenblatt, 1984; Rubin, Menniti, & Bridges, 1983). An antioxytocin given ICV which blocks MB in estrogen-treated pregnancy-terminated ZMSD rats has no effect on MB in CRSD rats (Fahrbach, Morrell, & Pfaff, 1985; Mayer & Rosenblatt, unpublished data). It should be noted, moreover, that the OXY effect occurs only when females are tested for MB in new, unfamiliar cages, not when they are tested in their home cages, and also that the

ZMSD strain of rats is normally highly responsive to pups even without hormone treatment.

Prolactin was designated early as the "maternal hormone" in the rat, but later studies disputed this claim because of failure to replicate the original findings. More recent studies using prolactin release blockers (Numan, Rosenblatt, & Komisaruk, 1977; Rodriguez-Sierra & Rosenblatt, 1977; Rosenblatt & Siegel, 1981c) are also ineffective in blocking estrogen stimulation of MB. These blockers (ergocornine hydrogen maleate, apomorphine hydrochloride, and ergokryptine [CB154-2 bromo-alpha-ergokryptine], when given to estrogen-treated pregnancy-terminated females without ovaries, have no effect on MB. Prolactin, therefore, does not mediate the effect of estrogen on MB. More recently, however, there is evidence that prolactin might play a role in MB. Hypophysectomized females failed to respond to progesterone and estrogen stimulation that normally elicits MB. A longer period was required from them to respond compared to females with their pituitaries. Pituitary gland replacement ectopically or administration of prolactin during 11 days followed by estrogen restored the short latencies (Bridges, Loundes, DiBase, & Tate-Ostroff, 1985). While these studies indicate that prolactin does play a role in MB, a later study in which pregnant rats were hypophysectomized at midpregnancy (and carried their young to term) resulted in no deficiency in MB. To explain these unexpected results, it was proposed that prolactin before midpregnancy and placental lactogen after midpregnancy may normally play a role in the initiation of MB. This hypothesis has not yet been tested, nor is it easy to design an experiment to do so.

### C. Hormonal Priming

Under normal conditions, the rise in estrogen at the end of pregnancy is preceded by a prolonged period of high circulating levels of progesterone and low levels of estrogen (see Fig. 2). These hormones serve to prime the female to respond to the acute rise in estrogen just prior to parturition: As noted earlier, if nonpregnant ovariectomized females are primed with these hormones or with progesterone alone for 16–17 days, they require a lower dose of estrogen or a shorter latency to initiate MB (Bridges, 1983; Bridges & Russell, 1981; Doerr, Siegel, & Rosenblatt, 1981). Nonpregnant females, lacking this hormonal priming, require higher doses of estrogen to initiate MB. An interesting series of problems for future study is presented by these findings: How is the priming effect represented in the brain regions responsive to estrogen mediating MB, and how do the higher doses of estrogen given to nonpregnant females produce their effects in the absence of priming by pregnancy hormones?

## II. Postpartum Phase: Maintenance of Maternal Behavior

The study of nonpregnant females exposed to pups for the first time revealed an unexpected initial aversion females have toward the odors of pups and a timidity to approaching a novel object in their cages (Fleming & Luebke, 1981; Fleming & Rosenblatt, 1974a, 1974b, 1974c; Terkel & Rosenblatt, 1972). After they have given birth, the aversion is transformed into an attraction, even to the pup odors that were previously aversive to them, and the timidity is very much reduced (Fleming & Rosenblatt, 1974a; Hård & Hansen, 1985). The first signs of this change are seen in the female's attraction to lactating mother's nesting material shortly before parturition (Bauer, 1983). In advance of delivery, therefore, females undergo changes which enable them to respond positively to their pups as they emerge from the birth canal, and these changes are based upon the hormones that stimulate MB. The hormonal situation that exists before parturition, however, undergoes a rapid change immediately after the female gives birth: She initiates an estrous cycle, exhibits lordosis, mates, and can become pregnant. After this postpartum estrus, estrous cycling is suppressed throughout lactation. High circulating levels of ovarian progesterone predominate, and lactation is maintained by the lactogenic complex including prolactin, growth hormone, and adrenocortical hormone. The hormonal basis for the *onset* of MB disappears, and the question is whether it is replaced by another hormonal stimulus for MB. Evidence indicates that this is not the case: Once MB is established hormonally prepartum, it appears to be maintained on a nonhormonal basis, that is, on the basis of stimulation that the female receives from her young (Rosenblatt, Siegel, & Mayer, 1979).

### A. Nonhormonal Basis of Maternal Behavior: Nonpregnant Females

It is necessary to introduce the concept of nonhormonally based maternal behavior as a preliminary to a discussion of the postpartum maintenance of MB. Nonpregnant, estrous-cycling females can be induced to exhibit MB by sensitization, exposing them continuously to pups for periods of 4–8 days (Cosnier & Couturier, 1966; Fleming & Rosenblatt, 1974a; Rosenblatt, 1967; Wiesner & Sheard, 1933). These females exhibit retrieving, crouching over pups as in nursing (but without nipple development and mammary gland function), nest building, and anogenital licking like lactating females, and they decline in their MB in the same manner (Reisbick, Rosenblatt, & Mayer, 1975). Several lines of evidence strongly suggest that this behavior is not elicited by pup-stimulated release of hormones. Hypophysectomized females can be sensitized as readily as intact females, and ovariectomy also does not prevent sensitization (Cosnier & Couturier, 1966; Rosenblatt, 1967). Moreover, high levels of prolactin do not affect sensitization (Baum, 1978), and cross-transfusion of blood from sensitized females to other nonpregnant females also does not induce MB as it does when newly parturient female blood is cross-transfused to a nonpregnant female (Terkel & Rosenblatt, 1971, 1972).

Although sensitization produces a behavioral "artifact," inasmuch as nonlactating maternal females, requiring several days of pup exposure to become maternal, do not occur naturally, nevertheless their occurrence enables us to conceive of MB which does not require a hormonal basis. Sensitized females continue to exhibit MB for as long as they have young pups, and they modify their behavior according to the age of the pups, finally declining in their "care" of them when the pups reach the age of weaning from normally lactating mothers (Fleming & Rosenblatt, 1974a; Reisbick, Rosenblatt, & Mayer, 1975).

## B.   Postpartum Maintenance: Nonhormonally Mediated

Following the pre- and early postpartum initiation of MB, pups are required to maintain this behavior, and in their absence, the female gradually loses her maternal responsiveness (Rosenblatt, 1965). The duration of persistence of MB in the absence of pups immediately postpartum varies from 2 days to more than a week, and some residual effects of having given birth may be evident even longer; but eventually, without pups, mothers show a waning of their responsiveness (Fleming & Orpen, 1986).

Further evidence of the nonhormonal nature of postpartum MB is the difficulty of interfering with it either by administering hormones to lactating females or by removing sources of hormones such as the pituitary gland, the ovaries, or the adrenal glands (Rosenblatt, Siegel, & Mayer, 1979). The implication is that these treatments are ineffective because the behavior is no longer dependent upon hormones. The neural basis of nonhormonal MB has been studied: Lesions of the MPOA or of lateral efferent fibers from this region severely reduce the ability of females to be sensitized (Numan, Rosenblatt, & Komisaruk, 1977). The MPOA is also the site of action of estradiol implants which stimulate females to exhibit MB. The lesions described above in the case of females not tested with hormones prevent females from responding to exposure to pups, that is, to the sensory stimuli normally associated with MB. The neural basis of estrogen-stimulated initiation of MB and pup-stimulated nonhormonal maintenance of MB may, therefore, be a neural organization centered in the MPOA but including other nuclei as well (Fleming & Orpen, 1986; Numan, 1985; see also Numan, chap. 12, this volume).

A recent study tested the possibility that OXY may be involved in the postpartum maintenance of MB in the ZMSD strain in which it has been shown that OXY stimulates MB in nonpregnant females and antioxytocin blocks estrogen effects in 16-day pregnancy-terminated estrogen-treated females (Fahrbach, Morrell, & Pfaff, 1985). On Day 5 of lactation, females were injected ICV with the antioxytocin agent, and their behavior before and after the injection was compared. There was little change and certainly no loss of any items of MB; as an example, the frequency of nursing contacts and the amount of time away from the litter were unchanged after the antioxytocin injection. Even when OXY may be involved in the onset of MB in the ZMSD strain, it is not involved in its maintenance.

We have speculated that it is adaptive for females to shift the maintenance of MB to a nonhormonal mechanism after parturition in order to speed up production of the next litter. Because she mates with a male immediatley postpartum, she is ready to implant the blastocysts as soon as suckling inhibition of gonadal estrogen secretion is relaxed, which is more than a week before she weans her current litter. She, therefore, speeds up her reproduction. This is possible because while the endocrine system is occupied with the next pregnancy, it is freed from maintenance of the current litter (except for the maintenance of lactation and other secondary functions related to maternal care of young).

C.  Postpartum Behavioral Synchrony between
    Mother and Young

The terms *synchrony, parasitism,* and *symbiosis* have been used to characterize the relationship between the mother and her young during the postpartum period that ends with weaning around 3–4 weeks of age (Alberts & Gubernick, 1983; Galef, 1981; Rosenblatt, 1965; Rosenblum & Moltz, 1983). Each emphasizes a different feature of the relationship: *Synchrony* was first used to describe the timing of MB and behavioral development during the MB cycle and to point to the fact that MB was continuously adapted to the behavioral and physical characteristics of the young through the stimulation the mother receives from the young during their interactions (Rosenblatt, 1965). *Parasitism* emphasizes the fact that many behavioral and physical features of the young can best be understood by considering the young as parasites in their relationship to the mother, needing to induce her to provide resources (i.e., food, heat, energy involved in retrieving, nest building, etc.) until they are capable of providing these for themselves (Galef, 1981). The concept *symbiosis* describing the relationship emphasizes the mutual exchange of resources between mother and young, in contrast to parasitism, and is exemplified by the role the young play in the mother's water economy, thermal regulation, and food intake, among other behaviors (Alberts & Gubernick, 1983; Rosenblum & Moltz, 1983).

We must distinguish between functional aspects of the mother–young relationship, both short term and long term, and causal aspects, though of course they are closely related. Anogenital licking is clearly in response to olfactory/gustatory stimuli from the pups; it even differs toward male and female pups (Moore, 1981; Moore & Morelli, 1979), and it functions to enable pups to eliminate and the mother to retrieve a major part of the water lost to the pups in the milk (Gubernick & Alberts, 1983). Contact with the young, most often nursing contact, functions to warm the young, and the causal mechanism is regulated, in part, by maternal thermoregulation (Leon, Croskerry, & Smith, 1978; Woodside & Leon, 1980).

Each of the above terms characterizing the mother–young relationship is intended, on the one hand, to suggest causal mechanisms underlying this relationship by referring to funcitonal aspects deriving from the interactions between the two and, on the other hand, to establish for these causal mechanisms functional contexts that point to their adaptive outcomes for one or both members of the interaction.

It would take us too far afield from our original purpose to discuss the rich literature on mother–young interactions in the rat. The reader is referred to several recent reviews (Hofer, 1981; Rosenblum & Moltz, 1983) and to chapters 1 and 11 in the present volume.

## III. Transition Period: A Unique Period in Maternal Behavior

The transition period is of variable duration and is not clearly delimited: It is defined theoretically as that period during which gestational hormones, having stimulated the onset of MB, gradually disappear and the nonhormonal, pup-stimulated maintenance of MB is established. This period is often called the *critical period* for the establishment of the mother–young bond among several species including sheep, goats, and humans. It bears a relationship to this period in these species insofar as maternal responsiveness per se is maintained by early contact with the young. It differs because this period often refers to the limited period of formation of individual attachment by the mother to her own young as compared to alien young (Rosenblatt & Siegel, 1980a).

Evidence of the uniqueness of the immediate postpartum period of mother–young contact for maintenance of MB was obtained by imposing on mothers a 4-day period of separation from the litter, starting either at parturition or at Days 4, 9, or 14 postpartum in different groups of mothers. Constant-age (5- to 9-day old) pups were given to mothers at the end of the period of separation. Only mothers whose litters were removed at parturition declined to nearly zero in responding to pups; those that had already had a period during which they could establish their maternal behavior on a nonhormonal basis were able to maintain maternal responsiveness during the separation (Rosenblatt, 1965).

Efforts have been made to isolate those features of the pups to which the mother initially responds and upon which her subsequent behavior toward them is based, that is, upon which is based the establishment and maintenance of maternal behavior during parturition and afterward. Newborn pups (0–2 days) and hamster young of equivalent size are optimal for eliciting maternal behavior without cannibalism from newly parturient females (Stern, 1985). Young that are larger and smaller than the mother's own newborn (older pups or very young hamster pups) are less effective in eliciting maternal behavior and stimulate cannibalism more often. Only females that have undergone parturition, as compared to near-parturient females delivered by cesarean section, are selectively responsive to newborn pups and show no cannibalism toward pups.

Females allowed different amounts and kinds of pup contact confined to the first 24 hr following cesarean section deliveries on Day 22 of pregnancy have been tested for their MB with pups 9 days later (Fleming & Orpen, 1986). Those females allowed either 24 hr of full exposure to pups which included retrieving, nursing, and otherwise interacting fully with them or only 30 min of exposure which included retrieving them were very responsive to pups 9 days later, in 65–75% of the cases. Fewer females responded maternally to the pups if they had spent only 15 min with the pups and retrieved them or if they were allowed only to retrieve them or to be exposed to them during the first 24 hr postdelivery. Most unresponsive were those females that had no contact with pups after delivery (Fleming & Orpen, 1986).

Another study investigated stimuli that maintain MB over the 1st week. Cesarean section–delivered females were exposed to pups confined to containers which allowed only selected pups' cues to be available to the females (Fleming & Orpen, 1986). Females were exposed either to pup vocalizations and odors, pup vocalizations, pup odors and visual cues, or all of the previous plus tactile stimulation; one group had no contact with the pups. Unless females were exposed to actual pups with all of their stimuli, their responsiveness to pups was minimal on Day 8, and they had long latencies to restore MB.

A further study in which pups were placed under the female's nest, but out of reach, for the first 24 hr after cesarean delivery and tested 9 days later showed varying degrees of responsiveness, with those females given full contact most responsive; those given partial exposure, as described above, much less responsive but more responsive than those given no exposure to pups (Fleming & Orpen, 1986). These studies confirm the findings of an earlier one (Stern, 1983) using a different method for evaluating the effectiveness of proximal and distal pup stimuli.

I have interpreted studies on the retention of maternal responsiveness for some period after parturition as a measure of the extent to which the nonhormonal basis of MB has been established on the assumption that simple arousal of MB by hormones does not leave any lasting effects. This assumption appears to be supported in the studies to be reviewed below (Bridges, 1975, 1977). Only the postpartum performance of MB which brings the female into contact with pups enables the female to retain the behavior even in the absence of further contact. Retention of maternal responsiveness is the retention of nonhormonally based MB.

The longest period of retention, 25 days after separation from pups, has been studied following various kinds of early contact at parturition and afterward as shown in Fig. 4 (Bridges, 1975, 1977). The females were tested for retention of earlier experience with pups while they were exhibiting estrous cycling, and their sensitization latencies were compared to those of inexperienced virgins that had never been hormonally or nonhormonally stimulated to exhibit maternal behavior. First to be noted in the middle of the figure is that females allowed no exposure to pups either during normal delivery or after cesarean section delivery were unresponsive to pups 25 days later and were no different than inexperienced virgins shown below.

In the studies cited earlier (Fleming & Orpen, 1986; Stern, 1983), some of the continued responsiveness to pups when females were tested only 7–9 days after parturition may have been based upon residual effects of hormonal stimulation.

Exposure to pups during parturition only was sufficient to enable females to respond to them with very short latencies 25 days later. These results, therefore, indicate that nonhormonally based maternal behavior begins to be established during parturition; it is likely that this continues for several days postpartum and is well established by 4 days.

## IV. Epilogue

The concept of phases, hormonal and nonhormonal, derives from early studies of MB in the mouse, studies in which it was shown that nest building in particular, but also other aspects of MB, continued after fe-

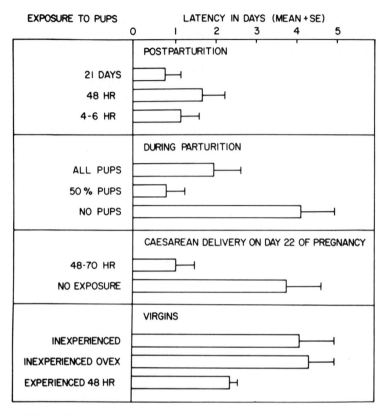

**Fig. 4.** Effects of parturition and postparturition contact with pups on latencies for induction of maternal behavior 25 days later. Period of exposure to pups shown on the ordinate and latencies on the upper abscissa. Cesarean section–delivered females and virgins shown for comparison. Based on data reported by Bridges (1975, 1977). From "Progress in the Study of Maternal Behavior in the Rat: Hormonal, Nonhormonal, Sensory, and Developmental Aspects" by J. S. Rosenblatt, H. I. Siegel, and A. D. Mayer. In J. S. Rosenblatt, R. A. Hinde, C. G. Beer, and M. C. Busnel (Eds.), *Advances in the Study of Behavior* (Vol. 10), New York: Academic Press, 1979. Copyright 1979 by Academic Press, Inc. Reprinted by permission.

males were hypophysectomized or ovariectomized postpartum (Leblond, 1938, 1940). The implications of this concept have been studied in the rat alone, although investigators of MB in sheep have employed a similar conceptual framework (Poindron & Le Neindre, 1980). It is not yet clear whether the concept applies broadly and also whether it will continue to be a fruitful hypothesis in studying the rat.

Its relevance in the present context of early behavioral development is to propose that the mother is bound to the young, in the first place, out of hormonal processes that arise endogenously during pregnancy. The high level of maternal responsiveness they engender, to be maintained, requires seeking stimulation from the pups which the mother avidly does during parturition and immediately afterward. The young are essential for her continued maternal responsiveness just as she is essential for their early development. The benefits that accrue to the young, in their interactions with the mother, in the areas of feeding, thermoregulation, water exchange, and the wide range of physiological functions, are in the last analysis the result of the mother's high level of maternal responsiveness.

## Acknowledgments

The research from this laboratory reported in this review was supported by National Institute of Mental Health Grant MH08604 to J.S.R. and B.R.S.G. and Busch grants to J.S.R. and is the product of colleagues and students, in particular Harold I. Siegel, Anne D. Mayer, Anthony Giordano, and Harry Ahdieh. I wish to thank Winona Cunningham for secretarial help and Cindy Banas for the figures. This is publication number 435 of the Institute of Animal Behavior.

## References

Alberts, J. R., & Gubernick, D. J. (1983). Reciprocity and resource exchange: A symbiotic model of parent–offspring relations. In L. A. Rosenblum & H. Moltz (Eds.), *Symbiosis in parent–offspring interactions* (pp. 7–44). New York: Plenum.

Bauer, J. H. (1983). Effects of maternal state on the responsiveness to nest odors of hooded rats. *Physiology and Behavior, 30,* 229–232.

Baum, M. J. (1978). Failure of pituitary transplants to facilitate the onset of maternal behavior in ovariectomized virgin rats. *Physiology and Behavior, 20,* 87–89.

Bolwerk, E. L. M., & Swanson, H. H. (1984). Does oxytocin play a role in the onset of maternal behaviour in the rat? *Journal of Endocrinology, 101,* 353–357.

Bridges, R. S. (1975). Long-term effects of pregnancy and parturition upon maternal responsiveness in the rat. *Physiology and Behavior, 14,* 245–249.

Bridges, R. S. (1977). Parturition: Its role in the long term retention of maternal behavior in the rat. *Physiology and Behavior, 18,* 487–490.

Bridges, R. S. (1983). A quantitative analysis of the roles of dosage, sequence, and duration of estradiol and progesterone exposure in the regulation of maternal behavior in the rat. *Endocrinology, 114,* 930–940.

Bridges, R. S., Feder, H. H., & Rosenblatt, J. S. (1977). Induction of maternal behaviors in primigravid rats by ovariectomy, hysterectomy, or ovariectomy plus hysterectomy: Effects of length of gestation. *Hormones and Behavior, 9,* 156–169.

Bridges, R. S., Loundes, D. D., DiBase, R., & Tate-Ostroff, B. A. (1985). Prolactin and pituitary involvement in maternal behavior in the rat. In R. M. MacLeod, M. O. Thorner, & U. Scapagnini (Eds.), *Prolactin: Basic and clinical correlates* (pp. 591–599). (Fidia Research Series, Vol. 1). Padua: Liviana.

Bridges, R. S., Rosenblatt, J. S., & Feder, H. H. (1978). Serum progesterone concentrations and maternal behavior in rats after pregnancy termination: Behavioral stimulation after progesterone withdrawal and inhibition by progesterone maintenance. *Endocrinology, 102,* 258–267.
Bridges, R. S., & Russell, D. W. (1981). Steroidal interactions in the regulation of maternal behaviour in virgin female rats: Effects of testosterone, dihydrotestosterone, oestradiol, progesterone and aromatase inhibitor 1,4,6-androstatriene-3,17-dione. *Journal of Endocrinology, 90,* 31–40.
Cosnier, J., & Couturier, C. (1966). Comportement maternal provoqué chez les rattes adultes castrées. *Comptes Rendus des Seances de la Societe de Biologie et de Ses Filiales, 160,* 789–791.
Doerr, H. K., Siegel, H. I., & Rosenblatt, J. S. (1981). Effects of progesterone withdrawal and estrogen on maternal behavior in nulliparous rats. *Behavioral and Neural Biology, 32,* 35–44.
Fahrbach, S. E., Morrell, J. I., & Pfaff, D. W. (1984). Oxytocin induction of short-latency maternal behavior in nulliparous, estrogen-primed female rats. *Hormones and Behavior, 18,* 267–286.
Fahrbach, S. E., Morrell, J. I., & Pfaff, D. W. (1985). Possible role for endogenous oxytocin in estrogen-facilitated maternal behavior in rats. *Neuroendocrinology, 40,* 526–532.
Fleming, A. S., & Luebke, C. (1981). Timidity prevents the virgin female rat from being a good mother: Emotionality differences between nulliparous and parturient females. *Physiology and Behavior, 27,* 863–868.
Fleming, A. S., & Orpen, G. (1986). Psychobiology of maternal behavior in rats, selected other species and humans. In A. Folgel & G. F. Melson (Eds.), *Origins of nurturance: Developmental, biological and cultural perspectives* (pp. 141–207). London: Erlbaum.
Fleming, A. S., & Rosenblatt, J. S. (1974a). Maternal behavior in the virgin and lactating rat. *Journal of Comparative and Physiological Psychology, 86,* 957–972.
Fleming, A. S., & Rosenblatt, J. S. (1974b). Olfactory regulation of maternal behavior in rats: I. Effects of olfactory bulb removal in experienced and inexperienced lactating and cycling females. *Journal of Comparative and Physiological Psychology, 86,* 221–232.
Fleming, A. S., & Rosenblatt, J. S. (1974c). Olfactory regulation of maternal behavior in rats: II. Effects of peripherally induced anosmia and lesions of the lateral olfactory tract in pup-induced virgins. *Journal of Comparative and Physiological Psychology, 86,* 233–246.
Friedman, M. I., Bruno, J. P., & Alberts, J. R. (1981). Physiological and behavioral consequences in rats of water recycling during lactation. *Journal of Comparative and Physiological Psychology, 95,* 26–35.
Galef, B. G., Jr. (1981). The ecology of weaning: Parasitism and the achievement of independence by altricial mammals. In D. J. Gubernick & P. H. Klopfer (Eds.), *Parental care in mammals* (pp. 211–242). New York: Plenum.
Grosvenor, C. E., & Mena, F. (1982). Regulating mechanisms for oxytocin and prolactin secretion during lactation. In E. E. Müller & R. M. MacLeod (Eds), *Neuroendocrine perspectives* (Vol. 1, p. 69). Amsterdam: Elsevier/North Holland.
Gubernick, D. J., & Alberts, J. R. (1983). Maternal licking of young: Resource exchange and proximate controls. *Physiology and Behavior, 31,* 593–601.
Hård, E., & Hansen, S. (1985). Reduced fearfulness in the lactating rat. *Physiology and Behavior, 35,* 641–643.
Hofer, M. A. (1981). Parental contributions to the development of their offspring. In D. J. Gubernick & P. H. Hofer (Eds.), *Parental care in mammals* (pp. 77–115). New York: Plenum.

Leblond, C. P. (1938). Extra-hormonal factors in maternal behavior. *Proceedings of the Society for Experimental Biology and Medicine, 38,* 66–70.

Leblond, C. P. (1940). Nervous and hormonal factors in the maternal behavior of the mouse. *Journal of Genetics and Psychology, 57,* 327–344.

Leon, M., Croskerry, P. G., & Smith, G. K. (1978). Thermal control of mother–young contact in rats. *Physiology and Behavior, 21,* 793–811.

Lisk, R. D., & Reuter, L. A. (1977). In vivo progesterone treatment enhances ($^3$H) estradiol retention by neural tissue in the female rat. *Endocrinology, 100,* 1652–1658.

Mayer, A. D., & Rosenblatt, J. S. (1984). Prepartum changes in maternal responsiveness and nest defense in *Rattus norvegicus. Journal of Comparative Psychology, 98,* 177–188.

Moltz, H., Levin, R., & Leon, M. (1969). Differential effects of progesterone on the maternal behavior of primiparous and multiparous rats. *Journal of Comparative and Physiological Psychology, 67,* 36–40.

Moltz, H., Lubin, M., Leon, M., & Numan, M. (1970). Hormonal induction of maternal behavior in the ovariectomized nulliparous rat. *Physiology and Behavior, 5,* 1373–1377.

Moore, C. L. (1981). An olfactory basis for maternal discrimination of sex of offspring in rats (*Rattus norvegicus*). *Animal Behaviour, 29,* 383–386.

Moore, C. L., & Morelli, G. A. (1979). Mother rats interact differently with male and female offspring. *Journal of Comparative and Physiological Psychology, 93,* 677–684.

Morishige, W. K., Pepe, G. J., & Rothchild, I. (1973). Serum luteinizing hormone (LH), prolactin and progesterone levels during pregnancy in the rat. *Endocrinology, 92,* 1527–1530.

Numan, M. (1985). Brain mechanisms and parental behavior. In N. Adler, D. W. Pfaff & R. W. Goy (Eds.), *Handbook of behavioral neurobiology: Vol. 7. Reproduction.* (pp. 537–605). New York: Plenum.

Numan, M., Rosenblatt, J. S., & Komisaruk, B. R. (1977). The medial preoptic area and the onset of maternal behavior in the rat. *Journal of Comparative and Physiological Psychology, 91,* 146–164.

Pedersen, C. A., Ascher, J. A., Monroe, Y. L., & Prange, A. J., Jr. (1982). Oxytocin induces maternal behavior in virgin female rats. *Science, 216,* 648–650.

Pedersen, C. A., & Prange, A. J., Jr. (1979). Induction of maternal behavior in virgin rats after intracerebroventricular administration of oxytocin. *Proceedings of the National Academy of Sciences, 76,* 6661–6665.

Pepe, G. J., & Rothchild, I. (1974). A comparative study of serum progesterone levels in pregnancy and various types of pseudopregnancy in the rat. *Endocrinology, 95,* 275–279.

Poindron, P., & Le Neindre, P. (1980). Endocrine and sensory regulation of maternal behavior in the ewe. In J. S. Rosenblatt, R. A. Hinde, C. G. Beer, & M. C. Busnel (Eds.), *Advances in the study of behavior* (Vol. 11, pp. 76–142). New York: Academic Press.

Reisbick, S., Rosenblatt, J. S., & Mayer, A. D. (1975). Decline of maternal behavior in the virgin and lactating rat. *Journal of Comparative and Physiological Psychology, 89,* 722–732.

Rodriguez-Sierra, J., & Rosenblatt, J. S. (1977). Does prolactin play a role in estrogen-induced maternal behavior in rats: Apomorphine reduction of prolactin release. *Hormones and Behavior, 9,* 1–7.

Rosenblatt, J. S. (1965). The basis of synchrony in the behavioral interaction between the mother and her offspring in the laboratory rat. In B. M. Foss (Ed.), *Determinants of infant behaviour* (Vol. 3, pp. 3–41). London: Methuen.

Rosenblatt, J. S. (1967). Nonhormonal basis of maternal behavior in the rat. *Science, 156,* 1512–1514.

Rosenblatt, J. S. (1984). Prolactin and parental behavior among selected species of mammals and birds. In F. Mena & C. Valverde-R. (Eds.), *Prolactin secretion: A multidisciplinary approach* (pp. 327–352). Orlando: Academic Press.

Rosenblatt, J. S., Mayer, A. D., & Siegel, H. I. (1985). Maternal behavior among the nonprimate mammals. In N. Adler, D. W. Pfaff & R. W. Goy (Eds.), *Handbook of behavioral neurobiology: Vol. 7. Reproduction* (pp. 229–298). New York: Plenum.

Rosenblatt, J. S., & Siegel, H. I. (1975). Hysterectomy-induced maternal behavior during pregnancy in the rat. *Journal of Comparative and Physiological Psychology, 89,* 685–700.

Rosenblatt, J. S., & Siegel, H. I. (1980a). Factors governing the onset and maintenance of maternal behavior among nonprimate mammals: The role of hormonal and nonhormonal factors. In D. J. Gubernick & P. H. Klopfer (Eds.), *Parental care in mammals* (pp. 14–76). New York: Plenum.

Rosenblatt, J. S., & Siegal, H. I. (1980b). Maternal behavior in the laboratory rat. In R. W. Bell & W. P. Smotherman (Eds.), *Maternal influences and early behavior* (pp. 155–199). Jamaica, NY: Spectrum.

Rosenblatt, J. S., & Siegel, H. I. (1981c). Physiological and behavioural changes during pregnancy and parturition underlying the onset of maternal behavior in rodents. In R. W. Elwood (Ed.), *Parental behaviour of rodents* (pp. 23–66). New York: Wiley.

Rosenblatt, J. S., Siegel, H. I., & Mayer, A. D. (1979). Progress in the study of maternal behavior in the rat: Hormonal, nonhormonal, sensory, and developmental aspects. In J. S. Rosenblatt, R. A. Hinde, C. G. Beer, & M. C. Busnel (Eds.), *Advances in the study of behavior* (Vol. 10, pp. 225–311). New York: Academic Press.

Rosenblum, L. A., & Moltz, H. (1983). *Symbiosis in parent–offspring interactions.* New York: Plenum.

Rubin, B. S., Menniti, F. S., & Bridges, R. S. (1983). Intracerebroventricular administration of oxytocin and maternal behavior in rats after prolonged and acute steroid pretreatment. *Hormones and Behavior, 17,* 45–53.

Shaikh, A. A. (1971). Estrone and estradiol levels in the ovarian venous blood from rats during the estrous cycle and pregnancy. *Biology of Reproduction, 5,* 297–307.

Siegel, H. I., & Rosenblatt, J. S. (1975a). Estrogen-induced maternal behavior in hysterectomized-ovariectomized virgin rats. *Physiology and Behavior, 14,* 465–471.

Siegel, H. I., & Rosenblatt, J. S. (1975b). Hormonal basis of hysterectomy-induced maternal behavior during pregnancy in the rat. *Hormones and Behavior, 6,* 211–222.

Siegel, H. I., & Rosenblatt, J. S. (1975c). Progesterone inhibition of estrogen-induced maternal behavior in hysterectomized-ovariectomized virgin rats. *Hormones and Behavior, 6,* 223–230.

Siegel, H. I., & Rosenblatt, J. S. (1978). Duration of estrogen stimulation and progesterone inhibition of maternal behavior in pregnancy-terminated rats. *Hormones and Behavior, 11,* 12–19.

Slotnick, B. M., Carpenter, M. L., & Fusco, R. (1973). Initiation of maternal behavior in pregnant nulliparous rats. *Hormones and Behavior, 4,* 53–59.

Smotherman, W. P., Bell, R. W., Hershberger, W. A., & Coover, G. D. (1978). Orientation to rat pup cues: Effects of maternal experiential history. *Animal Behaviour, 256,* 265–273.

Stern, J. M. (1983). Maternal behavior priming in virgin and ceasarean-delivered Long-Evans rats: Effects of brief contact or continuous esteroceptive pup stimulation. *Physiology and Behavior, 31,* 757–763.

Stern, J. M. (1985). Parturition influences initial pup preferences in later onset of maternal behavior in primiparous rats. *Physiology and Behavior, 35,* 25–31.

Terkel, J., & Rosenblatt, J. S. (1968). Maternal behavior induced by maternal blood plasma injected into virgin rats. *Journal of Comparative and Physiological Psychology, 65,* 479–482.

Terkel, J., & Rosenblatt, J. S. (1971). Aspects of nonhormonal maternal behavior in the rat. *Hormones and Behavior, 2,* 161–171.

Terkel, J., & Rosenblatt, J. S. (1972). Humoral factors underlying maternal behavior at parturition: Cross transfusion between freely moving rats. *Journal of Comparative and Physiological Psychology, 80,* 365–371.

Wiesner, B. P., & Sheard, N. M. (1933). *Maternal behavior in the rat.* London: Oliver & Boyd.

Wilson, N. E., & Stricker, E. M. (1979). Thermal homeostatis in pregnant rats during heat stress. *Journal of Comparative and Physiological Psychology, 93,* 585–594.

Woodside, B., & Leon, M. (1980). Thermoendocrine influences on maternal nesting behavior in rats. *Journal of Comparative and Physiological Psychology, 94,* 41–60.

Zarrow, M. X, Gandelman, R., & Denenberg, V. H. (1971). Prolactin: Is it an essential hormone for maternal behavior in mammals? *Hormones and Behavior, 2,* 343–354.

# 15

# Maternal Influences on the Developing Circadian System

STEVEN M. REPPERT, MARILYN J. DUNCAN,
and DAVID R. WEAVER
*Laboratory of Developmental Chronobiology*
*Children's Service*
*Massachusetts General Hospital*
*and Harvard Medical School*
*Boston, Massachusetts 02114*

## I. Introduction

The daily light–dark cycle synchronizes (entrains) circadian rhythms to the 24-hr period (Aschoff, 1981). Entrainment ensures a state of internal temporal order so that the rhythms are expressed in proper relationship to each other and to the 24-hr day. This temporal order enables an organism to function efficiently and to foresee and cope with predictable alterations in its environment.

In mammals, the suprachiasmatic nuclei (SCN) of the anterior hypothalamus are the site of a circadian pacemaker (biologic clock) generating a variety of hormonal and behavioral rhythms (Moore, 1983; J. S. Takahashi & Zatz, 1982). Photic information for entrainment reaches the SCN primarily by a monosynaptic retinohypothalamic pathway (Hendrickson, Wagonner, & Cowan, 1972; Moore & Lenn, 1972).

Studies in rats (Deguchi, 1975, 1977; Fuchs & Moore, 1980; Hiroshige, Honma, & Watanabe, 1982a, 1982b, 1982c; Reppert, Coleman, Heath, & Swedlow, 1984; Reppert & Schwartz, 1983; K. Takahashi & Deguchi, 1983; K. Takahashi, Hayafuji, & Murakami, 1982; K. Takahashi, Murakami, Hayafuji, & Sasaki, 1984; Yamazaki & Takahashi, 1983); hamsters (Davis & Gorski, 1985, 1986); mice (Viswanathan & Chandrashekaran,

Perinatal Development:
A Psychobiological Perspective

1984); and monkeys (Reppert & Schwartz, 1984a) show that a circadian clock is functioning during the perinatal period. Interestingly, the SCN clock of rodents is entrained to the light–dark cycle during late fetal and early neonatal life, before the retinohypothalamic pathway innervates the SCN (Fig. 1). During these early stages, the mother acts as a photic transducer between the environment and the fetal brain, coordinating the timing (phase) of the developing biologic clock to her own clock time, which, in turn, is entrained by ambient lighting. Maternal entrainment thus ensures that the developing circadian system is synchronized to prevailing light–dark conditions until the mechanisms for retina-mediated entrainment become functional. In this chapter, we review the studies showing maternal entrainment during both the pre- and postnatal periods.

## II. Prenatal Circadian Development

Although circadian rhythms are not overtly expressed until well into the postnatal period (Davis, 1981), the circadian pacemaker in the SCN is functional prior to that time (Fig. 1). Deguchi (1975) first provided evidence in rats suggesting that the developing biologic clock might be functional and entrainable by the mother during fetal life. In order to examine the circadian system before the overt expression of rhythmicity, he used the phase (timing) of the rhythm of pineal $N$-acetyltransferase (NAT) activity monitored under constant conditions during the postnatal period to infer what had happened to the central oscillator underlying the rhythm at an earlier stage of development; the NAT rhythm is one of the first circadian rhythms overtly expressed in rats (Reppert, 1982), and it accurately reflects circadian output from the developing SCN (Deguchi, 1982). He found that rat pups born and reared from birth under constant conditions express a synchronous population rhythm that is in phase with that of the dam. Furthermore, by fostering pups from birth (again under constant conditions) with dams whose circadian time is opposite that of the original dam, the phase of the pups' NAT rhythm shifts toward that of the foster dam. These findings suggest that a circadian clock is oscillating at or before birth and that its phase is influenced by the dam.

That a circadian clock is functioning in utero remained to be shown, however, because of the possibility that some rhythmic aspect of the birth process itself could start and set the timing of the developing clock. One such rhythmic event that might influence developing rhythmicity is the time of day of birth; this process is circadian in rats and can be manipulated over a 12-hr period, depending on the phase of the light–dark cycle

COMPONENT OR FEATURE                     DEVELOPMENTAL PERIOD
                                          ( days relative to birth )

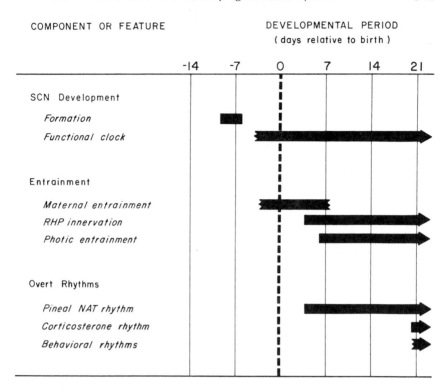

**Fig. 1.** Perinatal development of the circadian timing system in the rat. The solid bars represent the time that a component or feature is present. A jagged edge indicates that the component or feature may be present before or after that time. Behavioral rhythms refer to locomotor activity and drinking. Abbreviations: SCN, suprachiasmatic nuclei; RHP, retinohypothalamic pathway; NAT, *N*-acetyltransferase.

during pregnancy (Lincoln & Porter, 1976; Reppert, 1983; Sherwood, Downing, Golos, Gordon, & Tarbell, 1983).

A method proven useful for monitoring the oscillatory activity of the SCN itself in adult rats is the [14]C-labeled deoxyglucose (DG) technique (Schwartz, Davidson, & Smith, 1980; Schwartz & Gainer, 1977). This method allows for the simultaneous, in vivo determination of the rates of glucose utilization of individual brain structures after IV injection of tracer amounts of DG (Sokoloff *et al.*, 1977). Applying the DG procedure to study of the SCN in fetal rats, Reppert and Schwartz (1983) demonstrated that an entrainable circadian clock oscillates in the nuclei during late fetal development and that ambient lighting acts through the maternal circadian system to entrain the fetal clock.

For the DG experiments, timed pregnant Sprague-Dawley rats were exposed to various environmental lighting regimens and injected with DG at specified gestational ages and clock times. At 45 min after injection, the animals were sacrificed, fetal brains were removed and frozen, and serial coronal sections were cut and processed for autoradiography. The optical density of each SCN was measured, and optical densities of the SCN were compared between animals by using the optical density of the adjacent hypothalamus as an internal reference standard for each fetal brain.

In the first experiment, dams were exposed to diurnal lighting (12 hr of light per day) during pregnancy until Day 19 of gestation, when they were placed and thereafter maintained in constant darkness. The pregnant animals were then injected with DG either during the subjective night (the 12-hr period of the day that the lights would have been off had the animals remained in diurnal lighting) on Day 20 of gestation or during the subjective day (the 12-hr period of that day that the lights would have been on had the animals remained in diurnal lighting) on Day 21 of gestation. The resultant autoradiographs showed that the maternal and all fetal SCN were coordinated with one another at both injection times so that all SCN were metabolically active during the subjective day and relatively inactive during the subjective night. The fetal SCN thus exhibit a clear, consistent day–night variation in glucose utilization, and the fetal rhythm is synchronous with that in the mother. Next, a 12-hr phase shift in the lighting cycle during pregnancy, which shifted the maternal circadian system by 12 hr, resulted in a corresponding phase shift in the rhythm of fetal SCN metabolic activity. In a third experiment, blind dams were used to show that environmental lighting acts through the maternal circadian system to entrain the rhythm of fetal SCN metabolic activity; the fetal rhythm was synchronous with the circadian time of the blind mothers and not affected directly by ambient lighting.

Subsequent DG studies show that the fetal clock is oscillating as early as the 19th day of gestation (Reppert & Schwartz, 1984b). This early functional development is quite remarkable when compared with the SCN's morphological development. Based on autoradiographic studies using tritiated thymidine, the rat SCN are formed between gestational Days 13 and 16 (Altman & Bayer, 1978; Ifft, 1972). By electron microscopy, immature synapses are first evident within the SCN on gestational Day 18 (Koritsanszky, 1981); the vast majority of SCN synapses are formed postnatally (Lenn, Beebe, & Moore, 1977). The SCN thus begin functioning very early in development, and the oscillation of metabolic activity during fetal life is not dependent on the rich synaptic architecture characteristic of the adult nuclei.

Experiments in rodents show that the maternal SCN are essential for maternal entrainment of the fetal circadian clock. Davis and Gorski (1983) found in Syrian hamsters that complete lesions of the maternal nuclei on Day 7 of gestation disrupt the timing of the developing circadian system. These investigators monitored locomotor activity in individual pups reared under constant conditions. At the time of weaning, the phases of wheel-running behavior in pups born to and reared by SCN-lesioned dams were scattered, whereas the rhythms from pups of sham-operated dams were synchronous with one another.

In rats, complete ablation of the maternal SCN on Day 7 of gestation disrupts subsequent development of rhythms of SCN glucose utilization in fetuses and pineal NAT activity in 10-day-old pups (Reppert & Schwartz, 1986a). Because both rhythms were monitored from a population of animals, their disruption could indicate either loss of rhythmicity for individual animals or desynchronization of persistent rhythms among the individual animals within a litter. The latter interpretation is probably correct because individual rat pups born to and reared by SCN-lesioned dams and monitored under constant conditions express free-running rhythms of drinking behavior after weaning. These findings in rats and hamsters suggest that the maternal circadian system entrains the oscillation of an endogenous clock in the fetal SCN (Fig. 2), rather than maternal rhythmicity driving the fetal oscillation. In rats, entrainment of the fetus by the maternal SCN may occur by Day 10 of gestation (Honma, Honma, Shirakawa, & Hiroshige, 1984a, 1984b).

The nature of the maternal signal or signals used to entrain the timing of the fetal SCN is not yet known. The in utero environment provides a rich source of temporal signals from the mother. Since the rhythms of the concentrations of several hormones and nutrients in the maternal circulation cross the placenta and are reflected in the fetal circulation (Reppert, 1982), it is possible that one or a number of these in concert coordinates the timing of the fetal clock. Recent experiments have shown, however, that removal of the maternal pineal, adrenals, thyroid-parathyroids, pituitary, or ovaries does not abolish maternal coordination of the fetal circadian clock (Reppert & Schwartz, 1986b); all procedures were performed in separate experiments on or before Day 7 of gestation, the time when maternal SCN lesions are disruptive.

The phenomenon of prenatal maternal entrainment is not limited to rodents but also appears to occur in higher mammals. DG studies with pregnant squirrel monkeys (at 90% term gestation) suggest that the SCN are oscillating during late fetal life in the primate and that, as in the rat, the maternal circadian system coordinates the timing of the fetal primate clock to ambient lighting (Reppert & Schwartz, 1984a). The existence of

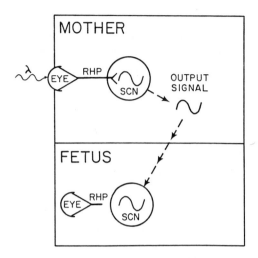

**Fig. 2.** Conceptual model of maternal–fetal coordination. Abbreviations: RHP, retinohypothalamic pathway; SCN, suprachiasmatic nucleus.

maternal entrainment in such diverse species as the rat and monkey suggests that the phenomenon is generalized among mammals and may also be present in humans.

## III.  Postnatal Circadian Development

Studies using pineal NAT activity (Deguchi, 1975, 1977; Reppert *et al.*, 1984; K. Takahashi & Deguchi, 1983); plasma corticosterone (Hiroshige *et al.*, 1982a, 1982b, 1982c; K. Takahashi & Deguchi, 1983; Yamazaki & Takahashi, 1983); and locomotor activity (Davis & Gorski, 1985; Deguchi, 1977; K. Takahashi *et al.*, 1984; Viswanathan & Chandrashekaran, 1984) to monitor the developing circadian system of rodents all show that maternal entrainment extends into the postnatal period. For these studies, the postnatal rhythm is monitored under constant conditions. Pups are fostered with a mother whose circadian time is out of phase with that of the original mother, in order to assess the postnatal influence of the maternal circadian system on the timing of the developing circadian system. The potency of the postnatal maternal influence reported by different laboratories is quite variable and may be due to differences in experimental design, strain or species differences, or a combination of the two. It has been consistently shown that the magnitude of the postnatal maternal influence changes throughout development, being greatest during the first week of life (Fig. 1) (Reppert *et al.*, 1984; K. Takahashi & Deguchi, 1983).

Our laboratory has studied postnatal maternal entrainment by monitoring the rhythm of pineal NAT activity in 10-day-old rat pups (Reppert *et al.*, 1984). This system was validated by showing that social interactions among pups do not contribute significantly to the maternal influence. When half the pups in a litter and the dam were blinded at birth and then the entire litter was exposed to a reversed light–dark cycle, the blind and intact pups expressed NAT rhythms 180° (12 hr) out of phase with each other. The rhythm of the blind pups was in phase with the circadian time of the blind dams (whose phase was set by the diurnal light–dark cycle during pregnancy), while the rhythm of intact pups was in phase with the postnatal (reversed) light–dark cycle. The clear segregation of these two groups, even though each litter was composed of the same number of blind and intact pups, indicates that social interactions among litter mates do not appreciably influence a pup's circadian system.

By fostering pups with a dam whose circadian time was out of phase with that of the original dam, we observed a variable postnatal maternal influence of the maternal circadian system on the developing circadian system; some litters were entrained to the original dam, some to the foster dam, and others showed an intermediate response. By cross-fostering at different ages, the maternal influence was found to be waning after postnatal Day 5. Cross-fostering per se did not contribute to the postnatal maternal influence observed in our studies, because fostering pups from birth with dams of the same circadian time as the natural dam did not alter the timing of the pups' NAT rhythm.

Maternal entrainment of the developing circadian system in the postnatal period depends on the maternal SCN, as it does in the prenatal period (Reppert & Schwartz, 1986a). The nature of the maternal output signal or signals that mediates entrainment during the postnatal period is not known. It is possible that different output signals are used during the pre- and postnatal periods. For example, prenatal entrainment may involve a maternal hormone, whereas the postnatal effect might involve some rhythmic aspect of maternal behavior, such as nursing (Levin & Stern, 1975).

As the postnatal maternal influence decreases, retina-mediated entrainment commences in the pups so that entrainment continues uninterrupted during the postnatal period (Fig. 1). By postnatal Day 4, the retinohypothalamic pathway has begun innervating the developing SCN (Stanfield & Cowan, 1976). Retina-mediated, light–dark entrainment is functional by Day 6 and capable of overriding any remaining postnatal maternal influence by Day 8 (Duncan, Banister, & Reppert, 1986).

Since the circadian clock in the SCN is oscillating before circadian rhythms are overtly expressed, the factor limiting the overt expression of rhythmicity must be maturation of the output pathways that couple the SCN to other structures that are ultimately responsible for rhythm expression. The different periods of maturation of output pathways for various rhythms most likely explain why different rhythms appear at different ages and why each undergoes some period of maturation. To cite some examples, pineal rhythms are manifested during the 1st week, whereas the corticosterone rhythm and most behavioral rhythms are not usually expressed until the 2nd or even 3rd weeks of life (Fig. 1).

## IV. Physiological Significance of Maternal Entrainment

Maternal entrainment assures that the developing circadian system is synchronized to prevailing lighting conditions until the time that maturation of the retina-mediated pathway permits direct photic entrainment. Such early entrainment must have considerable physiological significance.

One important function of maternal entrainment is to allow the young animal to assume its temporal niche. This is clearly exemplified in burrow-dwelling mammals in which the pups are probably not directly exposed to the daily light–dark cycle for the first few weeks of life, until they can crawl out of the burrow (Pratt, 1981). If the pups were not coordinated to the prevailing environmental conditions by the mother, they might exhibit disadvantageous behavioral patterns when they emerged from the burrow. For example, the pup's biologic clock might signal nocturnal behavior, such as foraging for food, during the daytime, rendering the pup more susceptible to predation. This deleterious situation could result in death or persistent danger until the time that the developing biologic clock could be directly synchronized to the solar day by environmental lighting.

One possible function of the developing clock and its entrainment during fetal life is that it might be involved in the initiation of parturition. As previously mentioned, the time of day of birth in the rat is coupled to the daily light–dark cycle by a circadian mechanism; most births occur during daylight hours of a light–dark cycle, and the distribution of births can be dramatically altered by changing the photoperiod. Since the circadian timing of parturition has been reported in a variety of other mammals, including horses (Rossendale & Short, 1967), monkeys (Jolly, 1972), and humans (Kaiser & Halberg, 1962), the possible role of the fetal SCN in this process may be applicable to many species.

In mammals, the fetuses of some species initiate parturition (Nathanielsz, 1976). This is an especially interesting phenomenon in a polytocous mammal such as the rat since all the fetal-placental units would have to be synchronized to function in unison to initiate birth. In this situation, maternal entrainment of each fetal clock to the external lighting cycle would synchronize all the fetal-placental units. Maybe that is why the timing of the fetal clock is set by the mother rat at least 3 days prior to the onset of labor. It is therefore conceivable that, at the appropriate time of gestational maturation, the circadian clock in the fetal SCN, which has been set by the mother to the outside world, initiates the cascade of events culminating in birth. For rhythmicity in fetal rats to initiate this process, specific outputs from the nuclei would have to exist even though none have so far been described.

## V.  Future Directions

### A.  Basic Science Issues

The studies reviewed in this chapter clearly demonstrate that the developing circadian system is entrained to maternal circadian rhythmicity. Several important issues pertaining to this maternal–fetal communication remain unanswered. The following list summarizes some of the areas we feel warrant further study.

1. How do metabolic oscillations occur in the morphologically primitive fetal SCN? The rhythm of DG uptake in the fetal SCN occurs despite the lack of anatomic specializations usually associated with interneuronal communication. Analysis of the metabolic basis for this rhythm should further our understanding not only of the development of the SCN but also of the mechanisms of neural circadian oscillators in general. A more detailed examination of the developmental anatomy of the fetal SCN is necessary, and brains should be examined from fetuses sacrificed both during the day and the night in the event that the metabolic activity rhythm is accompanied by a rhythm in SCN neuroanatomic development. For example, the degree of cell appositions/membrane contacts could show circadian variation, and cell apposition has been suggested as a mechanism of synchronizing cellular activity in other hypothalamic nuclei (Hatton, Perlmutter, Salm, & Tweedle, 1984).

2. What is the nature of the maternal signal or signals conveying circadian information to the developing circadian system? Elucidation of the maternal signal could provide a more general understanding of entrainment mechanisms, as well as allowing manipulations of circadian development through alteration of the levels or pattern of the maternal entraining signal. Several hormonal signals have been investigated as potential

signals during the prenatal period, but the endocrinologic approach has been unsuccessful so far (Reppert & Schwartz, 1986b). Other potential entraining signals, such as metabolic and behavioral rhythms, remain to be examined. It will also be important to delineate the maternal signal or signals used during the postnatal period. Are different maternal entraining signals used pre- and postnatally?

3. Can light transmitted into the uterus directly influence fetal development? Most obviously, this involves assessing the influence of light on the developing circadian system; for example, can external lighting serve as an entraining stimulus in utero? In rats, the retinohypothalamic pathway is immature prenatally, and light which is out of phase with the maternal rhythm does not override the maternal entrainment. In species in which the retinohypothalamic pathway is in place before birth, however, it is possible that the maternal entraining signal may be functionally replaced by the direct perception of light in utero. In such species, retina-mediated photic entrainment may begin, as in rats, prenatally instead of postnatally. Measuring transmission of light into the uterus of pregnant animals and comparing the ontogeny of the retinohypothalamic pathway innervation and SCN oscillations in several species is necessary. Naturalistic studies are clearly necessary in these species to determine the amount of light the dam is normally exposed to during pregnancy. Finally, the influence of light on the development of the primary visual system should be examined. For example, does light exposure during the prenatal period in some way facilitate the development of visual responsiveness? It should be possible to assess visual deficits that may result from photic deprivation in utero.

4. What is the physiological significance of maternal entrainment of the developing circadian system? While we have suggested that prenatal maternal entrainment serves to synchronize pups for the initiation of birth, little evidence is available in rats regarding the role of the fetal SCN in the timing or initiation of birth. We have also suggested that maternal entrainment is adaptive because it facilitates the developing animal's assumption of the appropriate ecological/temporal niche. While studies of burrow emergence behavior in hamsters demonstrate that hamster pups are coordinated to their environment before they have had the opportunity to become entrained by light directly (Pratt, 1981), other aspects of the "temporal niche" hypothesis, such as coordination with mother, should be tested. For example, does synchronization with the mother optimize weight gain and survival? We have also suggested that maternal entrainment of the developing circadian system is important because it coordinates physiological and behavioral rhythms and thus creates a state of "internal temporal order" as overt rhythms develop in the neonatal

animal. Studies are needed to address the adaptive significance of this internal temporal order. A final possible function of maternal entrainment is that it is essential for normal development of the SCN clock. Hamster and rat pups from dams with SCN lesions show normal circadian rhythms when raised in constant conditions, indicating that the development of circadian rhythms can occur normally in the absence of either maternal or environmental entrainment. However, we have not demonstrated whether animals raised in the absence of entraining stimuli truly have normal circadian rhythmicity. It would be interesting to see whether these animals show normal entrainment and respond appropriately to stimuli which induce phase shifts.

## B. Child Health Issues

The importance of circadian rhythms in humans is just beginning to be appreciated (Moore-Ede, Sulzman, & Fuller, 1982). Several disorders of the human circadian system have been described, and knowledge of the basic properties of circadian rhythms has led to successful treatment. Furthermore, knowledge of the circadian variations of certain biologic parameters can contribute to the proper interpretation of a diagnostic variable and improve diagnostic precision. Since the absorption, metabolism, and excretion of numerous drugs exhibit circadian rhythms, knowledge of these factors can also optimize better drug treatment schedules.

Compared to what we know about circadian rhythms in adults, relatively little attention has been directed at the developmental aspects of the circadian timing system. As previously discussed, the major reason for this deficiency is that in both rats and humans, circadian rhythms are not generally expressed until well into the postnatal period, and it has thus been thought that the circadian system is quiescent during early development. However, the studies cited in this review indicate in both rats and primates that a circadian pacemaker is already functioning during fetal life and that during pre- and early postnatal development this pacemaker is coordinated to the outside world.

These data, viewed in the context of limited developmental studies in humans, are consistent with the notion that a circadian clock is functioning in the human during fetal life (Reppert, in press). Furthermore, from its inception, this circadian clock probably is coordinated to prevailing environmental conditions (e.g., the daily light–dark cycle). The existence of a functioning circadian clock during early development brings several important questions to mind. Which environmental cues are important for entrainment during early development? When does light begin to directly influence the developing circadian system of humans? What are the biobehavioral consequences of temporal disarray in the human infant living in conditions (e.g., the nursery) in which lighting, auditory, and social cues are constant and uncoordinated? Answers to these questions will allow us to put the circadian timing system into proper perspective during early development and help us provide the human infant with better health care.

## Acknowledgments

Supported by March of Dimes Basic Research Grant 1-945 and Public Health Service Grant HD14427. S.M.R. is an Established Investigator of the American Heart Association.

## References

Altman, J., & Bayer, S. A. (1978). Development of the diencephalon in the rat: I. Autoradiographic study of the time of origin and settling patterns of neurons of the hypothalamus. *Journal of Comparative Neurology, 182*, 945–972.
Aschoff, J. (Ed.). (1981). *Handbook of behavioral neurology: Vol. 4. Biological rhythms.* New York: Plenum.
Davis, F. C. (1981). Ontogeny of circadian rhythms. In J. Aschoff (Ed.), *Handbook of behavioral neurobiology: Vol. 4, Biological rhythms* (pp. 257–274). New York: Plenum.
Davis, F. C., & Gorski, R. A. (1983). Entrainment of circadian rhythms in utero: Role of the maternal suprachiasmatic nucleus. *Society for Neuroscience Abstracts, 9*, 625.
Davis, F. C., & Gorski, R. A. (1985). Development of hamster circadian rhythms: I. Within litter synchrony of mother and pup activity rhythms at weaning. *Biology of Reproduction, 33*, 335–362.
Davis, F. C., & Gorski, R. A. (1986). Development of hamster circadian rhythms: II. Prenatal entrainment of the pacemaker. *Journal of Biological Rhythms, 1*, 77–85.
Deguchi, T. (1975). Ontogenesis of a biological clock for serotonin: Acetyl coenzyme A N-acetyltransferase in the pineal gland of rat. *Proceedings of the National Academy of Sciences, 72*, 2914–2920.
Deguchi, T. (1977). Circadian rhythms of enzyme and running activity under ultradian lighting schedules. *American Journal of Physiology, 232*, E375–E381.
Deguchi, T. (1982). Sympathetic regulation of circadian rhythm of serotonin N-acetyltransferase activity in pineal gland of infant rat. *Journal of Neurochemistry, 38*, 797–802.
Duncan, M. J., Banister, M. J., & Reppert, S. M. (1986). Developmental appearance of light-dark entrainment in the rat. *Brain Research, 369*, 326–330.
Fuchs, J. L., & Moore, R. Y. (1980). Development of circadian rhythmicity and light responsiveness in the rat suprachiasmatic nucleus: A study using 2-deoxy-(1-$^{14}$C) glucose method. *Proceedings of the National Academy of Sciences, 77*, 1204–1208.
Hatton, G. I., Perlmutter, L. S., Salm, A. K., & Tweedle, C. D. (1984). Dynamic neuronal–glial interactions in hypothalamus and pituitary: Implications for control of hormone synthesis and release. *Peptides, 5*, 121–138.
Hendrickson, A. E., Wagonner, W., & Cowan, W. M. (1972). An autoradiographic and electron microscopic study of retinohypothalamic connections. *Zeitschrift Zellforsch, 125*, 1–26.

Hiroshige, T., Honma, K., & Watanabe, K. (1982a). Ontogeny of the circadian rhythm of plasma corticosterone in blind infantile rat. *Journal of Physiology (London), 325,* 493–506.

Hiroshige, T., Honma, K., & Watanabe, K. (1982b). Prenatal onset and maternal modifications of the circadian rhythm of plasma corticosterone in blind infantile rats. *Journal of Physiology (London), 325,* 521–532.

Hiroshige, T., Honma, K., & Watanabe, K. (1982c). Possible zeitgebers for external entrainment of the circadian rhythm of plasma corticosterone in blind infantile rats. *Journal of Physiology (London), 325,* 507–519.

Honma, S., Honma, K., Shirakawa, T., & Hiroshige, T. (1984a). Effects of elimination of maternal circadian rhythms during pregnancy on the postnatal development of circadian corticosterone rhythm in blinded infantile rats. *Endocrinology, 114,* 44–50.

Honma, S., Honma, K., Shirakawa, T., & Hiroshige, T. (1984b). Maternal phase setting of fetal circadian oscillation underlying the plasma corticosterone rhythm in rats. *Endocrinology, 114,* 1791–1796.

Ifft, J. D. (1972). An autoradiographic study of the time of final division of neurons in rat hypothalamic nuclei. *Journal of Comparative Neurology, 144,* 193–204.

Jolly, A. (1972). Hour of birth in primates and man. *Folia Primatologica, 18,* 108–121.

Kaiser, I. H., & Halberg. F. (1962). Circadian periodic aspects of birth. *Annals of the New York Academy of Sciences, 98,* 1056–1068.

Koritsanszky, S. (1981). Fetal and early postnatal cyto- and synaptogenesis in the suprachiasmatic nucleus of the rat hypothalamus. *Acta Morphologica Academiae Scientiarum Hungaricae, 29,* 227–239.

Lenn, N. J., Beebe, B., & Moore, R. Y. (1977). Postnatal development of the suprachiasmatic nucleus of the rat. *Cell and Tissue Research, 178,* 463–475.

Levin, R., & Stern, J. M. (1975). Maternal influences on ontogeny of suckling and feeding rhythms in the rat. *Journal of Comparative and Physiological Psychology, 89,* 711–721.

Lincoln, D. W., & Porter, D. G. (1976). Timing of the photoperiod and the hour of birth in rats. *Nature, 260,* 780–781.

Moore, R. Y. (1983). Organization and function of a central nervous system circadian oscillator: The suprachiasmatic hypothalamic nucleus. *Federation Proceedings, 42,* 2783–2789.

Moore, R. Y., & Lenn, N. J. (1972). A retinohypothalamic projection in the rat. *Journal of Comparative Neurology, 146,* 1–14.

Moore-Ede, M. C., Sulzman, F. M., & Fuller, C. A. (1982). *The clocks that time us.* Cambridge: Harvard University Press.

Nathanielsz, P. (1976). *Fetal endocrinology: An experimental approach.* Amsterdam: Noord-Hollandsche.

Pratt, B. L. (1981). *Naturalistic studies of photoperiodism in Syrian and Djungarian hamsters.* Unpublished doctoral thesis, University of Connecticut, Storrs.

Reppert, S. M. (1982). Maternal melatonin: A source of melatonin for the immature mammal. In D. C. Klein (Ed.), *Melatonin rhythm generating system* (pp. 182–191). Basel: Karger.

Reppert, S. M. (1983). Time of birth in the rat is gated to the photoperiod by a circadian mechanism. *Pediatric Research, 17,* 154A.

Reppert, S. M. (in press). Circadian rhythms: Basic aspects and pediatric implications. *Clinical Endocrinology.*

Reppert, S. M., Coleman, R. J., Heath, H. W., & Swedlow, J. R. (1984). Pineal N-acetyltransferase activity in 10-day-old rats: A paradigm for studying the developing circadian system. *Endocrinology, 115,* 918–925.

Reppert, S. M., & Schwartz, W. J. (1983). Maternal coordination of the fetal biological clock in utero. *Science, 220,* 969–971.

Reppert, S. M., & Schwartz, W. J. (1984a). Functional activity of the suprachiasmatic nuclei in the fetal primate. *Neuroscience Letters, 46,* 145–149.

Reppert, S. M., & Schwartz, W. J. (1984b). The suprachiasmatic nuclei of the fetal rat: Characterization of a functional circadian clock using $^{14}$C-labeled deoxyglucose. *Journal of Neuroscience, 4,* 1677–1682.

Reppert, S. M., & Schwartz, W. J. (1986a). The maternal suprachiasmatic nuclei are necessary for maternal coordination of the developing circadian system. *Journal of Neuroscience, 6,* 2724–2729.

Reppert, S. M., & Schwartz, W. J. (1986b). Maternal endocrine extirpations do not abolish maternal coordination of the fetal circadian clock. *Endocrinology, 119,* 1763–1767.

Rossendale, P. D., & Short, R. V. (1967). The time of foaling of thoroughbred mares. *Journal of Reproduction and Fertility, 13,* 341–343.

Schwartz, W. J., Davidson, L. C., & Smith, C. B. (1980). In vivo metabolic activity of a putative circadian oscillator, the rat suprachiasmatic nucleus. *Journal of Comparative Neurology, 189,* 157–167.

Schwartz, W. J., & Gainer, H. (1977). Suprachiasmatic nucleus: Use of $^{14}$C-labeled deoxyglucose uptake as a functional marker. *Science, 197,* 1089–1091.

Sherwood, O. D., Downing, S. J., Golos, T. G., Gordon, W. L., & Tarbell, M. K. (1983). Influence of light–dark cycle on antepartum serum relaxin and progesterone immunoreactivity levels and on birth in the rat. *Endocrinology, 113,* 997–1003.

Sokoloff, L., Reivich, M., Kennedy, C., Des Rosiers, M. H., Patlak, C. S., Pettigrew, K. D., Sakurada, O., & Shinohara, M. (1977). The [$^{14}$C]deoxyglucose method for the measurement of local cerebral glucose utilization: Theory, procedure, and normal values in the conscious and anesthetized albino rat. *Journal of Neurochemistry, 28,* 897–916.

Stanfield, B., & Cowan, W. M. (1976). Evidence for a change in the retinohypothalamic projection in the rat following early removal of one eye. *Brain Research, 104,* 129–133.

Takahashi, J. S., & Zatz, M. (1982). Regulation of circadian rhythmicity. *Science, 217,* 1104–1111.

Takahashi, K., & Deguchi, T. (1983). Entrainment of the circadian rhythms of blinded infant rats by nursing mothers. *Physiology and Behavior, 31,* 373–378.

Takahashi, K., Hayafuji, C., & Murakami, N. (1982). Foster mother entrains circadian adrenocortical rhythm in blinded pups. *American Journal of Physiology, 243,* E443–E448.

Takahashi, K., Murakami, N., Hayafuji, C., & Sasaki, Y. (1984). Further evidence that circadian rhythm of blind rat pups is entrained by the nursing dam. *American Journal of Physiology, 246,* R359–R363.

Viswanathan, N., & Chandrashekaran, M. K. (1984). Mother mouse sets the circadian clock of pups. *Proceedings of the Indian Academy of Sciences (Animals Science), 93,* 235–241.

Yamazaki, J., & Takahashi, K. (1983). Effects of change of mothers and lighting conditions on the development of the circadian adrenocortical rhythm in blinded rat pups. *Psychoneuroendocrinology 8,* 237–244.

# V

# SOCIAL AND EMOTIONAL DEVELOPMENT

# 16

# Psychobiologic Consequences of Disruption in Mother–Infant Relationships

SEYMOUR LEVINE
*Department of Psychiatry and Behavioral Sciences*
*Stanford University School of Medicine*
*Stanford, California 94305*

The conceptual framework which provides the basic hypothesis of the work to be described in this chapter is that social variables have a profound effect in modulating psychological and biologic responses to stressful circumstances. In particular, the availability of familiar social partners results in an attenuated response to loss of primary social relationships, which in the case of the infant is loss of the mother. The data to be presented support the view by ethologists that one of the most important adaptations developed by higher primates is the ability for sustained social relationships involved in group living. As Hans Kummer has stated, "Primates seem to have only one unusual asset in coping with their environments: a type of society which, through constant association of young and old and through a long life duration, exploits their large brains to produce adults of great experience. One may, therefore, expect to find some specific primate adaptations in the way that primates do things as groups" (Kummer, 1971, pp. 37–38).

We have found that disruption of social relationships is one of the most potent psychological variables which results in the activation of neuroendocrine responses, particularly those of the hypothalamo-pituitary-adrenal axis, in nonhuman primates. Conversely, the presence of social partners can reduce, and at times completely eliminate (Stanton, Patterson, & Levine, 1985; Vogt, Coe, & Levine, 1981), the pituitary-adrenal response that occurs without such social support. This neuroendocrine response to the disturbance of social relationships emerges early in development.

Perinatal Development:
A Psychobiological Perspective

**359**

Relationship, of course, is best exemplified by the mother–infant relation-ship, which is the basis of the infant's first experience with any kind of social interaction. Beginning with the work of Harlow and Harlow (1969) using rhesus macaques, numerous studies have shown that the mother serves not only to provide sustenance but also to function as a source of emotional security. This latter role is evident in the behavioral observa-tions of even older, independent infants who will immediately seek prox-imity and make contact with the mother when a novel or fear-eliciting situation occurs. Once contact has been achieved, the infants no longer show signs of behavioral agitation. One such example of the influence of social variables on the response to separation has been demonstrated in the following experiment (Coe, Wiener, Rosenberg, & Levine, 1985; Wie-ner, Johnson, & Levine, 1987). In this study, infants were reared either in small maternal groups consisting of three mother–infant dyads or in indi-vidual cages with only their mothers. When the infants reared in social groups were removed from the mothers and placed in novel environments for 1 or 6 hr, there was a reliable elevation in plasma cortisol levels. However, if the same infants were allowed to remain in the home environ-ment during 1- and 6-hr separations, there was a significant diminution in the plasma cortisol response as well as a marked reduction in vocaliza-tion. This finding is consistent with previous reports on the squirrel mon-key regarding the beneficial effects of providing a familiar physical and social environment for separated infants (Coe, Wiener, & Levine, 1983). In contrast, when these same experimental conditions were imposed on infants reared alone with their mothers, the resulting pattern was differ-ent. No decrease in the adrenal response to separation was observed in the infants left alone in the home cage at either 1 or 6 hr. This experiment demonstrates that the adrenocortical response of group-reared infants to separation is not due primarily to a novel environment but to the loss of appropriate social support. The infant reared alone with its mother and separated, although remaining in a familiar environment, shows no ame-lioration in either the adrenocortical or behavioral response after loss of the mother. Therefore, a critical aspect of the home environment appears to be the presence of familiar conspecifics, which apparently functions to ameliorate the physiological and behavioral responses to maternal loss.

The next series of experiments performed with rhesus macaques fur-ther illustrate the importance of social variables on the response to sepa-ration. These studies highlight the importance of the mother, even when contact is not permitted, and further emphasize the significance of prese-paration social history on the separation response. The primary purpose for studying the separation response in the rhesus macaque, as well as in the squirrel monkey, was to provide an appropriate comparative base upon which to elaborate similarities and differences. Because the social organization and mother–infant interactions of the rhesus macaque are very different from those of the squirrel monkey, we felt it was important to conduct these parallel studies to be able to derive general principles concerning the parameters of separation. In addition, because depression is not usually observed in squirrel monkey infants, and insofar as most research using separation as an animal model for depression has used the macaque, we argued that if there were hormonal sequelae to the depressive response, we should be able to detect them in rhesus studies. Much to our surprise, throughout our experiments under a variety of separation paradigms, the characteristic depressive response described by other investigators (Mineka & Suomi, 1978) was rarely observed. There may be many valid reasons, such as genetic and rearing history, to account for the failure to observe this depressive response. In contrast to subjects used by other experimenters, our animals are always reared in stable social groups with their mothers.

The initial study (Smotherman, Hunt, McGinnis, & Levine, 1979) was designed to record the separation-induced effects on adrenocortical acitivity as well as to monitor ongoing behavior in group-living rhesus monkeys. Specifically, we had hoped to examine the possible relationships among the cortisol response to separation, the characteristics of the mother–infant interactions, and the social group structure. In this study, mother–infant pairs were captured and removed from the social group. They were then housed in standard primate cages for 3 hr either individually or as dyads. Individual housing was designated as the separation conditon, and paired housing as the control condition. During separation the mothers and infants were kept adjacent to the large outdoor cage and were permitted auditory and visual contact with each other and with the remaining members of the group. Each dyad was subjected to the separation (individual) and control (pair) conditions on three occasions.

The analysis of the cortisol levels between the separated and control conditions revealed a significant difference in the infants' corticoids. As most of our studies use a within-groups design due to the limited numer of subjects available, we can conclude that the infants show a greater cortisol response when separated in the presence of their mothers. Unfortunately, since the design of this experiment involved capture and immediate separation, it did not permit us to evaluate basal levels. Therefore, we were unable to ascertain whether the cortisol values of the infants in the control condition were equivalent to resting values. However, these data do suggest that social buffering occurred when the mother and infant were together in the control condition, as we have observed in previous experiments with squirrel monkeys (Mendoza, Smotherman, Miner, Kaplan, &

Levine, 1978). Further, within the context of this experiment, we could not dismiss the possibility that, when separated in the presence of their mothers, the infants showed a frustration-induced elevation in cortisol (Levine, Goldman, & Coover, 1972) rather than a response to separation per se.

There was significant individual variation in the plasma cortisol response. Variability in biologic and behavioral data does not occasion surprise. In this instance, however, we were able to determine at least one source of the variability. There was a significant correlation of infant steroid levels with maternal dominance status. The more dominant the mother, the higher the cortisol levels of her infant, both in the separation and control conditions. Dominance was determined by approach/avoidance behavior, a measure considered to be a reliable index of status in rhesus macaques (Bernstein, 1970; Rowell, 1972). High-dominance mothers ranked lowest on avoiding others and highest on being avoided by others. Low-dominance mothers ranked highest on avoiding others and lowest on being avoided by others. These data suggest that the maternal dominance status may have ramifications on the mother–infant interaction and that the nature of this interaction is then reflected in the infnat's response to separation. However, more systematic data on the relationship between the mother–infant interaction before separation and on the separation response itself would be required before such a hypothesis could be substantiated. Therefore, a subsequent study was conducted to more closely examine the relationship between aspects of the mother–infant relationship prior to separation and the infant's behavioral and pituitary-adrenal responses to separation and reunion.

Reunion following separation sometimes appears to be stressful for both mother and infant. Hinde and associates (Hinde & Davies, 1972; Hinde & McGinnis, 1977) found that high tension between mother and infant rhesus monkeys prior to separation predicted greater behavioral distress upon reunion. Thus, is this second study (Gunnar, Gonzales, Goodlin, & Levine, 1981), we introduced a number of procedural changes into the experiment in order to more appropriately examine both the behavioral and physiological responses to separation and the response to reunion. To obtain a basal sample, mothers and infants were removed as dyads and the pairs were placed in individual cages for 7 days. This procedure was based on the assumption that at the end of the 7-day habituation period the infants would show resting levels of plasma cortisol and the responses to separation could be compared to a valid base. Another major procedural change was the condition of separtion and the length of separation. Infants were separated by removing the mother from the home cage and rehousing her in another room, thereby preventing visual or auditory contact. Separated infants could see and hear other separated infants, and those housed in adjacent cages could achieve limited tactile contact. However, no form of contact between the separated infant and its mother was possible during this period. The length of separation was extended to 12 days. Since the depression response apparently takes several days to fully emerge, we lengthened the period of separation to observe the potential range of behavioral responses reported to occur in the separated infant. The Hinde index (number of infant approaches divided by the sum of mother and infant approaches, minus number of infant leaves divided by mother–infant interactions. This index of percentage of approach minus percentage of leave has been used as a measure of tension in the mother–infant relationship surrounding the maintenance of proximity. Values approaching 1.0 indicate that the infant does most of the approaching and the mother does most of the leaving; the reverse is indicated by values approaching −1.0. Values close to 0.0 indicate mother and infant engaged in about equal amounts of approaches and leaves, which is assumed to be a stable mother–infant relationship (Hinde & Spencer-Booth, 1967).

Three major findings emerged from this study. The first finding was related to the issue of social buffering. Following removal from the social group, where the mother and infant dyads were placed in individual cages, the mother showed a significant elevation in plasma cortisol as a result of this procedure. No such elevation was observed in the infants. Thus, whereas the mother appears to respond with a dramatic increase in plasma cortisol following removal from the social group, the infant appears to be buffered from this procedure, presumably as a consequence of contact and proximity with the mother. This finding of social buffering is consistent with those obtained in the squirrel monkey and has been reliably reproduced in subsequent experiments using the rhesus macaque. The second and third findings, concerning behavioral and physiological responses to separation, were surprising. Although there was a striking elevation in plasma cortisol during the early periods of separation, by 24 hr the cortisol levels were dramatically reduced and tended to remain stable throughout the rest of the period of separation. However, there tended to be a small but consistent elevation (approximately 10%) of plasma cortisol over preseparation basal levels throughout the period of separation when compared to the nonseparated control group. The behavioral responses to separation, although persisting somewhat longer than the cortisol response, also tended by the end of separation to return to the levels observed in the nonseparated infant. Thus, in contrast to our expectations of a profound and devastating effect on the separated infant, we were impressed with its resiliency following separation and the rapidity with which it was able to adapt to this new situation.

Rosenblum and Plimpton (1981) have identified specific vocalizations and locomotion as behaviors directed toward the reestablishment of maternal contact. These behaviors may show a short-term increase following separation during the period when the probability of relocating the mother is high (e.g., the first day or so). Reduction in these behaviors may signify that the infant has entered a second phase of separation, which may be characterized by an increase in behaviors indicative of despair or depression. However, whether depression or despair occurs appears to be highly idiosyncratic, and this second phase of separation may also be characterized as the infant primate's new adaptation to the absence of its mother. Individual differences in the appearance of the depressive response have been noted by many investigators. The factors which determine these individual differences are currently a subject of extensive investigation. Suomi (chap. 18, this volume) has hypothesized genetic variables to be a source of individual variation determining whether an infant primate will or will not become depressed following separation. In addition, we must also propose that the preseparation environment may be a very potent factor in determining the response of the infant primate to prolonged separation.

When dealing with the response of the pituitary-adrenal system to what is assumed to be a prolonged stress, the specter of physiological exhaustion is always raised. Exhaustion of the pituitary-adrenal system was proposed by Selye (1950) as the final phase of the general adaptation syndrome. Although there is little evidence that such exhaustion can occur within the context of this specific study, it is clear that a vigorous pituitary-adrenal response can occur in these separated infants following the 12-day period of separation. After the 12-day separation, the infant was brought into the room where the mother was present and placed for 1 hr in a cage placed 3 ft in front of cages occupied by adult females. Infants were exposed either to their own mother or to another female. The adrenal response to this procedure was equivocal, with the infant responding either to being presented to its own mother or to another adult female. Although cortisol did not discriminate between the different females to which the infant was presented, the behavioral response clearly showed a significant differentiation between whether the infant was exposed to its own mother or to another adult female. In particular, whoo calls were markedly increased over separation levels when presented with its own mother. Even though these data indicate that the primate infant can recognize its own mother (Rosenblum, 1968; Rosenblum & Alpert, 1974), it is possible that, with regard to the neuroendorcine response, the infant was responding maximally and that the distinction between the two conditions was overshadowed by the response to some aspect of the presentation procedure itself, such as novely of the room or transport. Finally, the data from this experiment confirmed the importance of the preseparation mother–infant relationship on the response to separation and reunion. Although there were no significant correlations observed between the Hinde index and the behavioral response following reunion with the mother, significant correlations were found between the Hinde index and the pituitary-adrenal response to both separation and reunion (Table I). Thus, the more stable the mother–infant relationship, the greater the cortisol response at 3 hr following separation. In contrast, the more unstable the mother–infant relationship, as indicated by the Hinde index, the higher the cortisol response 24 hr following reunion. Thus, not only do social variables modulate the response to separation during the separation process itself, but social interactions present before separation appear to be significant in determining the extent of the physiological response to separation and reunion.

Yet another aspect of the separation environment found to affect infant behavior is the degree of access to the mother during separation. The relation between infant distress and the degree of maternal access is not linear. Infants separated from their mothers by a wire mesh partition which allowed physical contact showed only minimal distress behavior. However, when members of the dyad were separated by a Plexiglas panel which prevented tactile contact, the usual infant "protest" behavior was observed (Suomi, Collins, Harlow, & Ruppenthal, 1976). Further, Seay and Harlow (1965) reported that infants with no access to the mother—those removed to a separate room—exhibited less protest behavior than infants separated from the mother by Plexiglas. In our laboratory, rhesus infants totally isolated from their mothers and other conspecifics emitted less vocalization than did those infants who were separated in view of the mother and/or social group (Levine, Franklin, & Gonzalez, 1984). Thus, visual contact with the mother in the absence of tactile contact appears to elicit more vocalization in infants than either limited tactile contact or total isolation from the mother. Since the early research relied heavily on vocalization as a measure of distress, it was assumed that exposure to the mother produced the greatest distress and that removal of the infant from the mother supported the "out-of-sight, out-of-mind" notion. However in view of the inverse relationship between cortisol and vocalization observed in squirrel monkeys, and by invoking the hypothesis of Rosenblum and Plimpton (1981) that the initial period of vocalization represents the infant's attempt to reestablish contact, we have argued that these initial vocalizations, particularly when visual access to the mother is available,

**Table I**

The Relationship between a Mother–Infant Dyad's Hinde Index Score
Prior to Separation and the Infant's Behavioral and Physiological
Responses to Separation and Reunion

| Separated pairs | % Approach–% leave (preseparation) | Whoo calls[a] | Separation | | Reunion | |
|---|---|---|---|---|---|---|
| | | | Movement | Agitation | Cortisol[b] | Cortisol[c] |
| 1 | 0.46 | 11.0 | 38.5 | 20.0 | + 9.3 | +27.1 |
| 2 | 0.31 | 36.5 | 216.0 | 77.5 | +13.7 | +12.7 |
| 3 | 0.29 | 13.0 | 75.0 | 22.5 | +26.5 | +20.5 |
| 4 | 0.19 | 13.5 | 80.0 | 1.5 | +27.3 | + 1.0 |
| 5 | 0.00 | 23.5 | 326.0 | 88.0 | +29.8 | − 0.7 |

[a] Levels of whoo calling, movement, and agitated state, Block 1 (Days 1 and 2).
[b] 3-hr separation value minus $\bar{X}$ Days 3 and 5 of adaptation expressed as $\mu g\%$.
[c] 24-hr reunion value minus $\bar{X}$ Days 3 and 5 of adaptation expressed as $\mu g\%$ (Gunnar et al., 1981).

represent active coping attempts on the part of the infant. In fact, the
physiological indexes of arousal indicate that the infants totally isolated
from the mother are indeed exhibiting greater distress.

To evaluate the relationship between availability of the mother during
separation and the behavioral and biologic responses under these different separation paradigms, we utilized both behavioral and adrenocortical
measures. Two experiments clearly support the hypothesis that visual
access to the mother produced different behavioral responses and modulated the physiological responses to separation. In the first experiment,
we evaluated the effects of degree of access to the mother on the psychobiologic response to separation by measuring infant vocalization and
adrenocortical activity (Levine, Johnson, & Gonzalez, 1985). Mother–
infant pairs were removed from the social group and permitted to habitu-
ate to individual cages for a period of 4 days. On the fifth day, the infants
were placed in adjacent cages under one of two conditions: (1) mother
present (MoPrs), mothers remained in an adjacent cage approximately 25
cm away, and (2) mother absent (MoAbs), mother was removed to a
separate area out of contact with the infant. The separation period lasted
for 3 days, after which the infants were reunited with the mother for 4
days and then separated into the other condition for 3 subsequent days.
The results obtained for the adaptation phase of this experiment were
similar to those obtained in previous studies emanating from our laboratory. Infants showed only a small or not cortisol response and showed no
behavioral signs of disturbance when removed from the social group in
the presence of the mother. We have called this phenomenon *social buf-*

*fering,* by which we mean the capacity of the presence of another organism or group of organisms within the environment to attenuate or eliminate the plasma cortisol response that would normally appear when animals are exposed to novel or stressful stimuli while they are alone. The behavioral data following separation shows a clear effect of presence or absence of the mother. Vocalization was more frequent in the presence of the mother; however, vocalization decreased significantly over the course of separation and occurred less frequently on Days 2 and 3 than on the initial separation day (Fig. 1). It should be noted that the frequency of vocalization appears less in these animals than what we have previously reported. However, these animals had been subjected to a brief prior separation, and we have reported that a previous history of separation does result in a reduced frequency of vocalization upon subsequent separations (Gunnar, Gonzalez, & Levine, 1980).

The presence of the mother during separation tended to ameliorate the cortisol response, and the only significant elevations of cortisol were within the first 3 hr following separation. In contrast, separation in the MoAbs condition led to a significant elevation of cortisol for as long as 3 days following separation (Fig. 2). It can be seen from Fig. 2 that there is an additional component to this cortisol response, namely, that there is a clear circadian rhythmicity and that the response tends to be more elevated in the morning. When included in an examination of the circadian aspects of the response based on the reports of Reite and Short (1978), the magnitude of the response to separation, both behaviorally and autonomically, appears to be greatest the morning after separation. The infant's cortisol levels, though elevated shortly after separation from the mother, have been reported to return to basal levels (Gunnar *et al.,* 1981) or at least to decline significantly 24 hr later (Gunnar *et al.,* 1980; Levine *et al.,* 1984). Blood samples in those studies were taken in the late afternoon; thus, the findings concur with the results of the present study, in which the infant's afternoon cortisol values were at basal levels by the 2nd day of separation. The current finding that in the mother's absence cortisol remained elevated in the mornings of the second and third separation days is the first evidence of elevated cortisol lasting more than 24 hr in separated rhesus infants. In fact, the adrenocortical response was recurrent, rather than persistent, since high levels were found only in the morning even when afternoon levels had returned to base. There are two possible interpretations for this recurrent morning cortisol elevation. It may be that spending the night without the mother is more stressful than being without her during the day. Studies of infant development have found that even as infant monkeys mature and increase the time spent away from the mother, they still sleep with her at night. Further, Reite and Short (1978)

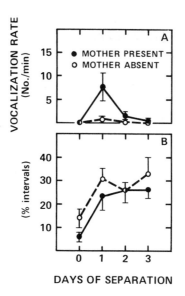

**Fig. 1.**  Behavioral responses following separation under different separation conditions. Data are means ± SE. From Levine *et al.*, 1985. Copyright 1985 by the American Psychological Association. Reprinted by permission of the publisher.

have reported disruptions of normal sleep patterns in separated rhesus infants.

What emerges thus far from these studies is a hierarchy of the physiological responses to separation conditions imposed upon rhesus monkey infants. Separation from the social group into a novel environment while in contact with the mother appears to be minimally arousing. The infants show little evidence of behavioral agitation and either very small, transient changes in plasma cortisol levels or no changes at all. Separation from the mother, but with visual access to her, results in an increase in vocalization which declines as a function of the length of separation, but the infants show very transient evidence of increased arousal by changes in plasma cortisol levels. The most physiologically arousing situation appears to be separation from the mother and from the social group simultaneously. Although the behavioral and physiological responses appear paradoxical, we have proposed that these events are highly related. Under conditions of stress, proximity and contact with the mother result in modulation and reduction of the infant's arousal levels; and the primary behavioral response that achieves proximity and contact in primates is vocalization. Thus, vocalization may function as a coping response on the part of the infant. When the cues from the mother are available, the infant

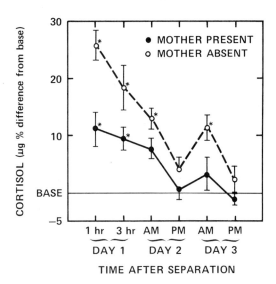

**Fig. 2.** Mean (± SE) plasma cortisol responses for infants at different times following separation. Asterisks indicate statistically significant differences from basal levels. From Levine *et al.*, 1985. Copyright 1985 by the American Psychological Association. Reprinted by permission of the publisher.

will vocalize in an attempt to achieve proximity. Although proximity and contact do not occur under the conditions of the present experiments, it appears that vocalization still serves an arousal-reducing function, leading either to reduced levels of plasma cortisol or to the elimination of the plasma cortisol response, which frequently occurs under other conditions of separation.

The final experiment we wish to report was conducted by Kevin Hayashi and Francoise Bayart-Leroy in our laboratory examining the effects of maternal access to the psychobiologic response to separation. This experiment primarily replicates the one previously discussed, with the addition of two important new dimensions. First, whereas we had previously discussed vocalization predominantly in terms of quantity, in this experiment we also measured the quality of vocalization by recording the calls under the two conditions of separation, MoPrs and MoAbs. In collaboration with Francoise Bayart-Leroy and Charles Snowdon, sonographic analyses were done on the vocalizations emitted under these two conditions. Second, in addition to examining plasma cortisol, we studied the activity of the monoamine system by obtaining samples of cervical cerebrospinal fluid (CSF). The fluid was obtained under basal conditions and at different times following separation under the two conditions. The reasons for examining the activity of the monoamine system were numerous. We wished to determine whether or not there was central representation of the response to separation that was concordant either with the behavior or the endocrinologic responses we observed. In addition, the monoamine system has been implicated in numerous psychiatric disorders, particularly those related to depression. Furthermore, insofar as the monoamine and endocrine systems have been shown to be intimately involved, we were interested in which aspects of the monoamine system were more closely related to either the behavior or the endocrine response observed following separation. Insofar as we had observed differences in both behavioral and endocrine responses under the two conditions of separation (MoPrs and MoAbs), this seemed an appropriate model by which to examine whether differential effects of monoamine activity could be observed as a consequence of the different experimental separation paradigms.

Both the behavioral and endocrinologic data were consistent with what has been previously reported. The frequency of vocalizations was greater when the infant was separated when the mother was present than when the mother was absent (Fig. 3). The plasma cortisol response was signifi-

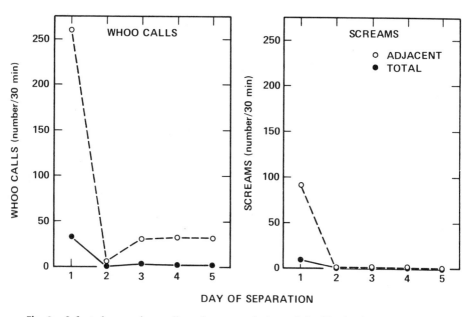

**Fig. 3.** Infant rhesus whoo calls and screams during a daily 30-min observation period following separation under two environments.

cantly greater and persisted for a longer period of time when the infant was totally isolated (Fig. 4). However, the sonographic analysis of the vocalizations revealed that rate of vocalization per se does not truly characterize the behavior of the infant rhesus under these two separation conditions. Vocalizations emitted under these two conditions were strikingly different. There appear to be two types of whoo calls which occur while the infant is adjacent to the mother, and a third, totally different type of whoo call emitted under total isolation (Fig. 5). These calls are exclusive to the separation condition. Whoo calls elicited when the mother was present are never emitted under total isolation, and vice versa. Thus, it appears that there may be specific calls related to communication and attempts to establish reunion, and other calls which may indeed be better characterized as distress vocalizations.

The data obtained in collaboration with Kym Faull and Jack Barchas of the Nancy Pritzker Laboratory of Behavioral Neurochemistry on the CSF metabolites following separation clearly discriminated between the two types of separation experiences. Although the metabolites related to dopamine (HVA and DOPAC) and serotonin (5-HIAA) appeared to be similar under both separation conditions, showing a transient elevation and return to baseline, the metabolite related to norepinephrine (MHPG) clearly discriminated between the two conditions (Fig. 6); MHPG was significantly elevated in total isolation and tended to persist, whereas in the MoPrs condition there was a transient elevation which returned to

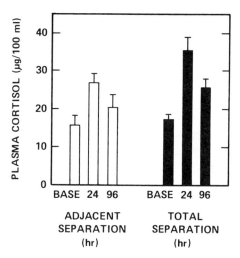

**Fig. 4.**   Plasma cortisol of infant rhesus monkeys prior to (BASE) and following separation (24 and 96 hr) under two environments.

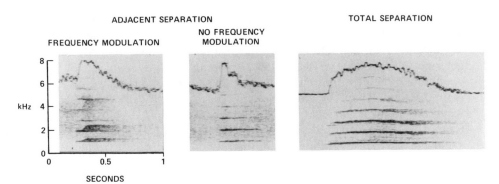

**Fig. 5.**  Sonograms of typical infant rhesus separation calls under two environments.

basal level. Although we had initially proposed that the monoamine metabolites would discriminate between the behavioral and endocrine responses to these different separation procedures, it is clear that such a discrimination is not possible at this time. The existence of specific whoo calls related to the adjacent and isolation separations indicates that the behavior is not only quantitatively different but clearly qualitatively different and that the whoo calls emitted by the infant when totally isolated are also reflected in neurochemical and endocrinologic differences. Insofar as these data have only just been obtained, we obviously have not done the appropriate experiments to manipulate the quality of the vocalization and determine the degree to which the physiological changes reflect these behavioral differences. We should point out, however, that we have seen similar changes in the neurochemical response to separation in the squirrel monkey. Dopamine and serotonin appear to show only transient changes, whereas the changes in those metabolites related to norepinephrine tended to remain persistently elevated for at least 24 hr (Coe *et al.*, 1985).

Throughout this chapter we have focused on the role of social variables in modulating the response to one type of stressful situation—separation—for the infant monkey. We have demonstrated that disruption of the social relationship, particularly within the context of the mother–infant interaction, is a potent psychological variable that causes increased pituitary-adrenal activity and results in changes in both neurochemical activity and behavior. Further, the presence of familiar conspecifics, or visual and auditory access to the maternal figure, can ameliorate the biologic and behavioral responses observed when these stimuli are not available to the isolated infant.

Although we have described several social variables which affect the enodcrine response to stress, we believe that these social factors can be

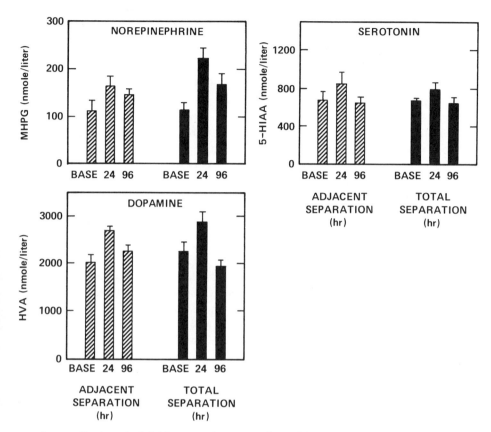

**Fig. 6.** Cerebrospinal fluid monoamine metabolites of infant rhesus monkeys prior to (BASE) and following separation (24 and 96 hr) under two environments.

subsumed within a more general theory of stress and coping.[1] For lack of a better term, one of the most potent psychological variables which results in an activation of the pituitary-adrenal system can be described as *uncertainty*. To understand the concept of uncertainty, it is important to appreciate that all situations vary along a continuum from highly certain, predictable events to highly uncertain, unpredictable events. Uncertainty can be evoked by novelty, by insuffcent information concerning the nature of forthcoming events, or by loss of control. For example, the adrenal response to a novel stimulus reflects the organism's respone to increased uncertainty because by definition there is little information that can be used to predict forthcoming events. We have hypothesized that

---

[1] For a more detailed analysis of coping theory in the context of the mother–infant relationship, see Garmezy and Rutter (1983).

any physical, informational, or cognitive operation that serves to reduce uncertainty, whether it be passive, such as habituation, or active, such as the utilization of control or predictability, will lead to a reduction or elimination of the endocrine response. We believe that it is possible to fit the data on social support within the general context of the proposition that uncertainty leads to activation of the pituitary-adrenal response and that reduction of uncertainty diminishes or eliminates this response. We therefore propose that the availability of stable and familiar social relationships provides a set of predictable outcomes due, in part, to the long history of previous interactions and experiences. Thus, the predictability of the social interactions in a group of familiar conspecifics tends by definition to reduce uncertainty.

The data presented in this chapter further extend this proposition to include highly salient social stimuli which, even in the absence of contact, provide the organism with the ability to make appropriate coping responses in order to reduce levels of arousal. This hypothesis would lead to the prediction that separation in an unfamiliar social group would provide none of these beneficial features but, in fact, should evoke a state of high uncertainty leading to a dramatic elevation of pituitary-adrenal activity. This hypothesis was substantiated in an experiment in which infant squirrel monkeys were separated from the mother and placed in an unfamiliar social group (Levine, unpublished data). We found no amelioration of the stress response under this condition. On the contrary, the data indicated that being placed with unfamiliar conspecifics following separation induced more dramatic behavioral and adrenocortical responses than did simply being isolated. In adult organisms, we have found that one of the most reliable elicitors of increased pituitary-adrenal activation is the formation of new social groups (Gonzalez, Hennessy, & Levine, 1981; Mendoza, Coe, Lowe, & Levine, 1979).

For a number of years our laboratory has been concerned with the specificity of psychological stimuli that activate the neuroendocrine systems regulating the pituitary-adrenal response. We have only begun to analyze the relationship between psychological stimuli and the activity of specific components of the monoamine system. Our data indicate that the various components of the monoamine system respond differentially to the psychological consequences of the separation procedure. Thus, along with the pituitary-adrenal system, the norepinephrine system appears to be sensitive to difference aspects of the separation paradigm, unlike the dopaminergic and serotinergic systems, which appear to only transiently respond to these psychological events. It is our hope that we will be able to describe the relationship among the norepinephrine system, the neuroendocrine systems regulating pituitary-adrenal activity, and behavior. At this time we are faced with the fact that specific behavioral sequelae and neurochemical and neuroendocrine events are associated with and sensitive to the social parameters of the separation environment. It is our ultimate goal to eventually specify the causal mechanisms within these systems. Only by systematically altering each facet of these systems can we determine which of these systems is regulating the others. This will require the use of sophisticated behavioral, neurobiologic, and pharmacological techniques in order to unravel this complex of biobehavioral phenomena.

## Acknowledgments

This research was supported by grants HD02881 from the National Institute of Child Health and Human Development, the MH23645 from the National Institute of Mental Health, and Research Scientist Award MH19936 from NIMH to S.L.; and by grant MH23861 from the NIMH to J. D. Barchas.

## References

Bernstein, I. S. (1970). Primate status hierarchies. In L. A. Rosenblum (Ed.), *Primate behavior* (Vol. 1, pp. 71–109). New York: Academic Press.

Coe, C. L., Wiener, S. G., & Levine, S. (1983). Psychoendocrine responses of mother and infant monkeys to disturbance and separation. In L. A. Rosenblum & H. Moltz (Eds.), *Symbiosis in parent–offspring interactions* (pp. 189–214). New York: Plenum.

Coe, C. L., Wiener, S. G., Rosenberg, L. T., & Levine, S. (1985). Physiological consequences of maternal separation and loss in the squirrel monkey. In L. A. Rosenblum & C. L. Coe (Eds.), *The handbook of squirrel monkey research* (pp. 127–148). New York: Plenum.

Garmezy, N., & Rutter, M. (Eds.). (1983). *Stress, coping, and development in children.* New York: McGraw-Hill.

Gonzalez, C. A., Hennessy, M. B., & Levine, S. (1981). Subspecies differences in hormonal and behavioral responses after group formation in squirrel monkeys. *American Journal of Primatology, 1,* 439–452.

Gunnar, M. R., Gonzalez, C. A., Goodlin, B. L., & Levine, S. (1981). Behavioral and pituitary-adrenal responses during a prolonged separation period in infant rhesus macaques. *Psychoneuroendocrinology, 6,* 65–75.

Gunnar, M. R., Gonzalez, C. A., & Levine, S. (1980). The role of peers in modifying behavioral distress and pituitary-adrenal response to a novel environment in year-old rhesus monkeys. *Physiology and Behavior, 25,* 795–798.

Harlow, H. F., & Harlow, M. K. (1969). Effects of various mother–infant relationships on rhesus monkey behaviors. In B. M. Foss (Ed.), *Determinants of infant behaviour* (Vol. 4, pp. 15–36). London: Methuen.

Hinde, R. A., & Davies, L. (1972). Removing infant rhesus from mother for 13 days compared with removing mother from infant. *Journal of Child Psychology and Psychiatry, 13,* 227–237.

Hinde, R. A., & McGinnis, L. M. (1977). Some factors influencing the effects of temporary mother–infant separation: Some experiments with rhesus monkeys. *Psychosomatic Medicine, 7,* 192–212.

376                                                                    Seymour Levine

Hinde, R. A., & Spencer-Booth, Y. (1967). The behaviour of socially living rhesus monkeys in their first two and a half years. *Animal Behaviour, 15,* 169–196.

Kummer, H. (1971). *Primate societies: Group techniques of ecological adaptation.* Chicago: Aldine-Atherton.

Levine, S., Franklin, D., & Gonzalez, C. A. (1984). Influence of social variables on the biobehavioral response to separation in rhesus monkey infants. *Child Development, 55,* 1386–1393.

Levine, S., Goldman, L., & Coover, G. D. (1972). Expectancy and the pituitary-adrenal system. In R. Porter & J. Knight (Eds.), *Physiology, emotion and psychosomatic illness* (pp. 281–296). Amsterdam: Elsevier.

Levine, S., Johnson, D. F., & Gonzalez, C. A. (1985). Behavioral and hormonal responses to separation in infant rhesus monkeys and mothers. *Behavioral Neuroscience, 99,* 399–410.

Mendoza, S. P., Coe, C. L., Lowe, E. L., & Levine, S. (1979). The physiological response to group formation in adult squirrel monkeys. *Psychoneuroendocrinology, 3,* 221–229.

Mendoza, S. P., Smotherman, W. P., Miner, M. T., Kaplan, J., & Levine, S. (1978). Pituitary-adrenal response to separation in mother and infant squirrel monkeys. *Developmental Psychobiology, 11,* 169–175.

Mineka, S., & Suomi, S. J. (1978). Social separation in monkeys. *Psychological Bulletin, 85,* 1376–1400.

Reite, M., & Short, R. A. (1978). Nocturnal sleep in separated infant monkeys. *Archives of General Psychiatry, 35,* 1247–1253.

Rosenblum, L. A. (1968). Mother–infant relations and early behavioral development in the squirrel monkey. In L. A. Rosenblum & R. W. Cooper (Eds.), *The squirrel monkey* (pp. 207–233). New York: Academic Press.

Rosenblum, L. A., & Alpert, S. (1974). Fear of strangers and specificity of attachment in monkeys. In M. Lewis & L. A. Rosenblum (Eds.), *The origins of fear* (pp. 165–193). New York: Wiley.

Rosenblum, L. A., & Plimpton, E. H. (1981). Adaptation to separation: The infant's effort to cope with an altered environment. In M. Lewis & L. A. Rosenblum (Eds.), *The uncommon child: Genesis of behavior* (Vol. 3, pp. 225–257). New York: Plenum.

Rowell, T. E. (1972). *Social behavior of monkeys.* London: Penguin.

Seay, B. M., & Harlow, H. F. (1965). Maternal separation in the rhesus monkey. *Journal of Nervous and Mental Disease, 140,* 434–441.

Selye, H. (1950). *Stress.* Montreal: Acta.

Smotherman, W. P., Hunt, L. W., McGuinnis, L. M., & Levine, S. (1979). Mother–infant separation in group-living rhesus macaques: A hormonal analysis. *Developmental Psychobiology, 12,* 211–217.

Stanton, M. E., Patterson, J. M., & Levine, S. (1985). Social influences on conditioned cortisol secretion in the squirrel monkey. *Psychoneuroendocrinology, 10,* 125–134.

Suomi, S. J., Collins, M. L., Harlow, H. F., & Ruppenthal, G. C. (1976). Effects of maternal and peer separations on young monkeys. *Journal of Child Psychology and Psychiatry, 17,* 101–112.

Vogt, J. L., Coe, C. L., & Levine, S. (1981). Behavioral and adrenocorticoid responsiveness of squirrel monkeys to a live snake: Is flight necessarily stressful? *Behavioral and Neural Biology, 32,* 391–405.

Wiener, S. G., Johnson, D. F., & Levine, S. (1987). Influence of postnatal rearing conditions on the response of squirrel monkey infants to brief perturbations in mother–infant relationships. *Physiology and Behavior,* in press.

# 17

## Influences of Environmental Demand on Maternal Behavior and Infant Development

LEONARD A. ROSENBLUM
*Health Science Center*
*State University of New York*
*Brooklyn, New York 11203*

It is the purpose of this chapter to explore the idea that in order to understand the nature of maternal patterns and their impact on the course of infant development, it is necessary to consider the total social and physical context within which these patterns emerge. Although it has long been recognized that complete social isolation or severe environmental restriction along other dimensions may markedly distort behavioral development in primates (e.g., Harlow, Harlow, Dodsworth, & Arling, 1966; Sackett & Ruppenthal, 1973), it is only recently that we have come to appreciate that there is a range of social and physical environmental influences that play important roles. As a consequence, we need to consider four broad dimensions which enfold the developing infant in a series of concentric layers of influence: the physical environment, the social group, the mother, and the infant's phenotypic characteristics. Each affects, interacts with, and is influenced by the others. After reviewing some aspects of the effects of the social environment on individual and sex-dimorphic patterns, the chapter will focus on recent work regarding the consequences of varied foraging demands for group and maternal response and their unfolding effects on developing infants. The perspective presented here suggests that it is ultimately the complex of strategic responses of the group and the mothers within it as they attempt to cope with the demands of their environment which, in conjunction with the infant's maturing capacities, shapes the course of infant development.

Perinatal Development:
A Psychobiological Perspective

## I.  Development of Discrimination of Mother from Nonmother

It has been fairly argued that the infant's relationship with its mother represents the model, or precursor at least, for all subsequent social relationships (Mason, 1978; Rosenblum & Alpert, 1977). However, for attachment or bonding to the mother to occur, the infant must be able clearly to differentiate mother from nonmother in its social world. Although early, and more proximate, discriminations in some species, including humans, may be olfactory (Kaplan, Cubicciotti, & Redican 1977), it is evident that, as in humans, when the nonhuman primate infant locomotes more widely in its environment, vision is the primary mode of connection with the mother. Experimental data, controlling for differential response by mother and other conspecifics toward the young infant, have made it clear in several species that group-reared monkeys cannot respond differentially to their mother in comparison to an unfamiliar conspecific on a visual basis before the 3rd month of life. This slowly developing discriminative response has been demonstrated in the bonnet and pigtail macaque and the squirrel monkey (Rosenblum & Alpert, 1977; Rosenblum, 1978). In the bonnet macaque, females attain this discrimination and preferential response earlier and more intensely than do males. Moreover, females develop a degree of "stranger anxiety" in the weeks following attainment of discrimination, whereas avoidance responses to strangers do not appear in males. Males of these species often seem more bold and show higher thresholds for avoidance of novelty (Rosenblum, 1974).

## II. Development of Filial Discrimination in Varied Environments

Since basic visual discriminations can be seen much earlier, by perhaps 2 weeks of age (Zimmerman & Torrey, 1965), development of this social discrimination (i.e., of mother from nonmother) must involve other factors. Our evidence suggests that the social milieu in which the dyad lives markedly influences the development of this basic social discrimination. In the bonnet macaque, social groups are unusually gregarious, with adults and independent juveniles spending a considerable part of the day and night in close proximity and contact with one another. The mother bonnet permits considerable access to her newborn beginning in the first minutes after birth. In the pigtail macaque, a closely related species, observed under identical laboratory conditions, adults are more aggressive, individual distances between unrelated subjects are consistently greater, and mothers markedly restrict access to their young during the first weeks of life. Discriminative responses to mother appear several weeks later in group-reared pigtails than in bonnets, and distinctions in response to mothers and strangers in pigtails are not nearly as definitive. Data of a more experimental nature which support this comparative difference have been obtained by raising bonnet infants with their mothers but outside of a group setting. In contradiction to hypotheses of early attachment theorists (Cairns, 1972) isolation of a primate infant with its mother after birth does not support the idea that "mutual discrimination develops most readily in the course of insulated and exclusive interactions" (p. 54). In fact, when infant bonnets are raised in this single-dyad situation, reliable discrimination of the mother does not appear before 7–8 months of age and in several infants was not present even at 1 year (Rosenblum & Alpert, 1977)!

It is instructive regarding the processes involved in the development of social discrimination that when the infant is raised with its mother and only one other adult female, discrimination between mother and the familiar female emerges during the 3rd month; the same infants cannot discriminate between their mother and a stranger until at least several months later. It appears that the course of development of infant social discriminations involves a period of specific negative learning at first, that is, who the mother is *not*. Only later, perhaps through a process akin to learning-set formation (Zimmerman & Torrey, 1965), a capacity for which does not emerge until several months of life, is the infant capable of learning the distinction between the class "mother" and the class "nonmother." It is clear that when the social environment is appropriate to the development of this discrimination, obviously a vital one, the differentiation between various conspecifics (and congenerics) is quite clear and may even be made on the basis of color-video stimuli alone (Rosenblum & Paully, 1980).

## III. Effects of the Social Environment on Behavioral Development

### A. Maternal Status and Infant Behavior

The developmental impact of the hierarchical nature of the normal social group in these species on developing infant and juvenile behavioral patterns has been demonstrated as well. When, for example, one creates a mixed group of pigtail and bonnet females, the larger, more aggressive pigtails rapidly emerge as dominant. The infant bonnets in such a group are reluctant to leave their mothers, play and explore relatively infrequently, and seem generally timid and restrained. Introduction of an adult bonnet male to this group immediately results in the shift of the bonnet females to dominant status. Their infants, freed of the restraint imposed by the subordinant status of their mothers, relax, move from the mothers more readily, and begin relatively high levels of exploration and play (Stynes, Rosenblum, & Kaufman, 1968). A variety of evidence from the field also indicates the importance of maternal status for the nature of the infant's early experience and possibly for the subsequent social roles different infants assume in adulthood (e.g., Cheney, 1977).

## B. Effects of Adults on Juvenile Patterns

Similarly, experimental studies with pigtail and bonnet macaques have demonstrated the impact of the adult group on peer interaction patterns and infant emotionality. In one study, the social behavior of bonnet juveniles was studied under one of three social conditions. Groups of unfamiliar 1-year-olds were formed either in the presence of their mothers, in the presence of a group of unrelated adult females, or in the complete absence of adults (Rosenblum & Plimpton, 1979). Using a within-groups treatment design, this study demonstrated that in the presence of their mothers, the juveniles were the most gregarious, mobile, and playful. In the presence of strange adult females, their movement around the pen was constrained, and markedly higher levels of emotional distress were present than in either the mother or peers-only situation.

Two interesting dimensions of this emotional and motoric restraint in the presence of adults suggest further the importance the complex species-characteristic social structure has for social development. First, as Golding dramatized so vividly in *The Lord of the Flies* (1959), aggressive patterns between the juveniles were most in evidence when no adults were present. Unlike more intimate and subdued patterns such as grooming, which were unaffected, the presence of either mothers or the other adults restrained infants from expressing all types of vigorous behavior including aggression and dominance-related displays. Since the more aggressive patterns are increasingly more characteristic of developing males (Maccoby & Jacklin, 1974), the impact of the social group in affecting the expression of different forms of behavior may well be differentiated along sexual lines.

## C. Ontogeny of Sexual Segregation in the Squirrel Monkey

Several other studies in the laboratory emphasize further the significant impact of various features of the social environment in influencing the course of infant development and in the emergence of sex-specific patterns. In squirrel monkeys of the Peruvian type (Rosenblum & Coe, 1984), adults form a sexually segregated social structure (Rosenblum, Coe, & Bromley, 1975) in which males and females remain within what we have termed a *sphere of potential interaction,* but the sexes remain relatively far from one another. Infants developing in a normal heterosexual group rarely interact with males during the 1st weeks of life. It is not until some time after the end of the 1st year that the developing offspring of a group begin to join together into their same-sex subgroups and cease the relatively frequent intersexual interactions which characterize younger peer groups. Experimental data indicate that the tendency for males and females to separate from one another develops slowly and is not manifested prepubertally unless a sexually segregated adult social structure is present in the environment (Coe & Rosenblum, 1974). Thus, the pattern of early social development, basic to the subspecies-specific social structure, involves interaction with an appropriate adult structure during early development.

## D. Sex Differences in Response to Early Rearing Conditions

Other studies, with environmental conditions ranging from complete deprivation of nondyadic social partners to settings of limited social interaction (Jensen, Bobbitt, & Gordon, 1968; Rosenblum, 1961; Sackett & Ruppenthal, 1973) have also suggested that infants of each sex may be differentially affected by the nature of the early environment. Even considering the most severe forms of environmental alteration, Sackett (1972) concluded: "These data suggest that deprivation rearing is much more devastating on the exploratory reactions of male monkeys. Thus generalizations concerning rearing condition effects must be tested on and qualified by sex differences" (p. 268).

This type of sex-related impact of environmental complexity on maternal behavior and infant development was also demonstrated in a study of development in squirrel monkeys in our laboratory. When infants raised in unstable social and physical environments were compared to those raised in stable settings, male infants showed more rapid development of infant independence than did females. This occurred in spite of the fact that, compared to stable-environment controls, the mothers of males in the varied setting rejected their infants less and attempted to restrain them more often (Rosenblum, 1974).

It is evident even from these limited examples that the earlier emphases on the mother–infant dyad as the basic context within which to understand infant development has provided a vital but too limited perspective from which to understand the array of forces acting on development.

Obviously, the infant is influenced in dramatic ways by its genetics, its prenatal environment, and the patterns of maternal behavior to which it is exposed. But the entire range of postnatal influences is also affected by the complex interplay of environmental features within which the dyad is found. As we have seen, the mother's behavior, particularly following the first weeks of life (Rosenblum, 1971), is affected by the nature of the social group and her position within it. The infant also is influenced both directly by the nature and structure of the group and in terms of its shaping of the mother's response. However, if we are to understand this process more fully, it is vital to consider the physical environmental factors which influence the social group itself, and thus all its members, including mothers and infants within it.

## IV. Feeding Ecology and Mother–Infant Relations

The enormous body of data that has appeared in the last several decades makes it clear that virtually no aspect of adult behavior is a fixed characteristic of a given species. In fact, even the most basic features of social structure (e.g., size and dispersion of groups, male–female ratios, hierarchical patterns, and peer relations in the young) vary as a complex function of key environmental conditions within which any given species group is found (S. A. Altmann, 1974; Baldwin & Baldwin, 1974; Crook & Gartlan, 1966). Although it would of course be absurd to discount the tremendous influence of phylogenetic and prenatal variables (Bernstein, 1971; Chalmers, 1973; Hainsworth & Wolf, 1979; Reinisch, 1983) in determining behavioral expression, comparisons across a number of species and across a number of dimensions of sociality suggest that more variance may be attributable to ecological than to phylogenetic factors (Berry, 1977; Rosenblum, 1979; Spuhler & Jorche, 1975).

The feature of the environment that is cited most often as influencing social structure to the greatest extent, both in contemporary and evolutionary terms, is the feeding ecology within which the group is found (i.e., the availability and type of foodstuffs and their distribution in time and space; Clutton-Brock, 1977; Dittus, 1974; and above). With only a few exceptions (e.g., J. Altmann, 1980), in spite of the acknowledged significance of the feeding ecology in influencing primate evolution and behavior, the available information on the impact of these factors on behavioral development has been sparse indeed, and until recent years experimentally controlled data on this topic have been absent altogether.

## A. Maternal Strategies in Demanding Environments

We wished to focus on the means through which the mother, in response to potentially difficult physical and social environmental factors, balances her life support needs with her efforts to promote a viable course of development in her offspring. It was assumed that mother who was concerned with a range of competing survival demands might, as a result, fail to provide her infant with a consistently available "secure base" for its excursions and explorations (Ainsworth, 1969). Based on the theoretical perspectives from the human child development literature, it was hypothesized that the infants would develop "insecure attachments" as a result of the fact that their mothers, though physically present, would not be reliably available for contingent responsivity to infant needs (Lewis & Goldberg, 1969). As a consequence, it seemed likely that such infants might show a number of disturbances in their early and subsequent behavior, including an enhanced susceptibility to affective response disorders, such as depression (Bowlby, 1977).

One additional point is in order before proceeding with a discussion of the specific findings of the study of the effects of environments which varied in their demand qualities. In keeping with modern optimal foraging theory (Pyke, Pulliam, & Charnov, 1977), feeding demands can be expected to compete strongly with many other types of behavior. However, this is not to suggest that all other functions will be sacrificed toward simply maximizing response to the foraging requirements. In any setting, reproduction and rearing of young must, to some degree, be figured into the equation of optimal foraging for the reproductively active female. Obviously the competition between these demands on the mother will be exacerbated in a sparse or otherwise difficult environment (J. Altmann, 1980) where the energy cost of obtaining food is relatively great. Given the considerable energy cost of lactation (Schwartz & Rosenblum, 1983) and the added costs of carrying the developing young with her through the environment during the search for food, it might be expected that high foraging demands would result in earlier and more vigorous rejection of the offspring. On the other hand, a demanding environment from which resources are difficult to obtain may have a negative impact on the capacity of a prematurely independent youngster to survive. This potential conflict between maternal and infant survival requirements is the focus of the classic views of the "weaning conflict" (Trivers, 1974) and goes to the heart of the sociobiologic concept of inclusive fitness (Hamilton, 1964; Wilson, 1975). The mother must, perhaps in active dispute with her infant, balance the demands of immediate personal survival, the survival of her current offspring, and the ultimate reproducive success of all past and potential future offspring she may bear. Certainly the dilemma and balancing act which confronts the human parent under similarly competing and difficult demand situations is no less severe nor any easier to solve.

## B. Principles of the Experimental Paradigm for Studying Ecology and Mother–Infant Relations

As a means of creating an experimental setting within which to systematically manipulate features of the feeding ecology in groups of nonhuman primate mothers and their infants, a paradigm for requiring different levels of work for the acquisition of food was created. The essential nature of this plan was to create an environment within which food might be dispersed and hidden so as to require mothers in experimental groups to spend varying periods of the day searching for food. Since food deprivation and its consequent nutritional impact would have confounded the results, adequate amounts of food were made available in this paradigm, with only the work load required for its acquisition being varied. Similarly, aggressive competition for limited or localized food was to be avoided, as the issue of dominance or aggressiveness between mothers was not a central concern in these studies. Rather, it was our goal to determine what the consequences of varied ecological demand were for group social interaction, patterns of maternal behavior, and the course of infant development.

In addition, our current program of research into the effects of foraging requirements has incorporated an extremely salient factor in relation to environmental demand and development, that is, the relative stability or predictability of the demand features of the environment. For the social group, the mother, and her developing infant, one key factor that will influence coping capacity is the predictability of environmental events and the relationship of each individual's actions to environmental outcomes (Levine, 1982; Mineka, 1982). An environment which does not provide perdictability necessarily reduces the quality of strategic response and has attendant upon it adverse effects on behavioral competence and affect. In human groups, chaotic environments may diminish the likelihood of competent parenting and normal mother–infant relations and can be the source of significant developmental pathology (Pavenstadt, 1965; Turnbull, 1973).

Our research approach builds upon a number of previous laboratory efforts to study the effects of varying foraging demand on primate groups (Plimpton, Swartz, & Rosenblum, 1981; Rosenblum & Smiley, 1984). The current study was designed to compare the effects of stable and unpredictably varying foraging requirements on normal and pathological paths of infant development in bonnet macaques.

## V. The Effects of Stable and Variable Feeding Environments

This study involved three groups of bonnet macaque (*Macaca radiata*) mothers and their infants, each group containing five dyads. The groups were age matched, with ages ranging from 4 to 17 weeks at the beginning of the study. Since one infant was born several weeks into the study, the youngest infants of each group were excluded from analyses to maintain age matching; all groups contained both male and female infants, although not in equal proportions. The groups were housed in similar double pens (connected via a pass-through doorway) of approximately 120 sq ft on each half, containing shelves at several heights, watering spigots for ad lib water, mesh ceilings, and overhead flourescent lighting. The groups were each observed through large one-way glass mirrors set into the front walls.

The groups differed in one pivotal feature of the environment: the extent of effort required to extract available food from the environment through foraging activity, a dimension we term *foraging demand*. In each group, subjects were required to extract monkey chow crackers hidden within special foraging devises distributed around the double pens. In all instances, on every day, more than enough food to sustain adult weights and normal growth of infants was available from these devises. In one group, designated low foraging demand (LFD), food was always available in abundance and could be found anywhere the subject sought it, with little effort. In the second group, high foraging demand (HFD), the food was more sparse and widely dispersed, and subjects were required to search for varying periods of time to obtain daily rations. The third group, designated variable foraging demand (VFD), alternated on a 2-week schedule between low-and high-demand schedules, with no obvious cues available to the animals as to which condition was in effect at any given time. All adults in each group easily accomplished the foraging task itself, and infants were observed to forage successfully by 3 months of age. Following 2 weeks of adaptation to the situation, groups were observed for 12 weeks, using a combination of time-sample and group-scan recording techniques.

As a reflection of the efficacy of the different demands imposed, food wastage was consistently higher during low-demand conditions, while frequency of foraging was higher during high-demand conditions. It is important to note however that in VFD there was a lag in response of at least several days following the unsignaled shifts in demand, and most differences in foraging patterns did not appear until the 2nd week of each condition. Overall, within the VFD group, mean scores for adult hierarchical behavior (e.g., threats, submissions, displacements), infant–mother contact, and the frequency with which mothers broke contact increased following shifts from low to high demand, whereas time spent by mother and infant in opposite pens, infant exploration of objects, and infant play decreased following these shifts to the more difficult foraging condition. Thus, it was clear that, both across the groups and within the VFD group itself from condition to condition (albeit with some days' lag), the differences in demand produced important alterations in behavior.

The essential differences between these groups that are of particular interest, however, emerged across the span of the entire study. It should be noted that for each of the behavioral patterns discussed below, there were no statistically significant differences between the groups under comparable conditions at the start of the study; thus, the differences which subsequently emerged were not a result of initial differences between these randomly assigned treatment groups. In keeping with the multidimensional perspective proposed here, we can consider the effects of the experimental manipulation of the physical environment at three levels: adult social behavior; mother–infant relations, and infant behaviors.

## A. Effects of Feeding Demand on Adult Behavior

The bonnet macaque has generally been identified in past studies as a particularly gregarious, nonaggressive species (Rosenblum, Kaufman, & Stynes, 1964). In the current study, of the three groups, the subjects in LFD, living under conditions most comparable to past ad lib feeding studies, did indeed engage in the lowest levels of hierarchical behavior and the highest levels of social grooming (a prominent affiliative pattern in most primates). It was the VFD group, however, that was the least gregarious, with the members of the stable HFD group falling at intermediate levels. Indeed, as reflected in Fig. 1, the VFD group developed into what was perhaps the most aggressive bonnet group we have observed during the last 24 years of study of this species.

In general, whereas each group started the study at low levels of hierarchical behavior, the LFD group stayed low throughout, the HFD group showed an initial sharp increase that gradually declined after 8 weeks, and the VFD group showed a steady and dramatic increase across the 14 weeks of observation. It was clear that the fluctuating and unpredictable changes in demand in the VFD condition had a cumulative effect and

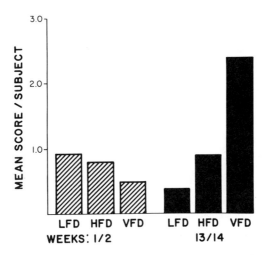

**Fig. 1.** Hierarchical behavior in the three treatment groups during the first and last 2 weeks of the study. Abbreviations: LFD, low foraging demand; HFD, high foraging demand; VFD, variable foraging demand.

sharply disrupted normal patterns of adult behavior in this species, notwithstanding periods of relatively easy access to food.

## B. Effects of Feeding Demand on Mother–Infant Interactions

The growing disruption in adult behavior in VFD relative to the two stable demand groups was also reflected in the patterns of mother–infant interaction. The dyads in the VFD group showed higher levels of mother–infant contact than the dyads in either of the other groups and showed, as well, significantly lower levels of time spent in opposite pens out of visual access to one another. The relatively "secure" infants of the LFD groups spent the most time out of sight of mother. The relatively insecure nature of the dyadic relationship in VFD was also reflected in the fact that as a result of heightened levels of maternal efforts to break contact and infant attempts to reestablish it, contact was made and broken more often in VFD than in the other groups. Indeed whereas the frequency of contact changes decreased over time in LFD and HFD as the infants of these groups spent longer and longer periods away from mother, the frequency of making and breaking dyadic contact actually increased in VFD as infants grew older. As illustrated in Fig. 2, HFD infants had initially long bout lengths off mother, which were sustained across the study; this was perhaps a result of initial maternal rejections which accompanied relatively high levels of hierarchical behavior as these subjects strategically

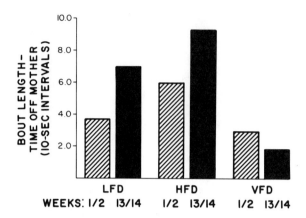

**Fig. 2.** Bout length of time off mother in the three treatment groups during the first and last 2 weeks of the study. Durations are in terms of the average number of contiguous 10-s intervals without contacting the mother. Abbreviations: LFD, low foraging demand; HFD, high foraging demand; VFD, variable foraging demand.

adapted to their high-demand schedule. LFD infants showed a gradual increase in bout lengths for time off mother, whereas in VFD, bout lengths of time off mother showed a slight decrease by the end of observations, even though subjects were, by that time, more than 3 months older.

The role of the mothers in VFD was quite crucial in producing this diminishing rather than growing independence of their young. In essence, mothers in VFD frequently attempted to break contact with their infants, while their infants made repeated efforts to maintain or reestablish contact with them. Mothers in VFD had significantly higher break-contact scores than those of either of the other two groups, and the infants of VFD showed the highest infant-return scores. Clearly the dyadic relationship in VFD was unstable and did not serve to mediate normal patterns of the development of infant independence.

## C. Effects of Feeding Demand on Affective Development

The growing disturbance of the VFD infants was manifest in a number of ways. When in close contact with their mothers, infant monkeys generally do not engage in active social interaction with others, nor can one readily discern any indications of emotional disturbance. Because infants in the three groups spent significantly different periods of time off their mothers as the study progressed, we analyzed the behaviors of the infants during the time spent off mother. The VFD infants showed significantly lower levels of social play and of object exploration than the members of

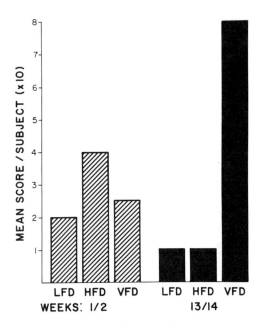

**Fig. 3.**   Levels of emotional disturbance in infants of the three treatment groups during the first and last 2 weeks of the study. Abbreviations: LFD, low foraging demand; HFD, high foraging demand; VFD, variable foraging demand.

either LFD or HFD. Because play behaviors are by far the most common patterns normally observed in monkey infants in this age range, and because social forms of play are particularly prominent in normal bonnet infants, this alteration in the developmental course in the VFD infants was particularly profound. It is clear from the remainder of our data that play behavior, which is generally viewed as a reflection of a positive, confident, and secure status in infants (Rosenblum, 1971), was incompatible with the affective status of the VFD infants when they were out of contact with their mothers. Behavioral disturbance in VFD infants, involving vocalizations, fear grimaces, cringing, and other postural changes, was significantly higher than that in either LFD or HFD infants and these differences were particularly manifest during the second half of the study (see Fig. 3).

The most surprising and dramatic indications of disturbance in VFD infants appeared particularly in two of the infants, and to a lesser degree in a third. With increasing frequency as the study progressed, when out of maternal contact as their mothers foraged, these infants displayed a pattern which has generally been labeled as "depression" in these species. In this pattern, the infants spent 10–20 min at a time relatively immobile, with their eyes closed and their bodies hunched over as they either clasped their own bodies or clung to or pressed against some other animal. This depressive pattern was observed in one or more of these subjects during virtually every one of the observations during the last 6 weeks of the study.

It is important to note that although a number of studies from this laboratory have described this type of depressive pattern in infant monkeys (Rosenblum, 1984), they have never been recorded *in the presence of the mother*. Moreover, even when the mothers of bonnet infants raised under LFD conditions have been totally removed, infants of this species generally transfer their attachment behavior to others in their group and, under these conditions of rearing, have never shown any depressive behavior whatsoever.

### D.   Response to Maternal Separation

In a follow-up study we examined the response to maternal separation in a number of these subjects. Unfortunately, before we could perform the separations in VFD, several of the mothers of this group grew ill, apparently from stress-related difficulties (no injuries or infections were present) and had to be removed for prolonged treatment. Separations were carried out in the LFD and HFD groups. Despite the apparent development of independent functioning in HFD, including relatively long bout lengths off mother, HFD infants were severely affected by the loss of mother as compared to comparably treated LFD infants. High foraging demand infants showed the highest levels of emotional disturbance during the 2-week separation, including some degree of the depressive pattern in several subjects, and recovered their emotional equilibrium significantly more slowly. Accompanying the heightened disturbance in the HFD subjects were sustained inhibitions of more positive patterns, including those of social play and exploration.

### E.   Pseudoindependence in Response to Maternal Rejection

This pattern of results from both the rearing and separation studies make several conclusions quite evident. Environmental conditions, in the form of increased or varying foraging demand, produce changes in adult, maternal, and infant patterns. Although sustained difficulty in extracting food from the environment can result in strategic adjustments in group and maternal patterns to avoid unremitting hostility and increasing infant debilitation, such conditions may nonetheless produce a kind of pseudoindependence in the developing young. There is no doubt that mothers can "train" or force their infants to stay out of contact and that during such periods, if mothers are not overly stressed themselves by the tasks at hand, they can still be somewhat responsive to immediate infant needs. Such was the case in HFD. But, as the separation data indicate, infants raised in such a setting may not be as secure in their movements to the outside world, nor as capable of independent functioning as infants raised by mothers who are virtually continuously responsive to fluctuating infant needs. The mothers in VFD, apparently unable themselves to increase their effectiveness in dealing with the unsignaled and uncontrollable variation in demand, not only were far less responsive to their infants' emotional needs but in fact increasingly forced their infants to function without them. Thus the VFD infants were in essence undergoing a form of severe separation reaction even though their mothers were visually, but not psychologically, available.

## VI. Conclusions and Hypotheses

What overall developmental hypothesis may help us to incorporate this rather complex and diverse body of data, and where should future research proceed? I would offer the following view of the interrelation between environmental properties, maternal response, and infant development. We have known for many years that the capacity of an organism to learn effective patterns of response in complex situations is negatively affected by heightened levels of motivation or arousal. That is, whereas the learning of simple discriminations, for example, may be aided by food deprivation procedures, the solving of more complex problems will, in fact, be disrupted when pronounced hunger or other motivational levels are produced. This is the so-called Yerkes-Dodson law. In monkey dyads living in complex situations, the same law may well apply as the infant attempts to cope with the extradyadic environment. In stable environments in which mothers allow infants to move from them when the infant feels secure enough to do so and in which mothers allow infants to return to them freely, the infants are able to modulate their arousal levels so as to permit learning of effective responses to the complex physical and social environment in which they and their mothers live. Forced to leave the mother, or forced to remain away despite heightened levels of arousal and disturbance, infants, though apparently operating apart from mother, are not in an appropriate emotional state to permit the formation of the skills necessary to function in that environment. Some learning and behavioral development does of course occur. But the limitation in coping ability that may result from the enforced confrontation with the environment was manifest in the relative inability of the HFD infants when their mothers were removed and, even more dramatically, was evident in the emotional disturbance and psychological withdrawal or depression seen in VFD infants even though their mothers were physically present.

Future laboratory research directed at this interplay between the strategic capacities of the mother in relation to specific environments and the emerging coping capacities of their infants should help us to discern major forces shaping infant behavioral development in "the real world." Moreover, an understanding of the diverse processes of normal adaptation in stable and less predictable and controllable settings will undoubtedly provide a significant entrée into a major research problem: the experimental production and subsequent alleviation of the pathology that may result when neither dyadic partner can cope effectively and efficiently with the strategic demands with which they are confronted in the struggle for survival and reproductive success.

## Acknowledgments

The research reported herein and the writing of the manuscript was supported by National Institute of Mental Health Grant MH15965 and support from the Harry Frank Guggenheim Foundation and the State University of New York.

## References

Ainsworth, M. D. S. (1969). Object relations, dependency and attachment: A theoretical review of the infant–mother relationship. *Child Development, 40,* 969–1025.

Altmann, J. (1980). *Baboon mothers and infants.* Cambridge: Harvard University Press.

Altmann, S. A. (1974). Baboons, space, time, and energy. *American Zoologist, 14,* 221–248.

Baldwin, J. D., & Baldwin, J. I. (1974). Exploration and social play in squirrel monkeys. *American Zoologist, 14,* 303–315.

Bernstein, I. S. (1971). Activity profiles of primate groups. In A. Scrier (Ed.), *Behavior of nonhuman primates.* New York: Academic Press.

Berry, J. (1977). Nomadic style and cognitive style. In H. McGurk (Ed.), *Ecological factors in human development.* New York: Elsevier North-Holland.

Bowlby, J. (1969). *Attachment and loss: Attachment.* New York: Basic Books.

Bowlby, J. (1977). The making and breaking of affectional bonds: Etiology and psychopathology in the light of attachment theory. *British Journal of Psychiatry, 130,* 201–210.

Cairns, R. B. (1972). Attachment and dependency: A psychobiological and social learning synthesis. In J. L. Gewirtz (Ed.), *Attachment and dependency* (pp. 29–80). Washington, DC: Winston.

Chalmers, N. R. (1973). Differences in behavior between some arboreal and terrestrial species of African monkeys. In R. R. Michaels & J. H. Crook (Eds.), *Comparative ecology and behavior of primates.* New York: Academic Press.

Cheney, D. L. (1977). The acquisition of rank and the development of reciprocal alliances in freeranging immature baboons. *Behavioral Ecology and Sociobiology, 2*, 303–317.

Clutton-Brock, T. H. (Ed.). (1977). *Primate ecology: Studies of feeding and ranging behavior in lemurs, monkeys and apes.* New York: Academic Press.

Coe, C. L., & Rosenblum, L. A. (1974). Sexual segregation and its ontogeny in squirrel monkey social structure. *Journal of Human Evolution, 3*, 551–561.

Crook, J. H., & Gartlan, J. S. (1966). Evolution of primate societies. *Nature, 210*, 1200–1204.

Dittus, W. (1974). *The ecology and behavior of the toque monkey (M. sinica).* Unpublished doctoral dissertation, Baltimore. University of Maryland.

Golding, W. (1959). *The lord of the flies.* New York: Capricorn Books.

Hainsworth, F. F., & Wolf, L. L. (1979). Feeding: An ecological approach. In *Advances in the study of behavior* (Vol. 9 pp. 53–89). New York: Academic Press.

Hamilton, W. D. (1964). The genetic evolution of social behavior. *Journal of Theoretical Biology, 7*, 1–52.

Harlow, H. F., Harlow, M. K., Dodsworth, R. O., & Arling, G. L. (1966). Maternal behavior of rhesus monkeys deprived of mothering and peer associations in infancy. *Proceedings of the American Philosophical Society, 110*, 58–66.

Jensen, G. D., Bobbitt, R. A. & Gordon, B. N. (1968). Effects of environment on the relationship between mothers and infant monkeys (M. nemestrina). *Journal of Comparative and Physiological Psychology, 66*, 259–263.

Kaplan, J. N., Cubicciotti, D. D., & Redican, W. K. (1977). Olfactory and visual differentiation of synthetically scented surrogates by infant squirrel monkeys. *Developmental Psychobiology, 12*, 1–10.

Levine, S. (1982). A psychobiological approach to the ontogeny of coping. In N. Garmazy & M. Rutter (Eds.), *Stress, coping, and development in children.* New York: McGraw-Hill.

Lewis, M. (1984). Social influences on development: An overview. In M. Lewis (Ed.), *Beyond the dyad* (pp. 1–12). New York: Plenum.

Lewis, M., & Freedle, R. (1977). The mother infant communication system: The effects of poverty. In H. McGurk (Ed.), *Ecological factors in human development.* New York: Elsevier North-Holland.

Lewis, M., & Goldberg, S. (1969). Perceptual-cognitive development in infancy: A generalized expectancy model as a function of mother–infant interaction. *Merill-Palmer Quarterly, 15*, 81–100.

Maccoby, E. E., & Jacklin, C. N. (1974). *The psychology of sex differences.* Stanford, CA: Stanford University Press.

Mason, W. A. (1978). Social experience and primate cognitive development. In G. M. Burghardt & M. Bekoff (Eds.), *The development of behavior: Comparative and evolutionary aspects.* New York: Garland.

Mineka, S. (1982). Depression and helplessness in primates. In H. E. Fitzgerald, F. A. Mullins, & P. Gage (Eds.), *Child nurturance: Studies of development in nonhuman primates.* New York: Plenum.

Pavenstadt, E. A. (1965). A comparison of the child rearing environment of upper-lower and very lower-lower class families. *American Journal of Orthopsychiatry, 35*, 89–98.

Plimpton, E. H., Swartz, K. B., & Rosenblum, L. A. (1981). The effects of foraging demand on social interactions in a laboratory group of bonnet macaques. *International Journal of Primatology, 2*, 175–185.

Pyke, G. H., Pulliam, H. R., & Charvov, E. L. (1977). Optimal foraging: A selective review of theory and tests. *Quarterly Review of Biology, 52*, 137–154.

Reinisch, J. M. (1983). Influence of early exposure to steroid hormones on behavioral development. In W. Everaerd, C. B. Hindley, A. Bot, & J. J. van der Werff ten Bosch (Eds.), *Development in adolescence* (pp. 63–113). Hingham, MA: Martinus Nijhoff.

Rosenblum, L. A. (1961). *The development of social behavior in the rhesus monkey.* Unpublished doctoral dissertation, Madison, University of Wisconsin.

Rosenblum, L. A. (1971). The ontogeny of mother–infant relations in macaques. In H. Moltz (Ed.), *The ontogeny of vertebrate behavior* (pp. 315–367). New York: Academic Press.

Rosenblum, L. A. (1974). Sex differences, environmental complexity and mother–infant relations. *Archives of Sexual Behavior, 11,* 117–128.

Rosenblum, L. A. (1978). *The development of visual discrimination of the mother in infant squirrel monkeys.* Unpublished manuscript.

Rosenblum, L. A. (1979). Monkeys in space and time: A situational taxonomy for the study of primates in the laboratory. In M. Lamb, S. J. Suomi, & G. Stephenson (Eds.), *Social interaction analysis: Methodological Issues* (pp. 269–290). Madison: University of Wisconsin Press.

Rosenblum, L. A. (1984). Monkeys' response to separation and loss. In M. Osterweis, F. Solomon, & M. Green (Eds.), *Bereavement: Reactions, consequences and care.* (pp. 179–198) Washington, DC: National Academy Press.

Rosenblum, L. A., & Alpert, S. (1977). Response to mother and stranger: A first step in socialization. In S. Chevalier-Skolnikoff & F. E. Poirier (Eds.), *Primate bio-social development* (pp. 463–478). New York: Garland.

Rosenblum, L. A., & Coe, C. L. (Eds.). (1984). *The handbook of squirrel monkey research.* New York: Plenum.

Rosenblum, L. A., Coe, C. L., & Bromley, L. (1975). Peer relations in monkeys: The influence of social structure, gender and familiarity. In M. Lewis & L. A. Rosenblum (Eds.), *Peer relations and friendships.* (pp. 67–98). New York: Wiley.

Rosenblum, L. A., Kaufman, I. C., & Stynes, A. J. (1964). Individual distance in two species of macaque. *Animal Behaviour, 12,* 338–342.

Rosenblum, L. A., & Paully, P. (1980). The social milieu of the developing monkey: Studies of the development of social perception. *Reproduction, Nutrition, Development, 20,* 827–841.

Rosenblum, L. A., & Paully, G. S. (1984). The effects of varying environmental demands on maternal and infant behavior. *Child Development, 55,* 305–314.

Rosenblum, L., & Plimpton, E. H. (1979). The effects of adults on peer interactions. In M. Lewis & L. A. Rosenblum (Eds.), *The child and its family* (pp. 195–218). New York: Plenum.

Rosenblum, L. A., & Smiley, J. (1984). Therapeutic effects of an imposed foraging task in disturbed monkeys. *British Journal of Child Psychology and Psychiatry, 3,* 485–497.

Sackett, G. P. (1972). Exploration behavior of rhesus monkeys as a function of rearing experiences and sex. *Developmental Psychology, 6,* 260–270.

Sackett, G. P., & Ruppenthal, G. C. (1973). Development of monkeys after varied experiences during infancy. In S. A. Barnett (Ed.), *Ethology and development* (pp. 52–87). Philadelphia: Lippincott.

Schwartz, G. G., & Rosenblum, L. A. (1983). Allometric influences on primate mothers and infants. In L. A. Rosenblum & H. Moltz (Eds.), *Symbiosis in parent–offspring interactions* (pp. 215–248). New York: Plenum.

Spuhler, J. N., & Jorche, L. B. (1975). Primate phylogeny, ecology, and social behavior. *Journal of Anthropological Research, 31,* 376–405.

Stynes, A. J., Rosenblum, L. A., & Kaufman, I. C. (1968). The dominant male and behavior in heterospecific monkey groups. *Folia Primatologica, 9,* 123–134.

Suomi, S. J., Kraemer, C. W., Baysinger, C. M., & DeLizio, R. D. (1981). Inherited and experiential factors associated with individual differences in anxious behavior displayed by rhesus monkeys. In D. F. Klein & J. Rakkin (Eds.), *Anxiety: New research and changing perspectives.* New York: Raven.

Trivers, R. L. (1974). Parent–offspring conflict. *American Zoologist, 14,* 249–264.

Turnbull, C. M. (1973). *The mountain people.* New York: Simon & Schuster.

Wilson, E. O. (1975) *Sociobiology: The new synthesis.* Cambridge: Harvard University Press, Belknap.

Zimmerman, R. R., & Torrey, C. C. (1965). Ontogeny of learning. In A. M. Schrier, H. F. Harlow, & F. Stolnitz (Eds.), *Behavior of nonhuman primates: Modern research trends* (Vol. 2, pp. 405–477). New York: Academic Press.

# 18

## Genetic and Maternal Contributions to Individual Differences in Rhesus Monkey Biobehavioral Development

STEPHEN J. SUOMI

*Laboratory of Comparative Ethology*
*Intramural Research Program*
*National Institute of Child Health and Human Development*
*National Institutes of Health*
*Bethesda, Maryland 20205*

## I. Introduction

This chapter will focus on recent studies of striking individual differences that are displayed early in life by both human children and rhesus monkey infants and which, in these species, appear to be relatively stable throughout development. These individual differences occur in the infants' behavioral and physiological reactions to changes and challenges in their physical and social environments. The differential reactions appear to be largely maintained throughout ontogeny in that individuals who as infants respond to unfamiliar and/or challenging stimuli with unusual behavioral and physiological perturbations, relative to those of their peers, generally continue to display extreme reactions to environmental change as they grow up.

The chapter will begin with a description of the basic differences in reactivity reported in human infants and children by a variety of investigators, not all of whom agree on the basis for such individual differences. Next, recent findings of seemingly similar patterns of developmentally stable individual differences among young rhesus monkeys in their behavioral and physiological responses to novelty and other environmental challenges will be presented. Results to data consistently suggest that these differences carry a strong genetic component but that their expression can be substantially influenced by specific environmental factors; these data will be briefly discussed. An ongoing study of monkey infants displaying differing characteristic reactivity patterns who are cross-fostered by multiparous females differing in their characteristic style of maternal care will next be described and the initial findings presented. Finally, a brief discussion of these results with respect to nature–nurture issues in development will be offered.

## II.  Developmental Stability of Individual Differences in Reactivity among Human Infants and Children

In the past few years a number of prospective longitudinal studies of social-emotional development in children have identified specific characteristics that seem to be relatively stable over time, at least under certain conditions. Studies of this genre include the now-classic work of Thomas, Chess, and their colleagues on infant temperament (Thomas, Chess, & Birch, 1968; Thomas, Chess, & Korn, 1982) and subsequent refinement of temperament assessment instruments by Carey (1970) and others, research by Sroufe and associates on long-term correlates of mother–infant attachment relationships (e.g., Sroufe, 1979; Sroufe, Fox, & Pancake, 1983), prospective twin studies by researchers in Colorado and Louisville (e.g., Plomin & Rowe, 1979; Matheny, Wilson, Dolan, & Krantz, 1981; Daniels & Plomin, 1985), and ongoing experiments by Kagan on the behavioral and physiological qualities of "behaviorally inhibited" toddlers (e.g., Kagan, 1982; Kagan, Reznick, Clarke, Snidman, & Garcia-Coll, 1984; Kagan, Reznick, & Snidman, 1987).

Interestingly enough, most of those measures described as developmentally stable by these different researchers seem to have had a common quality: Each one involves the differential reactions of individuals when confronted with novel stimuli and/or challenging situations. Thus, Thomas et al. (1982) found that some infants could be classified as "difficult" very early in life on the basis of their consistent withdrawal in the face of novelty, poor adaptability to environmental changes, a generally negative mood when challenged, and the extreme intensity of such reactions over time and in different situations. These tendencies were found to persist in some children even up to early adulthood. Sroufe (1984) reported that infants who were "anxiously attached" to their mothers at 12 and 18 months of age turned out to be highly dependent when they attended nursery school 3–4 years later. These children were rated very low on measures such as "can recover from stressful experiences," "is eager for new experience," "is curious and explorative," and "is resourceful in initiating activities"; they also tended to be whiney and required extra guidance and discipline from their nursery-school teachers. Plomin and Rowe (1979) determined that individual differences in the tendency to inhibit exploration in the face of novelty appeared to be genetically influenced, in that monozygotic twins were more similar in their reactions to strangers than were dizygotic twins, who were more similar in their reactions to strangers than were unrelated children. Wilson and Matheny (1983) reported parallel twin findings for their infant temperament measures of emotionality and adaptability. Finally, recent research by Kagan and his students (Kagan *et al.*, 1987; Kagan *et al.*, 1984; Garcia-Coll, Kagan, & Resnick, 1984) disclosed that individual differences in behavioral inhibition upon exposure to novelty were highly stable from 2 to 5 years of age. Moreover, "highly inhibited" children showed unusually low variability in heart rate under challenge conditions, while concomitant urinary measures of cortisol appeared to be relatively high for these individuals (Tennes, 1982). Earlier longitudinal research by Kagan and Moss (1962) revealed that individuals who had been judged to be extremely inhibited behaviorally when 3 years of age turned out to be shy and anxious in social situations when assessed in their mid-20s—and they also exhibited unusually stable heart rates while waiting for the adult test sessions. Taken as a whole, Kagan's old and new findings suggest that behavioral inhibition in the face of novelty may represent a personality characteristic that is inherently stable developmentally and that may have similarly stable physiological concomitants. However, such developmental stability is not apparently manifested in more "familiar" or "normative" environmental settings (Kagan, 1982).

It is to be emphasized that despite the apparently common thread of developmental stability of individual differences in reaction to novel and/ or stressful stimuli reported by the above investigators, their respective *explanations* of the basis for their observed phenomena have really been quite varied. For example, Plomin and Rowe (1979) and Wilson and Matheny (1983) attributed their findings largely to genetic factors, and Kagan argued for a genetic predisposition, possibly combined with prenatal influences. Sroufe, in contrast, considered the primary basis for his findings of developmental stability to lie in differences in the behaviors of mothers, which, in turn, differentially affected the subsequent attachment relationship these mothers formed with their infants (Sroufe, 1984). Finally, Thomas *et al.* (1982) viewed their reported individual differences to be the result of unique interactions or "transactions" among each infant's constitutional (genetic) predispositions, its emerging relationships with its caretakers, and various situational factors.

Of course, these different explanations of the basis for the observed stable differences are not necessarily mutually exclusive nor totally incompatible with one another. Nevertheless, it is very difficult to distinguish among these alternative explanations solely on the basis of the existing data. In part, this is because the various factors posited as largely responsible for the observed individual differences have not been manipulated independently in any of these generally excellent prospective longitudinal studies of human social-emotional development. Even in the twin studies it is difficult to disentangle nature from nurture or to describe how they might be interacting, in part because individuals who share genes, especially monozygotic twins, also tend to share rearing environments, so that in the absence of independent manipulations, these factors will always be confounded with each other to some degree (cf. West & King, in press). Still, difficulties in determining the basis for these individual differences should not detract from the consensus regarding not only their existence but also their apparent long-term developmental stability and their potential for affecting vulnerability to stress beyond childhood, through adolescence, and into adult life.

## III. Individual Differences in Reactivity among Rhesus Monkey Infants and Juveniles

Longitudinal studies of biobehavioral development in laboratory-born-and-reared rhesus monkeys have also revealed marked individual differences in response to environmental novelty and/or challenge. In these studies my colleagues and I have found a number of behavioral and physiological measures that consistently differentiate high-reactive subjects of various ages from those of their less reactive counterparts. The defining behavioral characteristics change with age in our rhesus monkeys, although the physiological characteristics seem quite stable, at least in the qualitative sense, over comparable periods of development. Thus, as neonates (1–4 weeks of age), high-reactive individuals display poor visual and auditory orienting responses to test stimuli, have relatively poor muscle tonus, and are slightly delayed developmentally in the initial appearance and subsequent disappearance of neonatal motor reflexes. They also tend to display difficult temperaments, are generally slow to explore novel stimuli, and typically have low predominant Prechtl state scores

(Schneider, 1984). As infants (1–6 months), high-reactive individuals show extreme and prolonged rises in plasma cortisol and adrenocortico-tropic hormone (ACTH) following short-term separation from their at-tachment objects (mothers, surrogates, or peers), along with high levels of self-directed behavior and low or nonexistent levels of locomotion, explo-ration, play, and vocalizations. Similar, although less extreme, behavioral and physiological responses, including elevated and stable heart rate, are displayed when high-reactive subjects are placed in novel physical set-tings, such as a test playroom.

As juveniles, (6 months–3 years), high-reactive subjects show similar responses to separation and introduction to novel environments, although their absolute levels of self-directed behavior, cortisol, and ACTH are lower than were displayed earlier in life in response to similar environ-mental challenges. High-reactive juveniles also display stereotypical mo-tor activity under these conditions, especially during Years 2 and 3 (Hig-ley, 1985). In addition, during periods of separation they have lower levels of CSF NE and higher levels of its metabolite MHPG than their less reactive cohorts, but relatively normal levels of dopamine metabolites (HVA and DOPAC) and the serotonin metabolite 5-HIAA (Suomi, Hig-ley, Kraemer, & Linnoila, 1987). As adolescents (4–5 years), high-reac-tive subjects continue to display the basic patterns of hypothalamic-pitui-tary-adrenal activation and increased CSF NE turnover in response to separation as in earlier life, but their behavioral reactions are now charac-terized by general agitation and excessive activity, usually involving sterotypical movements, rather than the behavioral withdrawal and rela-tive inactivity characteristic of their separation responses exhibited ear-lier in life (Guzzonato, Beattie, & Delizio, 1985; Higley, 1985). It should be pointed out that both the behavioral and physiological parameters differentiating high-reactive subjects of all ages from their normal cohorts are apparent only during times of environmental challenge. We have not yet found any behavioral or physiological indices that reliably differenti-ate high-reactive monkeys from their cohorts during baseline periods of stable group housing in familiar settings.

Thus, these patterns of individual differences among rhesus monkeys in their prototypical responses to challenge are quite similar to those re-ported for human infants and children, not only in terms of certain behav-ioral and physiological characteristics, but also in the general conditions in which such differences between subjects tend to be most pronounced. However, in both human children and rhesus monkeys the individual differences in response to challenge seem to disappear in familiar and nonthreatening situations.

## IV.  Factors Contributing to Individual Differences in Rhesus Monkey Reactivity

What is the underlying basis for the dramatic individual differences in behavioral and physiological responses to challenge shown by rhesus monkey infants, juveniles, and adolescents? What factors might contribute to the differences in reactivity that seem to be so ontogenically stable? The basic questions generated by these recent findings in rhesus monkeys are essentially the same as those raised by the human data regarding individual differences in reactivity—and the range of potential answers seems almost as broad. Most likely, multiple factors contribute to the individual differences observed to date in our rhesus monkey subjects. Prime candidates for major sources of influence include the caretaking and personality characteristics of the monkey infants' mothers and the subjects' own temperamental qualities—the same basic factors that routinely surface in discussions of the relevant human data.

Rhesus monkey mothers do not all rear their infants in identical fashion, and the relationships that these mothers establish with their respective infants can differ markedly in a number of respects. For example, not all mothers provide their infants with the same amount of milk, especially in feral environments, and some start weaning their infants to solid food earlier than do others (Altmann, 1980; Simpson, Simpson, Hooley, & Zunz, 1981). Rhesus monkey mothers also differ in the relative frequency and degree to which they physically restrain their infants and restrict their efforts to explore the environment early in life (e.g., Hinde & White, 1974; Simpson & Howe, in press). These efforts by the mothers may serve to buffer their offspring from at least some environmental stresses, so that differences in mothers' restraining activities might contribute to differences in their infants' early exposure to novelty and challenge.

Another difference in the characteristic maternal styles of rhesus monkey females that has attracted considerable attention in the primate literature concerns the frequency and intensity with which they physically reject and punish their offspring, especially around the time of weaning. All monkey mothers engage in this type of behavior at some point in the rearing of each infant, but there can be considerable variability in how early, how often, how severe, and for how long the punitive behavior is initiated and maintained by any one mother (e.g., Dienske & Metz, 1977; Hinde & White, 1974; Rosenblum, 1971; Suomi, 1976). While there have been disagreements in the literature regarding both the short- and long-term effects of maternal rejection and punishment on the infant's exploration of and interaction with its physical and social environment, virtually all investigators involved have agreed that differences in maternal punishment are likely to lead to differences in various aspects of the infant's subsequent social and emotional development (e.g., Arling & Harlow, 1967; Hinde, 1974; Jensen, Bobbitt, & Gordon, 1973; Kaufman & Rosenblum, 1969; Suomi, 1981). Moreover, the evidence to date suggests that after caring for their firstborn infants, rhesus monkey mothers become relatively consistent in the pattern of punishment they display toward subsequent offspring (Harlow, Harlow, Dodsworth, & Arling, 1966; Hinde & Spencer-Booth, 1971; Ruppenthal, Arling, Harlow, Sackett, & Suomi, 1976). Thus, individual mothers develop different characteristic styles in terms of their manner of rejecting and punishing offspring, and these differences can influence not only the mother–infant relationship itself but also the subsequent reactivity of the individual infants (cf. Stevenson-Hinde, Stillwell-Barnes, & Zunz, 1980; Suomi, 1983).

One other potential source of influence on observed infant reactivity attributable to differential characteristics of the infants' mothers lies in the mothers' own reactivity in the face of challenge. Stevenson-Hinde, Stillwell-Barnes, and Zunz (1980) reported that rhesus monkey females could be reliably classified by experienced observers according to a number of "personality" dimensions, including "anxious–confident" and "excitable–calm"; individual differences along comparable dimensions had previously been reported by Chamove, Eysenck, and Harlow (1972) for slightly younger rhesus monkeys. We have observed similar differences among our rhesus monkey mothers, especially following challenges such as short-term separation from offspring (Suomi, Mineka, & Delizio, 1983).

There are a number of ways in which a mother's distinctive reactivity to stress could affect not only her infant's own reactivity but also other aspects of its social-emotional development. The obvious prediction from most behaviorist perspectives is that offspring of high-reactive mothers should be more likely to develop high-reactive responses to novel and/or challenging environmental events than infants whose mothers displayed less extreme reactions to the same events. For example, infants of high-reactive mothers might be conditioned to react to certain events as a result of their mothers' predictable disruption following those specific events, whereas infants whose mothers failed to respond to the same events with equivalent behavioral and physiological disruption would be less likely to acquire a comparable CR to those events. Alternatively, infants of high-reactive mothers might model their mothers' characteristic responses to the same events, thus acquiring the pattern of extreme response to events that for infants of less reactive mothers remain essentially neutral. There are other plausible explanations that lead to the same general prediction. For example, neonates and infants might be unusually sensitive to the emotional (arousal) state of their mothers, with a tendency to ''match'' that state at the time (cf. Field, Woodson, Greenberg, & Cohen, 1982). In this case, a ''normal'' response to an extreme change in the mother's state of arousal would be an extreme change in the infant's emotional state at the time. On the other hand, infants with mothers who reacted to the same or similar circumstances with minimal changes in arousal would be less likely to show extreme reactions themselves if they were likewise ''matching'' their mothers' arousal levels at the time. Finally, high-reactive mothers should be more likely to rear high-reactive infants if this characteristic were highly heritable. In this case, the basis for the cross-generational similarity of relative reactivity would be genetic in nature, rather than through some sort of learning process.

In point of fact, an increasing body of evidence from our rhesus monkey breeding colony strongly suggests that relative reactivity in the face of challenge is indeed highly heritable. All of the rhesus monkey subjects whose reactivity has been assessed in our laboratory to date have come from the laboratory's breeding colony, so that for each of these subjects the identity of both its biologic mother and father are known. Furthermore, because monkeys in our breeding colony typically have spent most of their adult lives in circumstances promoting reproductive activities and, as in the wild, monogamy is clearly not the rule, most of these subjects have paternal half-sibs, maternal half-sibs, and occasionally full siblings whose relative reactivity has also been assessed, in many cases using the same measures obtained under the same experimental conditions in comparable physical and social settings. Comparisons between full siblings, half-sibs, and unrelated individuals have consistently shown that siblings and half-sibs are much more likely to share reactivity status than are individuals who are not close blood relatives. There is significantly less variability in levels of cortisol, ACTH, and both disturbance and coping behavioral patterns following challenge among siblings and half-sibs than among unrelated individuals (Scanlan, 1987; Scanlan, Suomi, Higley, Scallet, & Kraemer, 1982); similar results have been obtained using a measure of psychophysiological reactivity (Suomi, 1981).

Most of the comparisons between blood relatives have involved paternal half-sibs, largely because most breeding colony males have sired several offspring each year, while the interbirth interval for each female has never been less than 10–12 months, as in the wild. Nevertheless, findings to date do not suggest any major differences in concordance rate for the above measures of reactivity between paternal half-sibs and maternal half-sibs (there have been too few full siblings in these studies to make confident conclusions about their concordance rates relative to those of half-sibs). Some of these subjects were reared by their biologic mothers so that, as in most of the human studies reviewed earlier, genetic and maternal influences were confounded. However, in most of these cases paternal genetic contributions, shown to be substantial, were not confounded with the infants' caretaking experiences because the fathers were not present during rearing. More significantly, the majority of the monkey subjects whose reactivity we have studied longitudinally were separated from their mothers at birth and reared in identical fashion in the laboratory nursery, after which they were placed in social groups typically composed of like-reared peers who were not close relatives. Thus, for these subjects, genetic and environmental contributions have not been confounded, and it is among these subjects that the highest heritability ratios have been found.

An alternative strategy for evaluating the relative contributions of genetic and maternal factors to individual differences in reactivity involves the use of cross-fostering procedures in which infants of different genetic pedigree are not raised by their biologic mother but instead are foster-reared by unrelated multiparous females whose own reactivity and maternal style are known. This experimental strategy is currently being pursued in my laboratory.

## V.  A Cross-Fostering Experiment with Rhesus Monkey Infants of Differing Reactivity

This past year my graduate students at Wisconsin (Maribeth Champoux, J. D. Higley, James M. Scanlan, and Mary S. Schneider) and I followed the first cohort of rhesus monkey infants in a major cross-fostering longitudinal study from birth to 15 months of age. These infants were selected on the basis of their genetic pedigree in order to maximize individual differences in reactivity in the face of novelty or challenge. Half of the infants had biologic parents who in previous years had consistently produced offspring that throughout subsequent development exhibited extreme behavioral and physiological reactions to brief social separations and exposure to new environmental settings. The remaining infants in this cohort had parents whose previous offspring had generally displayed only mild reactions to similar or identical challenges at comparable ages. Put another way, half of the infants in this first cohort had older siblings and half-sibs who were highly reactive; the other half of the cohort had siblings and half-sibs who responded to environmental challenges with only moderate changes in their behavior and physiology. The majority of both subgroups among these previous offspring had been separated from their mothers at birth, reared in the laboratory nursery for their first month of life, then placed in groups of like-reared peers prior to most of these experimental challenges. Thus, the differences in reactivity displayed by these older siblings and half-sibs of the present infants could not be attributed to differential care by their biologic parents, because neither their mothers nor fathers took part in their rearing.

In the present cross-fostering study, both the high-reactive pedigree infants and those with less reactive relatives were separated from their biologic mothers within 96 hr of birth and immediately thereafter were introduced to their foster mothers. The foster mothers were selected on the basis of two dimensions: (1) their own relative reactivity in the face of earlier environmental challenges and (2) the patterns of maternal care they had displayed toward their own previous offspring, especially the frequency and duration of grooming behavior, on the one hand, and the relative incidence of rejecting and punishing behavior directed toward these offspring around the time of weaning, on the other hand. Half of the foster mothers could be characterized as high-reactive; the other half were more moderate in their typical responses to environmental challenge. In addition, half of the foster mothers ("nurturant" females) had displayed relatively high levels of grooming and extremely low levels of rejection and punishment of previous offspring. The remaining foster mothers ("punitive" females) had displayed much higher frequencies of rejecting and punitive behavior toward previous offspring, although these levels were not abnormally high (i.e., they were within 2 SD of mean levels for multiparous females in the laboratory breeding colony over the past decade). It should be pointed out that these two dimensions were essentially orthogonal to each other in that some high-reactive foster mothers were in the nurturant subgroup but others were in the punitive subgroup; the same was true for the less reactive foster mothers.

Unfortunately, for this first cohort in what will be a large, long-term cross-fostering study, there were not enough infants and foster mothers to fill all cells of the $2 \times 2 \times 2$ (Infant Reactivity $\times$ Foster Mother Reactivity $\times$ Foster Mother Maternal Style) design matrix for the long-term project, which is one major reason why we are currently following additional cohorts longitudinally. Nevertheless, although in the present cohort some cells in the $2 \times 2 \times 2$ matrix were empty and others contained only a single foster mother–infant dyad, it was still possible to make independent comparisons between dyads in which the infant was high versus moderately reactive, between dyads in which the foster mother was high versus moderately reactive, and between dyads in which the foster mother was relatively nurturant versus punitive.

In all dyads, the infants were first introduced to their respective foster mothers within 4 days of their own birth and within 7 days of the foster mothers' delivery of their own biologic infants, after which each dyad was subsequently housed as a pair in single caging units in a colony housing room. Here they were maintained without any experimental interruption for the next 6 months, with two exceptions. First, every infant was separated from its foster mother for a 20-min period once a week during its first month of life in order to be assessed on Schneider's (1984) neonatal test battery, after which time it was weighed and returned to its foster mother in its home cage. Second, each mother–infant dyad was observed for two 10-min periods 5 days per week throughout the infant's first 6 months of life. During these unobtrusive observation periods, the frequencies and durations of behaviors encompassed by an exhaustive category scoring system (described in detail by Suomi et al., 1983) were recorded for both the infants and their foster mothers.

Analysis of the neonatal test battery scores yielded a number of significant differences between high-reactive infants and their less reactive counterparts, which are summarized in the left-hand panel of Fig. 1. Over the first month of life, high-reactive infants achieved lower orienting scores, had somewhat ($p < .1$) poorer muscle tonus and were somewhat less advanced in their motor reflex patterns, displayed significantly greater degrees of behavioral inhibition, and had lower mean Prechtl state scores than the infants whose biologic parents had not produced high-reactive infants in previous years of breeding. These differences were consistent with earlier findings of differential neonatal test scores for high-versus low-reactive infants in the colony, including both those who had been raised by their biologic parents and those who had been hand-reared in the laboratory's neonatal nursery (e.g., Schneider, Suomi, Marra, Higley, & Brogan, 1984). In this respect, it appears that the selection of the present infants for the two experimental groups (high- vs. moderately reactive) on the basis of genetic pedigree was quite successful.

On the other hand, the status of these infants' foster mothers, both in terms of the foster mother's own reactivity and in terms of their relative maternal style, was not reflected in the infants' performance on the neonatal test battery. The center panel of Fig. 1 compares the scores of infants with high-reactive foster mothers with those of infants with moderately reactive foster mothers. No significant differences were disclosed on any neonatal measures except for muscle tonus, in which the infants with high-reactive foster mothers actually displayed better scores on average than those with moderately reactive foster mothers. Similarly, as indicated by the right-hand panel of Fig. 1, there were no significant differences in average neonatal test battery scores between infants whose foster mothers had displayed a more punitive maternal style toward their own previous offspring and those who had been more nurturant toward

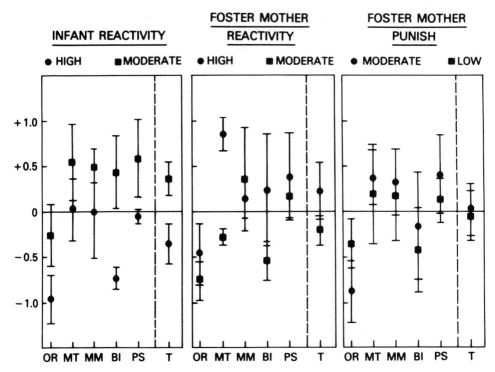

**Fig. 1.** Mean (+/− 1 SEM) Z-score values for five components of the rhesus monkey neonatal test battery (Schneider, 1984) plus a total composite score. Values are averaged over the four weekly test sessions during the infants' first month of life. Panel on the left plots infant scores grouped by infant reactivity pedigree (high-reactive vs. moderately reactive). The center panel plots infant scores grouped by foster mother reactivity (high vs. moderate). The panel on right plots infant scores grouped by foster mother caretaking style (moderately punitive vs. low-punitive). The ordinate is scaled in Z-score values derived from the population of both mother-reared and nursery-reared infants born in the laboratory colony 1982–1984. Abbreviations (on the abscissa) for components of neonatal test battery are as follows: OR, orienting responses; MT, muscle tonus; MM, motor maturity; BI, behavioral inhibition (high scores designate low behavioral inhibition); PS, predominant Prechtl state; T, total composite score.

previous infants. Thus, the genetic pedigree of the infants was a more powerful predictor of individual differences on these neonatal measures than were different characteristics of these infants' foster mothers.

In contrast, the genetic pedigrees of the infants were of little or no use in predicting differences in the infants' behaviors while in their home cages with their foster mothers throughout their first 6 months of life. Both high- and moderately reactive infants displayed initial levels and patterns of developmental change in mutual ventral contact with their foster mothers, in locomotion and exploration about their home cages, and in levels of self-directed "disturbance" behavior that were all well within the normative range of scores for the same behaviors shown by other rhesus monkey infants reared by their biologic mothers in dyad cages in our laboratory over the past decade. Indeed, as shown in the top panel of Fig. 2, infants with high-reactive pedigrees actually displayed slightly lower levels of ventral contact ($p < .10$) and higher levels of locomotion and exploration by 5–6 months of age than did their less reactive counterparts, exactly the opposite of what one would predict on the basis of the infants' relative reactivity alone (the pedigree differences in self-directed behavior at 3–4 and 5–6 months did not achieve statistical significance). Moreover, there were no significant differences in levels of any behavioral categories over the first 6 months between infants with high-reactive foster mothers and those whose foster mothers were less reactive. These results are illustrated in the center panel of Fig. 2.

On the other hand, there were significant differences in the infants' behavioral scores associated with the different caretaking styles of their foster mothers. Examination of the behavioral scores of the foster mothers revealed that the females classified as "punitive" rejected or punished their present adopted infants over three times as frequently as did the foster mothers classified as "nurturant" (there was no overlap between the two groups), but over the 6-month period, nurturant females groomed their foster infants twice as frequently as did the punitive females. Thus, in terms of caretaking styles displayed toward the present adopted infants, both groups of foster mothers were basically consistent with the caretaking patterns they had shown in rearing their own infants in previous years. Such differences were not without apparent consequences for the foster infants. As indicated in the lower panel of Fig. 2, infants with punitive mothers exhibited less ventral contact (during Months 3–4 and 5–6), more locomotion and exploration away from their mothers (during Months 1–2 and 3–4), and higher levels of self-directed disturbance (during Months 5–6) than did infants with more nurturant foster mothers, although all scores were well within the normative range of values for mother-reared infants in the laboratory. These differences essentially replicated findings from other laboratories comparing the behavioral development of macaque infants reared by mothers displaying different characteristic maternal styles (e.g., Berman, 1982; Hinde & Spencer-Booth, 1967; Hinde & White, 1974; Jensen *et al.*, 1973).

Thus, at least for the present infants, differences in reactivity attributable to differences in genetic pedigree were apparently of little or no consequence for their behavioral development under conditions of stable housing in familiar settings and in the presence of competent caretakers.

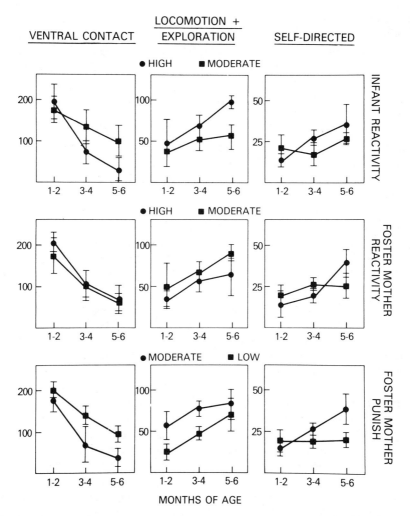

**Fig. 2.** Mean durations in seconds (+/− 1 SEM) of infant behaviors during the cross-fostering period. The top panel plots values grouped by infant reactivity pedigree, the center panel plots values grouped by foster mother reactivity, and the lower panel plots values grouped by foster mother maternal style.

To what degree the relative absence of developmental differences between high- and moderately reactive infants could be attributed to the ability of their foster mothers to buffer them from environmental challenges or to the relatively benign and stable nature of their rearing environments cannot readily be determined from these data alone. Nevertheless, it is noteworthy that under these rearing conditions, the most effective factor for predicting differences among the infants in their behavioral development was neither their own reactivity status nor that of their foster mothers but, rather, the differences in caretaking styles of the foster mothers.

Dramatically different results were obtained when, beginning at 6 months of age, these infants were separated from their foster mothers for four 4-day periods, interspersed between 3-day reunions back in the home cages. During separations, these young rhesus monkeys displayed reactions essentially consistent with that suggested by their respective genetic pedigrees. Infants whose biologic parents had previously produced high-reactive offspring consistently responded to the present separations with significantly greater behavioral and physiological disruption than did their cohorts with less reactive pedigrees. The top panel of Fig. 3 contrasts the mean separation levels of self-directed disturbance behavior, coping activities, incidence of passivity, and plasma cortisol displayed by infants of high-reactive pedigrees with those of their moderately reactive counterparts. It is apparent from the figure that the high-reactive pedigree subjects exhibited significantly more disturbance behavior, less coping activity, longer periods of passivity, and higher levels of plasma cortisol. Thus, during separation from their foster mothers, these high-reactive infants reverted back to their presumed biologic predispositions. In contrast, under identical conditions of separation, none of the infants predicted by pedigree to be only moderately reactive to environmental challenges actually displayed extreme reactions, either behavioral or physiological. Comparisons of separation reactions in the present subjects on the basis of the relative reactivity of their foster mothers, or on the basis of the foster mothers' maternal styles, failed to yield differences as dramatic, although they were generally in the direction one might well predict given the foster mothers' reactivity status or maternal style.

On the other hand, during periods of reunion between each separation, the infants' relative reactivity no longer was predictive of differences in levels of any categories of behavior. Figure 4 presents mean levels of mutual ventral contact, locomotion and exploration (coping), and self-directed disturbance during pairs of reunion periods and after the final separation and reunion period (postseparation). Reactive and nonreactive infants clung to their foster mothers for equivalent durations during reunions, they displayed similar amounts of coping activity, and the appearance of self-directed disturbance was not dramatically different in the two groups of infants. Thus, in the presence of their foster mothers, reactivity differences between these infants all but disappeared, even though major differences were exhibited just before and right after each reunion, that is, during the periods of separation. It appeared that the

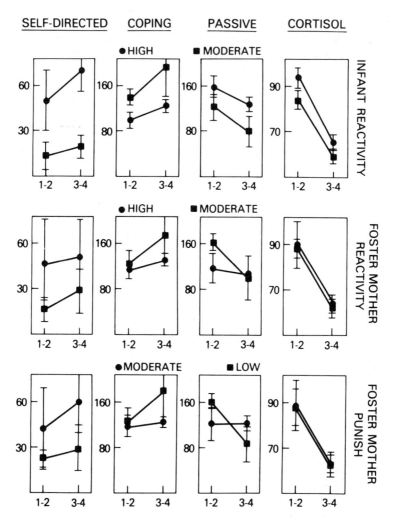

**Fig. 3.** Mean values (+/− 1 SEM) of infants' scores during separation periods. Scores are durations (in seconds) per 5-min observation period for self-directed, coping, and passive categories of behavior, and micrograms per deciliter for plasma cortisol collected 2 hr after the start of each separation. The top panel plots values grouped by infant reactivity pedigree, the center panel plots values grouped by foster mother reactivity, and the lower panel plots values grouped by foster mother maternal style.

availability and/or activities of the foster mothers overrode the different reactive tendencies of the infants.

Indeed, there was some evidence that the foster mothers contributed directly to the few major differences between individual infants in behavioral levels during reunions. This was most evident in infant levels of self-

LOCOMOTION +
**VENTRAL CONTACT          EXPLORATION          SELF-DIRECTED**

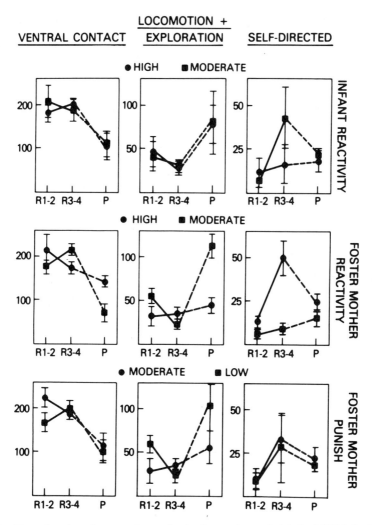

**Fig. 4.** Mean durations (in seconds) per 5-min observation period (+/− 1 SEM) for infant behaviors during reunion periods and over the 1-month period immediately following final separation and reunion. R1–2 = mean durations during first and second reunions, R3–4 = mean durations during third and fourth reunions, and P = mean durations during the 1-month postseparation period. The top panel plots values grouped by infant reactivity pedigree, the center panel plots values grouped by foster mother reactivity, and the lower panel plots values grouped by foster mother maternal style.

directed disturbance behavior. The highest levels of disturbance, especially during the third and fourth reunion periods, were shown by infants with high-reactive foster mothers. One factor almost certainly contributing to these differences derived from the behaviors of the foster mothers during the reunion periods as well as during the separations. High-reactive mothers, true to their subgroup assignment, displayed manyfold higher levels of self-directed disturbance behavior during separations than did the rest of the foster mothers, consistent with their reactions to previous separations experienced earlier in life. Their excessive levels of self-directed behavior carried over into the reunion periods, especially after the later separations. During these reunion periods, their foster infants also displayed their highest levels of self-directed behavior, although its incidence dropped to baseline levels during the postseparation period, as did the incidence of self-directed behavior in the high-reactive foster mothers.

When each infant was 9 months old, it was permanently separated from its foster mother and placed in a group of same-aged peers, some of whom had been reared by their biologic mothers, some of whom had been nursery reared and had since lived with like-reared peers, and the rest of whom had been reared by foster mothers. The present subjects have remained in these groups to this day, and we are continuing to study them longitudinally. Not surprisingly, virtually all of the high-reactive infants were relatively slow to adjust to their new situation, but having passed this initial period of adaptation, most of them are thriving in their new surroundings. Indeed, a few high-reactive subjects have since established strong ties with some older adults ("foster grandparents") who were recently added to some of these peer groups, and those particular high-reactive monkeys have become dominant over their less reactive peers. It is interesting that every one of these now-dominant high-reactive individuals had a nurturant foster mother. By way of contrast, the one high-reactive subject who also had a punitive and high-reactive foster mother is at the very bottom of the dominancy hierarchy of its group—but its low-reactive counterpart who also had a punitive and high-reactive mother now holds a much higher rank. These individual cases serve as reminders that knowledge of both an individual monkey's reactivity pedigree and the details of its rearing experiences and previous partners can be more useful in predicting and understanding its present situation than consideration of either factor by itself.

## VI.  Conclusions

The results from this rhesus monkey cross-fostering study are admittedly somewhat limited at this point in the larger long-term project of which it is a part. Nevertheless, they do provide some insights into efforts to determine the basis for observed differences in reactivity and into other aspects of an infant's emerging behavioral repertoire. The present data showed that differences in infant pedigree, in maternal reactivity, and in maternal caretaking style were each associated with specific patterns of intersubject variability in behavior and physiology displayed by rhesus monkey infants, but at different times during development and under different environmental circumstances. More interestingly, the particular patterns of influence associated with infant reactivity, foster mother reactivity, and foster mother caretaking style appeared to be systematic and conditionally predictable.

Thus under familiar, stable, and generally nonstressful circumstances, an infant's patterns of behavioral development were better predicted by the style of caretaking it received than by knowledge of its genetic pedigree or its caretaker's temperamental characteristics. However, when separated from its mother or foster mother, and therefore not only facing an environmental challenge but also no longer subject to the direct behavioral influence of its caretaker, the infant's characteristic behavioral and physiological responses were best predicted by knowledge of its genetic pedigree with respect to reactivity. When the infant was returned to its caretaker, but still under stomewhat stressful environmental circumstances, the reactivity status of the caretaker became the predominant influence on the infant's behavioral activity at the time, apparently overriding both infant reactivity and caretaking style factors. In a nutshell, these findings suggest that rhesus monkey infant reactivity most likely has a genetic basis that is clearly expressed under conditions of challenge but that is largely irrelevant in the absence of challenge and that can be overridden—even under stressful conditions—by the behavioral reactions of its caretaker, especially when the caretaker is physically present.

Thus, some factors attributable to nature and others to nurture appeared to be contributing to the individual differences in behavior and physiology displayed by the present monkey subjects, but in different ways and to differing degrees under different circumstances during their first 15 months of life. In this respect, no one factor—whether derived from nature or from nurture—served as "best predictor" across all situations for any of the many measures collected throughout the study. Instead, the observed individual differences seemed to be subject to multiple influences, some more powerful under certain conditions and/or during specific periods of development than others.

While the present cross-fostering data point to specific areas of influence attributable to each of the three factors experimentally manipulated during this study, they do not begin to reveal how these factors might interact and/or "transact" during the process of behavioral and physiological development. The limited number of foster mother–infant dyads studied to date precludes statistical evaluation of possible interactions between these variables. We do not yet know, for example, if high-reactive infants are less likely to exhibit severe separation reactions as a function of their caretakers' own reactivity and/or maternal style, or if moderately reactive infants' apparent resistance to severe separation reactions could be compromised by characteristics of their respective caretakers. These questions, and others like them, are being directly addressed in the larger, long-term longitudinal study of which the present data are merely a small initial component.

At any rate, it seems clear that both theoretical and empirical efforts to predict and understand individual differences in reactivity—be they monkey or human—must go beyond simple models and single-factor experimental designs if they are to realistically address the basic developmental issues at hand. These issues tend to become more complex with increasing scrutiny. Nevertheless, the discovery of such complexity in developmental phenomena should not discourage efforts to account for developmental diversity in our own and other primate species. Instead, recognition of ontogenic complexity should serve as a challenge to developmental researchers—one that most likely will generate marked individual differences in their respective responses to this scientific challenge.

## Acknowledgments

My colleagues in the rhesus monkey research described in this chapter are numerous and have ranged from senior research scientists to undergraduate student testers. They include the following individuals: Craig M. Baysinger, Virginia Burkes, Evan Byrne, Maribeth Champoux, Roberta D. Delizio, Wendi Erhman, Kristi Guzzonato, Dr. J. D. Higley, Regina M. Hirsch, William D. Hopkins, Dr. Gary W. Kraemer, Dr. Markku Linnoila, Lauren M. Marra, Sheryl A. Orman, Dr. A. S. Scallet, James M. Scanlan, Mary L. Schneider, Julie Sykes, and William Thompson.

## References

Altmann, J. (1980). *Baboon mothers and infants*. Cambridge: Harvard University Press.
Arling, G. L., & Harlow, H. F. (1967). Effects of social deprivation on maternal behavior of rhesus monkeys. *Journal of Comparative and Physiological Psychology, 64*, 371–377.
Berman, C. M. (1982). The ontogeny of social relationships with group comparisons among free-ranging infant rhesus monkeys: I. Social networks and differentiation. *Animal Behaviour, 30*, 149–162.
Carey, W. B. (1970). A simplified method for measuring infant temperament. *Journal of Pediatrics, 77*, 188–194.

Chamove, A. S., Eysenck, H. J., & Harlow, H. F. (1972). Personality in monkeys: Factor analyses of rhesus social behavior. *Quarterly Journal of Experimental Psychology, 24,* 496–504.

Daniels, D., & Plomin, R. (1985). Origins of individual differences in shyness. *Developmental Psychology, 21,* 118–121.

Dienske, H., & Metz, J. A. J. (1977). Mother–infant body contact in macaques: A time interval analysis. *Biology of Behaviour, 2,* 3–13.

Field, T. J., Woodson, R., Greenberg, R., & Cohen, D. (1982). Discrimination and imitation of facial expression by neonates. *Science, 218,* 179–181.

Garcia-Coll, C., Kagan, J., & Resnick, J. S. (1984). Behavioral inhibition in young children. *Child Development, 55,* 1005–1019.

Guzzonato, K., Beattie, J., & Delizio, R. D. (1985). *The effect of early rearing conditions on the imipramine treatment of adolescent rhesus monkeys* [Poster]. Presented at the biennial meeting of the Society for Research in Child Development, Toronto.

Harlow, H. F., Harlow, M. K., Dodsworth, R. O., & Arling, G. L. (1966). Maternal behavior of rhesus monkeys deprived of mothering and peer associations in infancy. *Proceedings of the American Philosophical Society, 110,* 58–66.

Higley, J. D. (1985). *Continuity of social separation behaviors from infancy to adolescence in rhesus monkeys (Macaca mulatta).* Unpublished doctoral dissertation, University of Wisconsin–Madison.

Hinde, R. A. (1974). *Biological basis of social behavior.* New York: Academic Press.

Hinde, R. A., & Spencer-Booth, Y. (1967). The behaviour of socially living rhesus monkeys in their first two and a half years. *Animal Behaviour, 15,* 169–196.

Hinde, R. A., & Spencer-Booth, Y. (1971). Effects of brief separations from mothers on rhesus monkeys. *Science 173,* 111–118.

Hinde, R. A., & White, L. E. (1974). The dynamics of a relationship. *Journal of Comparative and Physiological Psychology, 86,* 8–23.

Jensen, G. D., Bobbitt, R. A., & Gordon, B. N. (1973). Mothers' and infants' roles in the development of independence in *Macaca nemestrina. Primates, 14,* 79–88.

Kagan, J. (1982). Heart rate and heart rate variability as signs of temperamental dimension in infants. In C. E. Izard (Ed.), *Measuring emotions in infants and young children* (pp. 36–66). New York: Cambridge University Press.

Kagan, J., & Moss, H. A. (1962). *Birth to maturity.* New York: Wiley.

Kagan, J., Reznick, J. S., Clarke, C., Snidman, N., & Garcia-Coll, C. (1984). Behavioral inhibition to the unfamiliar. *Child Development, 55,* 2212–2225.

Kagan, J., Reznick, S., & Snidman, N. (1987). Temperamental variation in response to the unfamiliar. In N. A. Krasnegor, E. M. Blass, M. A. Hofer, & W. P. Smotherman (Eds.), *Perinatal development: A psychobiological perspective.* Orlando: Academic Press.

Kaufman, I. C., & Rosenblum, L. A. (1969). The waning of the mother–infant bond in two species of macaque. In B. M. Foss (Ed.), *Determinants of infant behaviour* (Vol. 4, pp. 41–59). London: Methuen.

Matheny, A. P., Wilson, R. S., Dolan, A. M., & Krantz, J. Z. (1981). Behavioral contrasts in twinships: Stability and patterns of differences in childhood. *Child Development, 52,* 579–588.

Plomin, R., & Rowe, D. C. (1979). Genetic and environmental etiology of social behavior in infancy. *Developmental Psychology, 15,* 62–72.

Rosenblum, L. A. (1971). The ontogeny of mother–infant relations in macaques. In H. Moltz (Ed.), *The ontogeny of vertebrate behavior* (pp. 315–368). New York: Academic Press.

Ruppenthal, G. C., Arling, G. L., Harlow, H. F., Sackett, G. P., & Suomi, S. J. (1976). A 10-year perspective of motherless mother monkey behavior. *Journal of Abnormal Psychology, 85,* 341–345.

Scanlan, J. M. (1986). *The inheritance of social dominance in rhesus monkeys.* Unpublished doctoral dissertation data, University of Wisconsin–Madison.

Scanlan, J. M., Suomi, S. J., Higley, J. D., Scallet, A. S., & Kraemer, G. W. (1982). Stress and heredity in adrenocortical response in rhesus monkeys (*Macaca mulatta*). *Society for Neurosciences Abstracts, 8,* 461–462.

Schneider, M. L. (1984). *Neonatal assessment of rhesus monkeys.* Unpublished master's thesis, University of Wisconsin–Madison.

Schneider, M. L., Suomi, S. J., Marra, L. M., Higley, J. D., & Brogan, N. (1984). *Neonatal behaviors as predictors of psychobiological response to stress in rhesus monkeys.* Paper presented at the Fourth Biennial Conference on Infant Studies, New York.

Simpson, M. J. A., & Howe, S. (in press). Changes in the rhesus mother–infant relationship through the first four months of life. *Animal Behaviour.*

Simpson, M. J. A., Simpson, A. E., Hooley, J., & Zunz, M. (1981). Infant-related influences on birth intervals in rhesus monkeys. *Nature, 290,* 49–51.

Sroufe, L. A. (1979). The coherence of individual development. *American Psychologist, 34,* 834–841.

Sroufe, L. A. (1984). Infant–caregiver attachment and patterns of adaptation in preschool: The roots of maladaption and competence. In M. Perlmutter (Ed.), *Minnesota symposium in child psychology* (Vol. 16, pp. 41–84). Hillsdale, NJ: Erlbaum.

Sroufe, L. A., Fox, N. E., & Pancake, V. R. (1983). Attachment and dependency in developmental perspective. *Child Development, 54,* 1335–1354.

Stevenson-Hinde, J., Stillwell-Barnes, R., & Zunz, M. (1980). Subjective assessment of rhesus monkeys over four successive years. *Primates, 21,* 66–82.

Suomi, S. J. (1976). Mechanisms underlying social development: A re-examination of mother–infant interactions in monkeys. In A. Pick (Ed.), *Minnesota Symposium on Child Psychology* (Vol. 10, pp. 201–230). Minneapolis: University of Minnesota Press.

Suomi, S. J. (1981). Genetic, maternal, and environmental influences on social development in rhesus monkeys. In A. B. Chiarelli & R. S. Corruccini (Eds.), *Primate behavior and sociobiology* (pp. 81–87). Heidelburg: Springer-Verlag.

Suomi, S. J. (1983). Social development in rhesus monkeys: Consideration of individual differences. In A. Oliverio & M. Zappella (Eds.), *The behavior of human infants* (pp. 71–92). New York: Plenum.

Suomi, S. J., Higley, J. D., Kraemer, G. W., & Linnoila, M. (1987). Manuscript in preparation.

Sumoi, S. J., Mineka, S., & Delizio, R. D. (1983). Short- and long-term effects of repetitive mother–infant separations on social development in rhesus monkeys. *Developmental Psychology, 19,* 770–786.

Tennes, K. (1982). The role of hormones in mother–infant transactions. In R. N. Emde & R. J. Harmon (Eds.), *Development of attachment and affiliative systems.* New York: Plenum.

Thomas, A., Chess, S., & Birch, H. G. (1968). *Temperament and behavior disorders in children.* New York: New York University Press.

Thomas, A., Chess, S., & Korn, S. J. (1982). The reality of difficult temperament. *Merrill-Palmer Quarterly, 28,* 1–20.

West, M. J., & King, J. A. (in press). Settling nature and nurture into an ontogenic nich. *Developmental Psychobiology.*

Wilson, R. S., & Matheny, A. P. (1983). Assessment of temperament in infant twins. *Developmental Psychology, 19,* 172–183.

# 19

## Temperamental Variation in Response to the Unfamiliar

JEROME KAGAN, J. STEVEN REZNICK,
and NANCY SNIDMAN
*Department of Psychology*
*Harvard University*
*Cambridge, Massachusetts 02138*

## I. Introduction

The relation between biologic processes and behavioral systems assumes three major forms in contemporary research. The first is illustrated by the effects of specific environmental manipulations on neural structures and their related behaviors. The changes in the distribution of neurons and in discriminatory capacities of kittens that follow early occlusion of one eye provide a well-known example (Hubel & Wiesel, 1965). A second class of investigation seeks correlations between the time of emergence of behavioral milestones in juvenile organisms and changes in the CNS (Bateson, 1978; Goldman-Rakic, 1981). A third domain of inquiry involves study of intraspecific covariation in particular behavioral and biologic characteristics. In children these covariations have acquired the adjective *temperamental*. The current interest in temperamental qualities is attributable, in part, to the pioneering work of Thomas and Chess (1977) and, in part, to recent discoveries in behavioral physiology, psychopharmacology, and behavioral genetics.

Of the many candidates for status as temperamental variables, the initial tendency to approach or to avoid unfamiliar people, contexts, and objects appears to be the most viable (Goldsmith & Campos, 1985). Although individual differences in the probability of approach to or withdrawal from unfamiliar events are subtle before 7 months of age, such

Perinatal Development:
A Psychobiological Perspective

**421**

differences are unambiguous by the middle of the 2nd year. It is easy to distinguish between those 18-month-old infants who become quiet and wary and those who approach an unfamiliar adult quickly and with positive affect. The situations that reveal these individual differences best during the 2nd year are unfamiliar persons, contexts, and objects. Many investigators have found that these behavioral differences can be preserved from late infancy to the preschool and early school years and from early to late childhood (Moskowitz, Schwartzman, & Ledingham, 1985; Backteman & Magnusson, 1981; Elder, Liker, & Cross, 1984; Coie & Dodge, 1983; G. W. Bronson, 1970; G. W. Bronson & Pankey, 1977; W. C. Bronson, 1981; Emmerich, 1964). On occasion, these differences persist into adolescence and adulthood, where they can assume the form of caution and social introversion, in contrast to spontaneity and extraversion (Kagan & Moss, 1962; Waldrop & Halverson, 1975).

Follow-up investigations of clinical cases also reveal modest preservation into adulthood of extreme forms of withdrawal behavior in childhood. A group of 66 children diagnosed as school phobic when they were between 4 and 11 years of age were assessed by a psychiatrist when they were 12–21 years old. About one quarter of the group had no symptoms and were regarded by the clinician as well adjusted. Although another 40% were no longer phobic, these adults displayed one or more other symptoms, including poor school achievement and dependency upon others. An additional one third of the original group was still extremely anxious (Coolidge, Brodie, & Feeney, 1964). As might be expected, extremely shy, phobic, or withdrawn children are likely, as adults, to select bureaucratic jobs with minimal risk (Morris, Soroker, & Burruss, 1954).

Although the modest preservation of these two classes of behavior does not require the assumption of any biologic influence, recent research implicates genetic factors. Studies of monozygotic and dizygotic twins—infants, adolescents, and adults—reveal that the psychological characteristics with the best evidence for heritability appear to be related to approach or withdrawal from the unfamiliar. For example, examiners rated, six times between 3 and 24 months-of-age, the test behavior of a large number of twins growing up in the same homes. Factor analysis revealed a factor labeled timidity and inhibition which showed evidence of heritability at 6, 12, and 24 months-of-age (Matheny, 1980). In a similar investigation, behavioral ratings were made on 350 twin pairs at 8 months and 4 and 7 years (Goldsmith & Gottesman, 1981). Differences in fearfulness, which were most evident in reluctance to separate from the mother at 7 years of age, were among the most heritable of the behavioral variables, especially for boys. Indeed, the difference in intraclass correlation between monozygotic and dizygotic 7-year-old twins was greater for fearfulness than for IQ score at 4 years of age. Finally, the heritability of the social introversion score on the Minnesota Multiphasic Personality Inventory (MMPI) in adolescent twin pairs, which is likely to be a developmental derivative of extreme withdrawal in childhood, was the highest of the MMPI scales, especially for male twins (Gottesman, 1963; see also Eaves & Eysenck, 1975; Loehlin, 1982).

## II.  Longitudinal Study

Our laboratory has been following two independent groups of Caucasian children, middle- and working-class, who were selected at either 21 or 31 months to be timid and cautious (inhibited) or socially outgoing and bold (uninhibited) when exposed to unfamiliar rooms, people, and objects. Classification into one of the two groups required that the child show consistent withdrawal from or approach to a variety of incentives. We screened over 400 children to find initial groups of 60 behaviorally inhibited and 60 behaviorally uninhibited children, with equal numbers of boys and girls in each group. It may not be a coincidence that when German kindergarten teachers in Munich were asked to select only those children who were extremely shy, only 15% of the total school population of 1,100 was chosen—about the same proportion we found in our screening (Cranach, Grote-Dahm, Huffner, Marte, Reisbeck, & Mittelstadt, 1978).

The index of inhibited or uninhibited behavior in Cohort 1 seen initially at 21 months was based on the child's behavior with an unfamiliar female examiner, unfamiliar toys, a woman displaying a trio of acts that were difficult to recall, a metal robot, and temporary separation from the mother. The signs of behavioral inhibition were long latencies to interact with or retreat from the unfamiliar people or objects, clinging to the mother, and cessation of play or vocalization. The uninhibited children showed the opposite profile. They approached the unfamiliar quickly, rarely played close to their mothers, and talked early and frequently.

The original index of inhibited behavior in Cohort 2 seen at 31 months was based primarily on behavior with an unfamiliar peer of the same sex and age and secondarily on behavior with an unfamiliar woman. The indexes of inhibition were similar to those used with Cohort 1—long latencies to interact with the child, adult, or toys; retreat from the unfamiliar events; and long periods of time proximal to the mother. Each of our two longitudinal samples has been seen on two additional occasions since the original selection, the latest being at 5½ years of age with about 10% attrition in the samples (see Garcia-Coll, Kagan, & Reznick, 1984;

Kagan, Reznick, Clarke, Snidman, & Garcia-Coll, 1984; Reznick, Kagan, Snidman, Gersten, Baak, & Rosenberg, 1986; Snidman, 1984). At 4 years of age for Cohort 1 and at 3½ years for Cohort 2, the indexes of inhibition were based primarily on behavior with an unfamiliar child of the same sex and age. At 5½ years of age, the index was based more broadly on behavior with an unfamiliar peer in a laboratory setting, in a school setting, with an examiner in a testing situation, and in a room that contained unfamiliar objects mildly suggestive of risk (a balance beam, a black box with a hole). An aggregate index of inhibition for Cohort 1 was a mean standard score across the separate situations presumed to index an inhibited disposition. (The analyses of the data for Cohort 2 are not yet complete.)

The behaviors that characterize inhibited and uninhibited children were preserved from the original assessment to the later assessments at 4 and 5½ years of age. The correlation for Cohort 1 between the index of inhibition at 21 months and the aggregate index at 5½ years was .52 ($p <$ .001). The correlation between the indexes at age 4 and 5½ was .67 (see Table I). One of the scores in the aggregate index at 5½ years was derived from observation of each child in his or her kindergarten during the 1st week of school. An observer who did not know the child's prior classification noted every 15 s the occurrence of a small number of variables reflecting the child's physical proximity to other children and social interaction with them. The children classified as inhibited at 21 months were more often isolated from their peers and not in any form of social interaction. The correlation between the index of inhibition at 21 months and low sociability during the 1st week of kindergarten was .39 ($p < .05$) (Gersten, 1986).

However, there was more obvious preservation of uninhibited than inhibited behavior in both cohorts. This asymmetry in stability is reasonable because American parents, reflecting the values of their society, regard bold, sociable behavior as more adaptive than shy, timid behavior. About 40% of the original groups of inhibited children became much less inhibited at 5½ years, although none was as spontaneous as the average uninhibited child. By contrast, less than 10% of the uninhibited children became more timid. There was, however, a gender asymmetry in the direction of change. More boys than girls changed from inhibited to uninhibited, while the small number of uninhibited children who became more inhibited were usually girls from working-class families. This pattern is in accord with the supposition that a proportion of working-class American parents value an obedient, quiet daughter, a standard less common among middle-class families of daughters or sons.

**Table I**

The Stability of Behavioral Inhibition, Heart Period, and Heart Period Variability across Three Assessments (Cohort 1)

| Dependent variables | 21-month variables | | | 4-year variables | | |
|---|---|---|---|---|---|---|
| | Index of inhibition | Heart Period[a] | Heart period variability | Index of inhibition | Heart period | Heart period variability |
| Age 4 | | | | | | |
| Index of inhibited behavior | .51** | -.12 | .15 | — | — | — |
| Heart period | -.47** | .23 | .29* | -.33* | — | — |
| Heart period variability | -.36* | .12 | .49** | -.39** | .77*** | — |
| Age 5½ | | | | | | |
| Index of inhibited behavior | .52*** | .03 | -.06 | .67*** | -.39** | -.39** |
| Heart period | -.44** | .15 | .19 | -.46*** | .58*** | .54*** |
| Heart period variability | -.39** | .11 | .39** | -.44** | .44** | .64*** |

[a] A higher heart period reflects a lower heart rate.
* $p < .05$.
** $p < .01$.
*** $p < .001$.

There are more inhibited children who are later born rather than first-born—about two thirds of the group—and more uninhibited children who are firstborn—a result affirmed by Snow, Jacklin, and Maccoby (1981). We interpret this fact to mean that later born status may represent a chronic stress for those infants who are born with a biologic disposition to be inhibited, but not for the average infant who does not begin life with this temperamental quality.

Because any behavioral surface can be the result of different mediating processes, the reasonableness of the argument that claims a biologic influence on inhibition requires evidence suggesting that more inhibited than uninhibited children display some peripheral physiological signs that might be interpreted as reflecting altered thresholds of excitability in those parts of the CNS that normally respond to novelty and challenge. These include the sympathetic nervous system, the reticular activating system, and the hypothalamic-pituitary-adrenal axis. Because we quantified the child's heart rate and heart rate variability at every assessment, we are able to make the firmest statement about these two parameters which are influenced, in part, by sympathetic activity.

## A.  Heart Rate and Variability

Heart rate and heart rate variability, which in our data are always negatively correlated under both relaxed conditions and mild cognitive stress (correlations between $-.6$ and $-.7$), are under the joint influence of sympathetic and parasympathetic activity, with sympathetic discharge making a greater contribution to cardiac acceleration and parasympathetic activity a greater contribution to cardiac deceleration (Chess, Tam, & Calaresu, 1975; Porges, McCabe, & Yongue, 1982; Porges & Raskin, 1969). Inhibited children had higher and more stable heart rates than uninhibited children at every age of evaluation, with the magnitude of the correlation between behavior and cardiac profile higher at 5½ years than at 21 months. Further, differences in heart rate and heart rate variability in Cohort 1 were preserved across the period from 4 to 5½ years, while differences in variability were preserved from 21 months to 5½ years (see Table I). More important, the inhibited children who had consistently higher and more stable heart rates over the first two assessments were more likely to remain inhibited than the inhibited children who had lower and more variable heart rates. The former children were significantly more inhibited with the unfamiliar peer at 5½ years and had more unusual contemporary fears. Additionally, more of these children had one or more of the following symptoms during infancy: chronic constipation, allergy, extreme irritability, or sleeplessness. These data imply that inhibited children with high and stable hearts rates are under high sympathetic arousal. This conclusion is supported by spectral analyses of heart rate data. Respiration exerts the major influence on heart rate variability, especially at rest, and this variability, called respiratory sinus arrhythmia, is mediated primarily by vagal activity (Katona & Jih, 1975). Variations in blood pressure and temperature regulation, which can affect heart variability and whose cycles are at lower frequencies than respiratory rate, are monitored by sympathetic activity, even when parasympathetic activity remains unchanged. More inhibited than uninhibited children in Cohort 2 showed greater power in the heart rate spectrum at these lower frequencies when they were placed under mild cognitive stress. This result suggests that the higher, more stable heart rates of inhibited children are mediated by greater sympathetic tone and are not just the result of a loss in parasympathetic tone.

Both inhibited and uninhibited behavior can be influenced by socialization experiences. As indicated earlier, about 40% of behaviorally inhibited children became much less inhibited by 5½ years of age. Several such children who had a high and stable heart rate when evaluated originally, displayed a low and variable heart rate at the last assessment. Evaluations of recorded individual interviews with each of the mothers—about a half hour long—suggest that the parents of the inhibited children who became less inhibited had self-consciously helped their children to overcome their inhibition by using techniques like introducing peers into the home and encouraging the child to cope with stressful situations, whereas parents of the inhibited children who did not change intervened less in their child's behavior. Because American parents are more threatened by fearful sons than by fearful daughters, it is not surprising that more boys than girls changed their behavioral surface from early inhibition to uninhibited behavior by school entrance. A much smaller group of uninhibited children, about 10% and typically girls, became mildly inhibited at later ages. The interviews suggested that these mothers wanted a more cautious child. In two cases, these 5-year-olds began to show a high and stable heart rate for the first time, suggesting it is possible for experience to alter both the behavioral and physiological characteristics that define the two temperamental categories. However, because these inferences come from interview data, this conclusion should be regarded with some caution.

B.  Pupillary Dilation

Additional support for the hypothesis that the temperamentally inhibited children have a lower threshold for sympathetic activation comes from data on pupillary dilation gathered while the children were administered a series of cognitive tasks that included recall memory for words and digits, a mental comparison of the relative size of objects, inferring an object from its features, and listening to a story. The inhibited children had significantly larger pupillary diameters than uninhibited children under both baseline and task conditions, even though the differences between the two groups were less striking for pupil size than for heart rate or heart rate variability. Additionally, more inhibited than uninhibited children in Cohort 1 at 5½ years maintained a large pupil across a series of cognitive episodes (67 vs. 36% of each group). The combination of a tonically large pupil together with a high and stable heart rate across a series of cognitive episodes invites the inference that more of the inhibited children are under greater sympathetic tone.

This suggestion is affirmed by the consistent tendency among inhibited children to show more brief phasic accelerations to the initial stimulus items in a test series, even when an item required attention to a visual stimulus. It should be noted that past work by many investigators reveals that most children and adults show a cardiac deceleration to the presentation of visual stimuli requiring perceptual analysis. This reaction is one of the most robust in autonomic psychophysiology. Nevertheless, at 5½ years we administered a task to Cohort 2 children that required them to decide if the members of a pair of black-and-white pictures projected on a screen were identical or different with regard to a single subtle feature. Half of the 32 pairs were identical and half were different. Although most of the children, inhibited and uninhibited, did show more initial decelerations than accelerations to the presentation of the pictures (however, three inhibited children actually showed more accelerations than decelerations), the ratio of the number of decelerations to accelerations was significantly smaller for inhibited children. Nine uninhibited children had ratios greater than 4.0; not one inhibited child had a ratio that high.

The 5½-year-old children in Cohort 1 watched a series of 20 slides accompanied by a taped narration of a story about a fearful and a fearless child. Although cardiac deceleration was a typical reaction to the appearance of the picture on the screen, inhibited children showed twice as many accelerations as uninhibited children, and the number of accelerations was significantly associated with behavioral inhibition at every age of assessment.

Further, inhibited children typically had a higher heart rate at the end of the 60-min testing session than at the beginning, while uninhibited children had a lower heart rate at the end of the testing battery. The combination of frequent phasic accelerations to a stimulus, as well as the gradual acceleration over the longer period, is in accord with the suggestion of greater reactivity in those parts of the sympathetic chain serving the heart.

## C. Muscle Tension

The reticular activating system sends axons to nuclei in skeletal motor tracts, one of which is the nucleus ambiguus serving the muscles of the larynx and the vocal folds. Increased tension in these skeletal muscles is usually accompanied by a decrease in the variability of the pitch periods of vocal utterances (Lieberman, 1961; Stevens & Hirano, 1981). The increased muscle tension can be due not only to activity of the nucleus ambiguus but also, indirectly, to sympathetic activity that constricts arterioles serving the muscles of the larynx and vocal folds (Vallbo, Hagbarth, Torebjork, & Wallin, 1979).

In the production of human speech, the vocal cords of the larynx open and close at a rapid rate during the process of phonation to produce a sequence of puffs of air. The rate at which the vocal cords open and close defines the fundamental frequency of phonation (Fo). But the duration of each period of the phonatory cycle, which varies around a mean of 4 ms, varies even when a person is maintaining a steady average fundamental frequency. This variation—called perturbation—appears to be a consequence of the interplay of aerostatic, aerodynamic, and tissue forces involved in phonation; and it decreases when the laryngeal muscles are under tension (Lieberman, 1961). If the expected increase in muscle tension in limbs and trunk that often occurs under task demands also occurs in the vocal cords and laryngeal muscles, one acoustic consequence would be less microvariation in the duration of the successive cycles of the fundamental Fo (i.e., less variability). The index of variability we used was the standard deviation of the normalized distribution of twice the difference between two successive periods divided by the sum of the periods.

In the research for her doctoral dissertation, Coster (1986) has found that inhibited 5½-year-old children in Cohort 1, compared with uninhibited children, showed less variability in single-word utterances spoken under mild psychological stress (the words were *bed, cake, dog, goat, pipe,* and *tub*). The child first spoke each of the words singly (no stress) and then repeated the same words in a series of four or six words (mild stress). A second stressful condition required the child to guess which of the six words just repeated was the correct answer to a particular question (e.g., "What does a man smoke?"). Under this last condition, not only did inhibited children show a lower average variability in the pitch periods, but also a larger number of them showed a linear decrease in variability from the first through the sixth reply. (The correlation between the index of inhibition at 21 months and the index of variability was −.43, $p < .01$.) Although there was no relation between fundamental frequency and the variability of the pitch periods of the single-word utterances, the standard deviation of the fundamental frequency values across all the words (about 22 values), whether spoken under low or high stress, was a little smaller for inhibited than for uninhibited children ($r = -.28$). Data collected from Cohort 2 at 43 month of age also revealed that inhibited children showed a greater decrease in variability than uninhibited children when single words were spoken under cognitive stress; in this case the stress was repeating the words as part of a series of four, five, and six words. It is also of interest that in a brief interview between the examiner and the child during the testing session, inhibited children gave shorter answers ($r = -.49$, $p < .001$), reflecting a lack of spontaneity with the examiner.

## D. Cortisol

Secretion of cortisol is enhanced following encounter with an unfamiliar or unpredictable event to which the organism has no coping reaction. Radioimmunoassays of salivary cortisol levels in Cohort 1 at 5½ years, before and after a laboratory session, as well as during the early morning before the stress of the day had begun, revealed significantly higher cortisol levels for inhibited than for uninhibited children. The correlation between mean laboratory cortisol, on the one hand, and the index of behavioral inhibition at 21 months, on the other hand, was .45 ($p < .01$); and with the index of inhibition at 5½ years, the correlation was .37 ($p < .05$). Further, cortisol levels gathered early in the morning were correlated with the index of inhibition at 5½ years ($r = .39$, $p < .05$).

## E. Norepinephrine

An index of total NE activity, based on a single urine sample obtained at the end of the laboratory session, was available for 21 inhibited and 21 uninhibited children in Cohort 1 at 5½ years of age. The NE index was computed by averaging the concentration of four products (in micromoles per gram of creatinine): NE, normetanephrine, 3-methoxy-4-hydroxyphenyglycol (MHPG), and vanillylmandelic acid (VMA). The inhibited children had a higher index of total NE activity. The correlation with the index of inhibition at 5½ years was .31 ($p < .05$). The children who were consistently inhibited over all three assessments had the highest total NE values.

F.  Aggregate Index

In sum, the inhibited children are more likely than the uninhibited ones to show three characteristics to be expected from a hypothesis of lower thresholds in the limbic system. However, only one third of the inhibited children showed evidence of high reactivity in all of the peripheral indexes, and most of the intercorrelations among the peripheral physiological variables were low. In order to assess the degree of concordance in responsivity, we computed a mean standard score for eight physiological variables gathered in Cohort 1 at 5½ years of age: (1) cortisol level in the morning at home, (2) cortisol level obtained in the laboratory, (3) heart period during cognitive tasks, (4) heart period variability during cognitive tasks, (5) pupillary dilation during cognitive tasks, (6) variability of pitch periods under cognitive stress, (7) standard deviation of all fundamental frequency values, and (8) the index of NE. We reversed the values for Variables 3, 4, and 7 so that a high score reflected higher arousal.

The correlation between the aggregate index of the eight physiological variables and the index of inhibited behavior at 21 months was .70 ($p <$ .001); the correlation with the index of inhibition at 5½ years was .58 ($p < .001$).

## III.  Supporting Data

The suggestion that children and adults vary in the responsivity of the sympathetic nervous system and that this variation is associated with behavior finds support in other investigations (Manuck & Garland, 1980). Twin studies of heart rate and blood pressure reveal heritability for both variables (Shapiro, Nicotero, Sapira, & Scheib, 1968). Additionally, investigations of adult personality attributes typically reveal a relation between scores on scales purporting to measure social introversion, on the one hand, and, on the other, a higher and more stable heart rate (Thackray, Jones, & Touchstone, 1974), larger cardiac accelerations (Gange, Geen, & Harkins, 1979; Hinton & Craske, 1977), and larger pupillary dilations (Stelmack & Mandelzys, 1975). Women admitting to conscious feelings of anxiety showed a more stable heart rate under cognitive stress than women reporting low levels of anxiety (Holroyd, Westbrook, Wolf, & Badhorn, 1978).

Similar differences have been noted in animals. A laboratory study of obvious relevance involved 21 pigtail infant monkeys studied from birth to 5 months (Reite & Short, 1980). The infants with highly variable heart rates spent more time away from their mothers than those with minimally variable heart rates. This finding matches our data, for in both cohorts the inhibited children, who have lower heart rate variability, spent more time proximal to their mother than the uninhibited children when in an unfamiliar playroom or with an unfamiliar peer (see Suomi, 1984).

Over 20 years ago Scott and Fuller (1965/1974) published the results of a longitudinal study of behavioral and physiological differences among five species of dogs: wire-haired terriers, beagles, basenjis, Shetland sheepdogs, and cocker spaniels. The basenjis, beagles, and terriers showed more frequent behavioral signs of emotionality to novelty than did shelties or cocker spaniels, especially muscle tremor and attempts to escape from a novel stimulus or constraint. Additionally, when the unfamiliar experimenter entered the dog's perceptual field, the basenjis, beagles, and terriers showed heart rate acceleration, while the cocker spaniels and shelties showed cardiac deceleration—a finding exactly parallel to our data on inhibited and uninhibited children. A factor analysis of the data from 53 dogs revealed two major factors. The first was called activity level. The second reflected the relation between behavioral inhibition and sympathetic activation of the heart, for the three variables with the highest loadings were a high and a stable heart rate and timid behavior.

In a more recent study, puppies from four species (Labradors, Australian kelpies, boxers, and German shepherds) were tested from birth in ecologically natural situations (Goddard & Beilharz, 1985). Discriminant analysis revealed that a factor called alertness was unrelated to the dogs' pedigree. But a second factor, defined best by the "tendency to avoid unfamiliar objects during a walk on a noisy street," revealed significant differences among the breeds, with the German shepherds most and the labradors least fearful.

Comparable relations have been found among different strains of rats. An original population of Long-Evans rats was bred over 20 generations to be either good or poor at ease of learning an avoidance response in a shuttle box. A rat with poor performance shows extreme motor inhibition to shock; hence, it fails to learn the avoidance response. The good and poor performance groups did not differ in visual acuity or pain threshold, but the "poor" learners showed frequent defecation in an open field test, which is one sign of arousal in part of the limbic system (Brush et al., 1985).

In a comparison of Wistar-Kyoto and Brown-Norway rat strains, the former secreted more NE and epinephrine following intermittent foot shock (McCarty, Kirby, & Garn, 1984), although there were no strain differences in catecholamine secretion under nonstress conditions. In a subsequent experiment, the Wistar and Norway rats were first shocked in a compartment and then returned to the compartment 24 hr later. The Wistar-Kyoto rats, who typically respond with high epinephrine and NE to shock, waited longer than Norway rats before placing all four paws in the shock compartment (McCarty *et al.,* 1984).

Blizard and his colleagues (Blizard, 1981; Blizard, Liang, & Emmel, 1980; Liang, Dunlap, Freedman & Blizard, 1982) studied rats bred over many generations to be either high- or low-reactive in an open field defecation test. The reactive strain had higher systolic and diastolic blood pressure, higher heart rate, larger cardiac accelerations to stress, and a larger number of $\beta$-adrenergic receptors on the heart. The relation between the behavioral index of defecation to novelty and the indexes of cardiac sympathetic activity is congruent with our interpretation of the bases for the differences in heart rate and variability between inhibited and uninhibited children. Perhaps the best support for these ideas comes from comparison of the excitability of the amygdala and hypothalamus of consistently defensive, nonaggressive versus aggressive domestic cats. The defensive cats show evidence of lower thresholds of neuronal activity in the amygdala and larger evoked potentials in the ventromedial nucleus of the hypothalamus as a result of electical stimulation of the amygdala (Adamec & Stark-Adamec, 1986). These results imply that a stable disposition to withdraw from novelty, which is characteristic of the defensive cats, is associated with lower thresholds in these limbic structures.

## IV. Behavior in the Strange Situation

The centrality of the concept of attachment in developmental theory has led to the widespread use of a particular procedure, called the *Strange Situation,* to classify 1–2-year-olds as securely or insecurely attached. The two classifications are based primarily on the child's behavior in an unfamiliar laboratory setting during two 3-min periods when the child is left first with a stranger and later completely alone in the unfamiliar room. The children who cry with mild intensity following maternal departure but who greet her and are soothed easily upon her return are called securely attached. Infants who show little distress upon maternal departure and do not greet her when she returns, as well as those who show extreme distress and are not easily soothed, are classified as insecurely attached. As might be expected, the child's behavior following reunion with the mother is correlated with the degree of distress displayed immediately following her departure (Connel, 1985). Thus, the vulnerability to becoming upset by the unpredicted maternal departure in an otherwise unfamiliar room will affect the child's attachment classification. Infants classified as resistant and insecurely attached at 1 year were different from securely attached infants during the opening weeks of life. The former were more irritable, more prone to sleep problems, and harder to manage (Chen & Miyake, 1982/1983; Crockenberg, 1981; Miyake, Chen, & Campos, 1985; Waters, Vaughn, & Egeland, 1980).

Further, 1-year-old boys who showed extreme distress in the Strange Situation (and classified as resistant and insecurely attached) were behaviorally withdrawn when evaluated at 6 years of age, while the 1-year-old girls who reacted with distress became minimally aggressive 6-year-olds. (Lewis, Feiring, McGuffog, & Jaskir, 1984). More persuasive affirmation of the role of temperamental inhibition in the classification of attachment types is the finding that the disposition to show timidity and caution during the first minutes in a strange room with the mother present is a better predictor of a resistant-insecure classification than a prior history of maltreatment by the mother (Schneider-Rosen, 1984). Similarly, infants (11–14 months old) who showed withdrawal and lack of spontaneity to a stranger were most likely to be classified as Type C resistant-insecure in the Strange Situation (Sagi, Lamb, & Gardner, in press).

It appears that the temperamental characteristics that lead a 1-year-old child to show inhibition in unfamiliar contexts makes a significant contribution to the classification of an insecure attachment. Of course, these temperamental qualities influence the way parents interact with their children; hence behavior in the Strange Situation should reflect, in part, the history of parent–child encounters. But the classification represents some complex product that simultaneously involves the child's temperament and his or her relation to the parent, produced, in part, by the parents' behavior.

## V. Summary

The variation in the tendency to approach or avoid unfamiliar events appears to be a moderately stable individual characteristic in young children and one which is associated with peripheral physiological signs that imply a special state of CNS functioning.

The existing data are relevant to an important philosophical issue, namely, the most fruitful way to conceptualize the relation of states of physiological arousal to the varied empirical indexes of those states. One view assumes a generalized state of physiological arousal with each measurement—be it behavior, cortisol, or heart rate—reflecting that state with differential fidelity. There is sometimes the additional, tacit assumption that an average of all the physiological measurements is the best estimate of the general state.

An alternative, but less popular, stance is to reject the theoretical utility of a general arousal state and posit instead families of related states but no core, or central, actualization. Each class of empirical measurement probably reflects an aspect of the state of one component of the family. If two empirical indexes are highly correlated, it is likely that they reflect the same state; if not, it is likely they index components of different families. We can never know the related states, only infer them from the measurements. The circulatory system provides an analogy. There is no average state of the circulatory system. Members of the family of states include blood pressure, heart rate, vagal tone, and concentration of oxygen in the blood. Further, each family (blood pressure, for example) has no single, ideal value, but assumes different values at different sites in the body and under different physical conditions. Thus, a useful way to conceptualize inhibited and uninhibited children is to regard each group as a product of different profiles of related states. All inhibited children do not show the same physiological profile, but more inhibited than uninhibited children display at least one member of the family.

A second theoretical issue concerns the degree of change in the profile of qualities that differentiates the two groups over the period of infancy and childhood. A static position assumes a set of biologic characteristics that changes very little (for example, excitability in the limbic lobe), even though the surface behaviors are transformed. However, an alternative strategy assumes that the profile of biologic and behavioral qualities in each group can change dramatically with development. Hence, the names applied to each category of child should not be the same at different developmental stages. Consider, as an analogy, the different names we use for gender across the lifespan. Even though girls and women differ from boys and men in biologic and psychological characteristics we use the terms *girl* and *woman* to differentiate the profiles associated with childhood and adulthood.

The categories of inhibited and uninhibited behavior were first discovered when the children were 1–3 years of age, a time when clinging to mother and cessation of playing and vocalization in response to the unfamiliar, or the opposite qualities, are prominent features that differentiate the two groups. However, during the first 6 months of life these responses are not as differentiating. It is possible that differences among infants in irritability and sleeplessness might be sensitive signs of these dispositions; hence, a different construct should be applied to these children. Similarly, at age 6, when most inhibited children are much less timid in unfamiliar rooms or with unfamiliar adults, the more obvious signs of this temperamental disposition include caution in situations of risk and vigilance with unfamiliar children. It might be wise, therefore, to call one of our groups "irritable to stress" during the period of infancy; "inhibited to the unfamiliar" during early childhood; and "vigilant toward others" during later childhood. One reasonable retort to this suggestion is to argue that if the central quality of excitability in the limbic lobe remains stable, then that single construct should be applied to children at all of the stages. However, it is not clear that this assumption is valid; for example, some children showed changes in heart rate and variability over time. For these reasons, we believe it is theoretically useful to assume dynamic changes in both groups and to name the two psychological categories differently at different phases of development, as we do for the stages of metamorphosing animals, like frogs and butterflies. *Inhibited* and *uninhibited* are apt names for early childhood, and even though the two groups of children are likely to be different from each other during adolescence, they will have different biologic and psychological profiles from those displayed when they were 3 years old. The error of a static view is similar to the pre-Darwinian error of positing the fixity of species since creation. The horse that lived 15,000 years ago in North America is not the same horse that lives today on a Kentucky farm, even though it was then and is now easily distinguishable from a goat.

Although psychologists accept the fact of genetically based differences in emotionality among strains of animals, they have been more reluctant to assume similar processes in humans without psychosis, with the exception of the complex quality called intelligence. Even though individuals can, through effort and academic study, improve their cognitive skills, there is a pessimism, shared with Kant, over the malleability of fears and emotionality. Put plainly, to suggest that some infants—like German shepherds—will be vulnerable to states of uncertainty and anxiety throughout their lives rubs against our egalitarian ethic. However, the data we have summarized suggest that shyness and timidity, like intelligence, are malleable characteristics. Further, in an industrialized society, there are adaptive aspects to both inhibited and uninhibited behavior, whereas this symmetry does not apply to IQ scores. Because extremely inhibited children tend to avoid social relationships with peers, they are likely to invest more effort in school work and, if successful, may choose a career that involves intellectual work. Such careers typically enjoy challenge, high status, and economic reward in industrialized societies. Finally, the individual's life course is under the influence of many factors, including the will to change one's characteristics; hence, a biologic disposition to be inhibited or uninhibited does not determine in any fixed way the variation among adults in the characteristics our society values.

## Acknowledgments

The research for this chapter was supported in part by a grant from the John D. and Catherine T. MacArthur Foundation. The work on muscle tension is part of a continuing collaboration with Philip Lieberman, Department of Linguistics, Brown University. The work on cortisol in collaboration with Peter Ellison and Terrence Deacon of Harvard University, is part of Pamela Lutz's Senior Honors Project at Radcliffe College, 1985. The analyses of norepinephrine were performed by Dr. Farouk Karoum and Richard J. Wyatt of the Intramural Research Program, National Institute of Mental Health, St. Elizabeth's Hospital, Washington, DC.

## References

Adamec, R. E., & Stark-Adamec, C. (1986). Limbic hyperfunction, limbic epilepsy and interictal behavior. In B. K. Doane & K. E. Livingston (Eds.), *The limbic system* (pp. 103–145) New York: Raven.

Backteman, G., & Magnusson, D. (1981). Longitudinal stability of personality characteristics. *Journal of Personality, 49,* 148–160.

Bateson, P. P. G. (1978). How does behavior develop? In P. P. G. Bateson & P. H. Klopfer (Eds.), *Perspectives in Ethology* (Vol. 3, pp. 55–66) New York: Plenum.

Blizard, D. A. (1981). The Maudsley reactive and nonreactive strains. *Behavioral Genetics, 11,* 469–489.

Blizard, D. A., Liang, B., & Emmel, D. K. (1980). Blood pressure, heart rate, and plasma catecholamines under resting conditions in rat strains selectively bred for differences in response to stress. *Behavioral and Neural Biology, 29,* 487–492.

Bronson, G. W. (1970). Fear of visual novelty. *Developmental Psychology, 2,* 33–40.

Bronson, G. W., & Pankey, W. B. (1977). On the distinction between fear and wariness. *Child Development, 48,* 1167–1183.

Bronson, W. C. (1981). *Toddlers' behaviors with age mates.* Norwood, NJ: Ablex.

Brush, F. R., Baron, S., Froehlich, J. C., Ison, J. R., Pellegrino, L. J., Phillips, D. S., Sakellaris, R. C., & Williams, V. N. (1985). Genetic differences in avoidance learning: In Rattus norvegicus. *Journal of Comparative Psychology, 99,* 60–73.

Chen, S., & Miyake, K. (1982/1983). Japanese versus United States comparison of mother–infant interactions and infant development. In K. Miyake, (Ed.), *Annual report of the research and clinical center for child development* (pp. 13–26). Hokkaido: Hokkaido University.

Chess, G. F., Tam, R. M., & Calaresu, F. R. (1975). Influence of cardiac neural inputs on rhythmic variations of heart period in the cat. *American Journal of Physiology, 228,* 775–779.

Coie, J. D., & Dodge, K. A. (1983). Continuities and changes in children's social status: A five-year longitudinal study. *Merrill-Palmer Quarterly, 29,* 261–282.

Connell, J. P. (1985). *Emotion and social interaction in the Strange Situation.* Unpublished manuscript.

Coolidge, J. C., Brodie, R. B., & Feeney, B. (1964). A ten year follow-up study of 66 school phobic children. *American Journal of Orthopsychiatry, 34,* 675–684.

Coster, W. J. (1986). *Aspects of voice and conversation in behaviorally inhibited and uninhibited children.* Unpublished doctoral dissertation, Harvard University, 1986.

Cranach, B. V., Grote-Dahm, R., Huffner, U., Marte, F., Reisbeck, G., & Mittelstadt, M. (1978). Das social Gehemmte Kind im Kindergarten. *Praxis der Kinderpsychologie und Kinderpsychiatrie, 27,* 167–179.

Crockenberg, S. B. (1981). Infant irritability, mother responsiveness, and social support influences on the security of infant–mother attachment. *Child Development, 52,* 857–865.

Eaves, L., & Eysenck, H. J. (1975). The nature of extroversion: A genetical analysis. *Journal of Personality and Social Psychology, 32,* 102–112.

Elder, G. H., Liker, J. K., & Cross, C. E. (1984). Parent–child behavior in the Great Depression. In P. B. Baltes & O. G. Brim, Jr. (Eds.) *Lifespan development, and behavior* Vol. 6 (pp. 109–158). Orlando: Academic Press.

Emmerich, W. (1964). Continuity and stability in early social development. *Child Development, 35,* 311–332.

Gange, J. J., Geen, R. G., & Harkins, S. G. (1979). Autonomic differences between extraverts and introverts during vigilance. *Psychophysiology, 16,* 392–397.

Garcia-Coll, C., Kagan, J., & Reznick, J. S. (1984). Behavioral inhibition in young children. *Child Development, 55,* 1005–1019.

Gersten, M. (1986). *The contribution of temperament to behavior in natural contexts.* Unpublished doctoral dissertation, Harvard Graduate School of Education.

Goddard, M. E., & Beilharz, R. G. (1985). A multivariate analysis of the genetics of fearfulness in potential guide dogs. *Behavior Genetics, 15,* 69–89.

Goldman-Rakic, P. S. (1981). Development and plasticity of primate frontal cortex. In F. O. Schmitt, F. G. Worden, S. G. Dennis, & G. Adelman (Eds.), *Organization of the cerebral Cortex.* (pp. 69–97). Cambridge, MA: MIT Press.

Goldsmith, H. H., & Campos, J. J. (1985). Fundamental issues in the study of early temperament. In M. E. Lamb & A. Brown (Eds.), *Advances in developmental psychology* (pp. 231–283).

Goldsmith, H. H., & Gottesman, I. I. (1981). Origins of variation in behavioral style: A longitudinal study of temperament in young twins. *Child Development, 52,* 91–103.

Gottesman, I. I. (1963). Heritability of personality. *Psychological Monographs,* (Whole No. 372), 1–26.

Hinton, J. W., & Craske, B. (1977). Differential effects of test stress on the heart rates of extraverts and introverts. *Biological Psychiatry, 5,* 23–28.

Holroyd, K. A., Westbrook, T., Wolf, M., & Badhorn, E. (1978). Performance, cognition, and physiological responding in test anxiety. *Journal of Abnormal Psychology, 87,* 442–451.

Hubel, D. H., & Wiesel, T. N. (1965). Receptive fields and functional architecture in two nonstriate visual areas (18 and 19) of the cat. *Journal of Neurophysiology, 28,* 229–289.

Kagan, J., & Moss, H. A. (1962). *Birth to maturity.* New York: Wiley.

Kagan, J., Reznick, J. S., Clarke, C., Snidman, N., & Garcia-Coll, C. (1984). Behavioral inhibition to the unfamiliar. *Child Development, 55,* 2212–2225.

Katona, P. G., & Jih, F. (1975). Respiratory sinus arrhythmia. *Journal of Applied Physiology, 39,* 801–805.

Lewis, M., Feiring, C., McGuffog, C., & Jaskir, J. (1984). Predicting psychopathology in six-year-olds from early social relations. *Child Development, 55,* 123–136.

Liang, B., Dunlap, C. E., Freedman, L. S., & Blizard, D. A. (1982). Cardiac B receptor variation in rat strains selectively bred for differences in susceptibility to stress. *Life Sciences, 31,* 533–539.

Lieberman, P. (1961). Perturbations in vocal pitch. *Journal of Acoustical Society of America, 33,* 597–603.

Loehlin, J. C. (1982). Are personality traits differentially heritable? *Behavior Genetics, 12,* 417–428.

Manuck, S. B., & Garland, F. N. (1980). Stability of individual differences in cardiovascular reactivity. *Physiology and Behavior, 24,* 621–624.

Matheny, A. P.. (1980). Bayley's infant behavior record: Behavioral components in twin analyses. *Developmental Psychology, 51,* 1157–1167.

McCarty, R. R., Kirby, R. F., & Garn, P. G. (1984). Strain differences in sympathetic-adrenomedullary responsiveness in behavior. *Behavioral and Neural Biology, 40,* 98–113.

Miyake, K., Chen, S., & Campos, J. J. (1985). Infant temperament, mother's mode of interaction, and attachment in Japan. *Monographs Society Research Child Development. 50,* 276–297.

Morris, D. P., Soroker, E., & Burruss, G. (1954). Follow-up studies of shy, withdrawn children: I. Evaluation of later adjustment. *American Journal of Orthopsychiatry, 24,* 743–754.

Moskowitz, D., Schwartzman, A. E., & Ledingham, J. E. (1985). Stability and change in aggression and withdrawal in middle childhood and early adolescence. *Journal of Abnormal Psychology, 94,* 30–41.

Porges, S. W., McCabe, P. M., & Yongue, B. G. (1982). Respiratory–heart rate interactions: Psychophysiological implications for pathophysiology and behavior. In J. Cacciopo & R. Petty (Eds.), *Perspectives in cardiovascular Psychophysiology.* New York: Guilford.

Porges, S. W., & Raskin, D. C. (1969). Respiratory and heart rate components of attention. *Journal of Experimental Psychology, 81,* 497–503.

Reite, M., & Short, R. (1980). A biobehavioral developmental profile for the pigtailed monkey. *Developmental Psychobiology, 13,* 243–285.

Reznick. J. S., Kagan, J., Snidman, N., Gersten, M., Baak, K., & Rosenberg, A. (1986). Inhibited and uninhibited behavior: A follow-up study. *Child Development, 57,* 660–680.

Sagi, A., Lamb, M. E., & Gardner, W. (in press). Relations between strange situation behavior and stranger sociability among infants on Israeli kibbutzim. *Infant Behavior and Development.*

Schneider-Rosen, R. (1984). *Quality of attachment and the development of the self-system.* Unpublished doctoral dissertation, Harvard University.

Scott, J. P., & Fuller, J. L. (1974). *Dog behavior: The genetic basis.* Chicago: University of Chicago Press, Phoenix. (Originally published 1965).

Shapiro, A. P., Nicotero, J., Sapira, J., & Scheib, E. T. (1968). Analysis of the variability of blood pressure, pulse rate, and catecholamine responsivity in identical and fraternal twins. *Psychosomatic Medicine, 30,* 506–520.

Snidman, N. (1984). *Behavioral restraint and the central nervous system.* Unpublished doctoral dissertation, University of California, Los Angeles.

Snow, M. E., Jacklin, C. N., & Maccoby, E. E. (1981). Birth order differences in peer sociability at 33 months. *Child Development, 52,* 589–595.

Stelmack, R. M., & Mandelzys, N. (1975). Extraversion and pupillary response to affective and taboo words. *Psychophysiology, 12,* 536–540.

Stevens, K. N., & Hirano, M. (Eds). (1981). *Vocal fold physiology.* Tokyo: University of Tokyo Press.

Suomi, S. J. (1984). The development of affect in rhesus monkeys. In N. A. Fox & R. J. Davidson (Eds.), *The psychology of affective development* (pp. 119–159). Hillsdale, NJ: Erlbaum.

Thackray, R. I., Jones, K. N., & Touchstone, R. M. (1974). Personality and physiological correlates of performance decrement on a monotonous task requiring sustained attention. *British Journal of Psychology, 65,* 351–358.

Thomas, A., & Chess, S. (1977). *Temperament and development.* New York: Brunner/ Mazel.

Vallbo, A. B., Hagbarth, K. E., Torebjork, H. E., & Wallin, B. G. (1979). Somatosensory, proprioceptive, and sympathetic activity in human peripheral nerves. *Psychological Review, 59,* 919–957.

Waldrop, M. F., & Halverson, C. F. (1975). Intensive and extensive peer behavior: Longitudinal and cross-sectional analyses. *Child Development, 46,* 19–26.

Waters, E., Vaughn, N. B., & Egeland, B. R. (1980). Individual differences in infant–mother attachment relationships at age one. *Child Development, 51,* 208–216.

# Index

# H

Habituation, 57, *see also* Behavior
Hindbrain, 179, 188, *see also* Brain
Hinde index, 363
Hippocampus, 189, 211–212, 224, *see also* Brain
Hormone, 6, 200, 299, 329, *see also* Antiestrogens; Estradiol benzoate; Estrogen; Growth hormone; Lactase; Neuroendocrinologic; Oxytocin; Pituitary–adrenal system; Placental lactogen; Progesterone; Prolactin
Horseradish peroxidase (HRP), 287, 289
Huddling, 51, 78, 264
Human offspring, 1, *see also* Baby
Hyperactivity, 256, *see also* Behavior
Hypothalamo–pituitary–adrenal axis, 359
Hypothalamus, 426, *see also* Brain; Ventromedial nucleus
Hysterectomy, 325, 327

# I

Individual differences, 8, 397–399, 401–402
Infant, 3, 406, *see also* Baby; Neonate
Inferior olive (IO), 237, *see also* Brain
Ingestion, 86, 88, 97, *see also* Behavior system, 170
Inhibited-unhibited, 8, 423–424, 426
Interaction, 2
Interdisciplinary approach, 2, 5
Intermodal transfer, 3, 83, 88–89, 95–96
Intersensory transfer, 88, 92, 97, 105–106
Intraoral milk infusion, 151
Intrauterine sound, 112–113
Intrauterine environment, 41–42, 44, 51, 57
Introversion-extroversion, 422–423, 431
Isolation, 264, 379

# L

Lactase, 20, *see also* Nursing; Suckling
Lactation, 321, *see also* Nursing; Suckling
Lateral hypothalamus, 284, 287, 289, 292, *see also* Brain
Lateral preoptic area (LPOA), 277, 284, 286, 287, 289, *see also* Brain
Learning, 2–5, 26, 30, 40–41, 44, 47, 63, 84–85, 88, 98–99, 107, 169–170,
187–188, 209, 224, 379, *see also* Behavior; Conditioning; Conditioning, classical; Discrimination; Early learning; Extinction; Fetal learning; Reinforcement; Reward
Licking, 322–323
Limbic system, 431–432, 436, *see also* Brain
Locomotion, 256
Long-term potentiation, 211

# M

Maltreatment, p. 434, *see also* Maternal aggression
Mammary duct, 257, *see also* Nursing, Nipple seeking
Maternal aggression, 321, 323, *see also* Maternal behavior
Maternal behavior (MB), 6–7, 299–301, 303, 305–309, 311–317, 337, 321–322, 324, 327–328, 330, *see also* Full maternal behavior; Licking; Nest building; Retrieving
  dominance, 362
  strategy, 383
Maternal odor, 145–146
Maternal punishment, 402
Maternal rejection, 402
Maternal status, 379–380
Maternal voice, 115, 118, 121
Maturation rate, 256
Maze, 206
Medial forebrain bundle, 173–175, 184, *see also* Brain
Medial preoptic area (MPOA), 6, 276–279, 281, 283–284, 286–287, 289, 292, 294, 331, *see also* Brain
Memory, 3, 64, 66, 206, 224, *see also* Memory trace
Memory trace, 223
Metabolic
  activity, 176–177
  mapping, 186, 190
  state, 185
Midbrain, 187–188, *see also* Brain
Milk infusion, 170–171, 173, 183–184, *see also* Conditioning
Model system, 225
Monoamine, 369, *see also* Catecholamines

## W

Water exchange, 337
Weaning, 22, 28, 383, *see also* Nursing;
    Suckling; Nipple seeking
Whoo call, 364
Withdrawal, 421

## Y

Yerkes-Dodson law, 391

## Z

$Z$ scores, 179
Zinc sulfate ($ZnSO_4$), 260, 268